PHARMACOLOGY C[

INTRODUCTORY NURSING CARE OF ADULTS

SECOND EDITION

Adrianne Dill Linton, PhD, RN
Associate Professor
Department of Chronic Nursing Care
University of Texas Health Science Center at San Antonio
School of Nursing
San Antonio, Texas

Judith A. Harris, MSN, RN
Assistant Professor/Clinical
Department of Family Nursing Care
University of Texas Health Science Center at San Antonio
School of Nursing
San Antonio, Texas

W.B. Saunders Company
A Division of Harcourt Brace & Company
Philadelphia   London   Toronto   Montreal   Sydney   Tokyo

W.B. SAUNDERS COMPANY

A Division of Harcourt Brace & Company

The Curtis Center
Independence Square West
Philadelphia, PA 19106-3399

NOTICE

Nursing is an ever-changing field. Standard safety precautions must be followed, but as new research and clinical experience broaden our knowledge, changes in treatment and drug therapy become necessary or appropriate. Readers are advised to check the product information currently provided by the manufacturer of each drug to be administered to verify the recommended dose, the method and duration of administration, and the contraindications. It is the responsibility of the treating licensed prescriber, relying on experience and knowledge of the patient, to determine dosages and the best treatment for the patient. Neither the publisher nor the editor assumes any responsibility for any injury and/or damage to persons or property.

The Publisher

PHARMACOLOGY COMPANION FOR
INTRODUCTORY NURSING CARE OF ADULTS, 2ND EDITION

ISBN 0-7216-8332-0

Printed in the United States of America

Last digit is the print number: 9 8 7 6 5 4 3 2 1

To Barry. I admire your determination.
To Dorris and Louis, my in-laws, who have given unfailing support and
encouragement through all my ventures.

—ADL

To Pat, who patiently lived with stacks of books and piles of paper for the
duration of the project. And many thanks for letting me appropriate the
laptop!

—JAH

ACKNOWLEDGMENTS

*W*e would like to thank the editorial team at W.B. Saunders for their support for this concept. They include Thomas Eoyang, Editorial Manager; Terri Wood, Senior Editor; Catherine Ott, Editorial Assistant; Barbara Cicalese, Associate Developmental Editor; and freelancers Annette Ferran and Lisa Hernandez. The manuscript reviewers are from schools across the nation and provided invaluable feedback that enabled us to produce a book that we believe fills an important void. Dr. Nancy Maebius provided feedback about the scope of the book. The students who have studied pharmacology with us over the years have been the source of inspiration for this work. Last, we want to express appreciation to our families and friends who tolerated our inattention to them while this work was in progress.

ADL
JAH

CONTENTS

PREFACE

*D*rug therapy is an important aspect of the nurse's role. Nurses need to know how drugs work in order to understand expected outcomes and possible adverse reactions. They also must recognize safe dosage ranges, be aware of potential interactions, recognize patient factors that affect drug actions, know the specifics of safe drug administration, and educate patients for self-medication. This is a challenge, as each year brings dozens of new drugs and no nurse can remain current with all of them.

Safe administration of drugs requires:

- a basic understanding of the actions and effects of each drug classification.
- knowledge of the specifics related to each prescribed drug.
- the ability to accurately calculate drug dosages.
- skill in administration by the prescribed route.

Pharmacology Companion for Introductory Nursing Care of Adults addresses the first requirement, an overview of the major drug classifications, and provides an introduction to drug dosage calculation. For each drug classification, information is presented about the actions, uses, interactions, and contraindications. General nursing implications for the classification are derived. At least one prototype is presented for each classification. Specific information is provided about that prototype as an example for the student nurse. There is no intent to include all important drugs. The student should learn the prototypes as examples of the classifications and transfer knowledge of the classifications to other examples.

The book is organized to be used with the second edition of *Introductory Nursing Care of Adults* by Linton, Matteson, and Maebius. The first unit introduces basic concepts of pharmacology with an explanation of how drugs work and why nurses need to study this area. Unit 2 identifies classes of drugs used to treat physiologic responses to illness and injury: anti-inflammatory agents, anti-infectives, immunizing agents, antihistamines, and analgesics. Unit 3 covers drugs used in the care of the surgical patient. Unit 4 addresses pharmacologic issues in long-term and home health care.

The relationship of drugs to falls, immobility, and confusion is explored. Based on concepts of palliative care, drug therapy during terminal illness is also included. Unit 5 covers drugs used to treat cancer. Units 6 through 16 are organized by body systems and present drug classifications used to treat disorders affecting each system. Every effort has been made to be efficient and to refer the reader to earlier coverage of material rather than repeating it. Unit 17 explains drugs used to treat mental illness. Unit 18 is a brief introduction to dosage calculation. Students will require additional practice problems to assure competence with this skill.

Most chapters are very short, allowing the student to focus on a small portion of content at a time. Each unit is followed by study questions that encourage the student to review the material. Some questions are related to case studies presented in the companion textbook. However, adequate information is included in this book to allow the student to answer the questions without referring back to the companion textbook. The answer key for the study questions is in Appendix A.

There are additional requirements for safe drug therapy that are not specifically covered in this text. It is the authors' belief that every nursing student needs not only a general text such as this *Pharmacology Companion,* but also a drug handbook. This general text introduces basic concepts that remain useful over time. The drug handbook provides details about individual drugs including dosage range, interactions, contraindications, and specific nursing implications. To be current, every nurse should have access to an updated drug handbook each year.

A Note to the Faculty

This text may have a different conceptual approach than other pharmacology textbooks that you have used. However, we encourage you to evaluate how using this text to integrate pharmacology into the medical-surgical and psychiatric nursing curriculum makes the content more meaningful to students. We believe it will enhance student understanding of drug therapy at a more conceptual level which provides the tools for critical thinking. The printed and electronic test banks that are available to adopters of the companion textbook contain specially coded pharmacology questions appropriate for testing the students on this content.

Adrianne Dill Linton
Judith A. Harris

CONTRIBUTOR

Mark D. Soucy, MS, RN, CS
Clinical Instructor
University of Texas Health Science Center at San Antonio
School of Nursing
San Antonio, Texas

REVIEWERS

Rebecca Lynn Agnew, RN, MSN
Campbell/Philbin and Associates
Pittsburgh, Pennsylvania

Donna Cartwright, APRN, MS
College of Eastern Utah at Price
Price, Utah

Marilyn Collins, RN, BSN, PHN
Citrus Community College
Glendora, California

Karen Kathryn Haagensen, RNC
Howard College–San Angelo
San Angelo, Texas

Joyce Harris, RN, BS.Ed, MA.Ed
Butler County Program of Practical Nurse Education
Hamilton, Ohio

Nancy B. Henry, MSN, RN
Delaware Technical and Community College
Georgetown, Delaware

Patricia M. Jacobsen, RN, BSN, MSN
Bullard Havens Regional Vocational-Technical School
Bridgeport, Connecticut

Patricia Laing-Arie, RN
Program of Practical Nursing
Meridian Technology Center
Stillwater, Oklahoma

Mary L. Marquardt, RN, BA
Central Lakes College
Brainerd, Minnesota

Rita Michelson, RN, BS
Howell Cheney Vocational-Technical School
Manchester, Connecticut
Middlesex Community Technical College
Middletown, Connecticut

Sally Johnson O'Neil, RN, BS, MS.Ed
Formerly Kaynor Vocational-Technical School
Waterbury, Connecticut

Sharon S. Romine, RN, BSN, MSN
Bessemer State Technical College
Bessemer, Alabama

Lyndi C. Shadbolt, BSN, RN
Amarillo College
Amarillo, Texas

Cynthia A. Steury-Latz, MSN, RN, CS
Kankakee Community College
Kankakee, Illinois
Olsten Health Services
Bourbonnais, Illinois

Deborah Toth, RN, MSN, AOCN
EHOVE School of Practical Nursing
Milan, Ohio

Marilyn Tyhonas, RN, M.Ed
Practical Nursing Program
Fayette County Area Vocational-Technical School
Uniontown, Pennsylvania

Patricia P. Wickham, RN, BSN, MSN
Practical Nursing Program
Center for Arts and Technology, Brandywine Campus
Coatesville, Pennsylvania

INTRODUCTION TO PHARMACOLOGY

OBJECTIVES

1. Define *pharmacology*, *pharmacodynamics*, and *pharmacokinetics*.

2. Explain drug sources and names.

3. Describe the forms of drug preparations.

4. Identify how drug legislation and regulation protect the public.

5. Explain drug actions and uses.

6. Discuss the factors that affect drug dosage and actions.

7. Discuss the implications of drug therapy during pregnancy and lactation.

8. Describe nursing responsibilities in drug therapy.

CHAPTER 1

WHAT IS PHARMACOLOGY?

Pharmacology is the study of chemicals that act on living tissues. *Drugs* are chemicals used in the prevention or treatment of diseases or other disorders. Naturally occurring substances (plants, minerals) have been used throughout history for their physiologic effects. Five-thousand-year-old Chinese records document the medicinal uses of senna and ginseng. Ancient Egyptians compiled considerable drug information and employed such agents as opium and castor oil. Pharmacology as a science, however, did not emerge until the 19th century.

DRUG SOURCES

Drugs were first obtained from natural sources: plants, animals, and inorganic chemicals. Now they are more often manufactured in laboratories. Some are completely synthetic, some are natural products that are altered, and some are the products of DNA technology. In recombinant DNA technology, genetic material from a substance is inserted into living organisms such as *Escherichia coli* or yeast. The organisms then produce large amounts of the substance, which can be harvested for use as a drug. "Human" insulin is obtained in this manner.

DRUG NAMES

Drugs have chemical, generic, and trade names. *Chemical names* describe the exact structural make-up of the drug. These names are usually too complicated for practical use. Imagine having to ask for 7-(D-q-amino-α-phenyl-aceamido)-3-methyl-3-cephem-4-carboxylic acid, monohydrate. A *generic name* is derived from the chemical name of the drug in most cases. The generic name is the same regardless of the manufacturer. However, generic names are sometimes complicated also. The generic name of the drug mentioned above is cephalexin. For convenience and for marketing purposes, each manufacturer assigns a unique *trade name* to the drug; in this case, Keflex. The trade name is protected by copyright. Note that the chemical and generic names are all lower case and the trade name begins with a capital letter. When a drug is manufactured by several companies, the drug will have multiple trade names. For example, trade names for tetracycline include Achromycin, Sumycin, and Panmycin.

DRUG PREPARATIONS

Oral Drug Preparations

Drugs come in a variety of forms best suited for the intended route of administration. Oral drugs are available as liquids, tablets, capsules, powders, granules, and troches. For liquid oral forms, the drug is dissolved in a solvent, often water with flavorings and coloring. When sugar is added to improve the taste, the liquid is called a *syrup*. A *tincture* contains a drug in an alcohol solvent. When alcohol and aromatic flavorings are used, the liquid is called an *elixir*.

Tablets are compressed forms of the drug usually mixed with an inactive ingredient (called a vehicle) that helps hold it together. Some tablets have a coating that improves taste or protects the drug from deterioration. Others have an *enteric coating* that prevents the drug from dissolving until it passes into the small intestine where the pH is less acidic. This can be important when giving drugs that irritate the stomach or drugs that are destroyed by gastric acids.

Troches, also called *lozenges*, are tablets that are allowed to dissolve in the mouth. Examples are cough drops, which dispense a local anesthetic to tissues of the mouth and throat as they dissolve.

Capsules are solid or liquid drugs that are encased in gelatin shells. When it is desirable for the drug to be absorbed slowly over time, a capsule may contain beads of the drug that dissolve at different rates. These are called *sustained release capsules*.

Topical Drug Preparations

Topical drugs may be applied to external structures for local effects or may be absorbed for systemic effects. Topical drugs may be packaged as lotions, creams, ointments, and patches. Patches resemble Band-Aids, with the gauze pad containing a drug that can be absorbed through the skin.

Parenteral Drug Preparations

Drugs intended for injection may come in liquid form or in powders that must be reconstituted before use. To reconstitute a drug, a liquid diluent (solvent) is added according to the manufacturer's directions. It is critical to use the correct diluent and the correct amount for reconstitution. Always be sure you have a preparation that is labeled for the route ordered.

DRUG LEGISLATION AND REGULATION

Once drug manufacturing began, it became evident that standards were needed to ensure safety and effectiveness. Important legislation is summarized in Table 1–1. Of special importance to nurses are the requirements related to controlled substances. *Controlled substances* are drugs that have the potential for physical or psychological dependence. Controlled substances are kept in a double-locked cabinet and each dose dispensed must be properly documented.

TABLE 1–1

Drug Legislation

Date	Law	Provisions
1906	Federal Pure Food and Drug Act	Restricted manufacture and sale of drugs. Designated the *U.S. Pharmacopeia* and *The National Formulary* as official standards for drug strength and purity.
1938	Food, Drug, and Cosmetic Act	Mandated tests for toxicity (first law to regulate for safety). Charged FDA (Food and Drug Administration) with reviewing tests for toxicity prior to approval for marketing.
1962	Kefauver-Harris Amendment to the Food, Drug, and Cosmetic Act	Required proof of effectiveness of new drugs, as well as old drugs approved since 1938. Increased requirements for testing of new drugs.
1970	Federal Comprehensive Drug Abuse Prevention and Control Act. Includes the "Controlled Substances Act"	Established rules for manufacture and distribution of substances with abuse potential. Classified substances as Schedule I, II, III, IV, or V depending on abuse potential (see Table 1–4). Abuse potential is highest with Schedule I drugs and lowest with Schedule V drugs.

TABLE 1–2

Schedules of Controlled Substances

Schedule	Examples	Abuse Potential
I	Heroin, lysergic acid diethylamide (LSD), peyote, mescaline, tetrahydrocannabinol, marijuana	No accepted medical use; high potential for abuse.
II	Opioids: analgesics: codeine, hydromorphone (Dilaudid), methadone (Dolophine), meperidine (Demerol), morphine, oxycodone (OxyContin), oxymorphone	Accepted medical use; high abuse potential; risk of psychological or physical dependence.
	Central nervous system stimulants: cocaine, dextroamphetamine (Dexedrine), methamphetamine, phenmetrazine, methylphenidate (Ritalin) Barbiturate sedative/hypnotics: amobarbital, pentobarbital (Nembutal), secobarbital (Seconal)	
III	Mixtures containing small amounts of controlled substances (e.g., codeine). Barbiturates not on other schedules. Paregoric Central nervous system stimulants: benzphetamine, phendimetrazine Male sex hormones: androgens, anabolic steroids	Some appropriate medical uses; less abuse potential than Schedule I or II drugs; risk of psychological or physical dependence.
IV	Benzodiazepines: chlordiazepoxide (Librium), diazepam (Valium), lorazepam (Ativan), flurazepam (Dalmane), temazepam (Restoril). Sedative/hypnotics: phenobarbital, chloral hydrate (Noctec) Some prescription appetite suppressants: diethylpropion, fenfluramine, mazindol, phentermine	Have appropriate medical uses; some potential for abuse.
V	Opioids: buprenorphine, diphenoxylate plus atropine	Some potential for abuse. Can be dispensed without prescription under certain regulations.

REFERENCES FOR DRUG INFORMATION

As a licensed vocational nurse, you must know about the drugs you are giving. This book and other basic pharmacology texts provide information about categories of drugs. They provide general information about groups of drugs and some specific examples called *prototypes*. However, a drug handbook is needed for you to check specific drug implications and dosages. Eventually, you will become familiar with drugs that you give often, but you will frequently encounter new drugs in your practice. When you have an order for a drug that is unfamiliar, you must take time to look it up before you give it. Every patient care setting should have current drug references readily available. Recommended sources are the *American Hospital Formulary Service* and *Drug Facts and Comparisons*. The *Physicians' Desk Reference (PDR)* is another useful resource that compiles information from manufacturers' drug inserts. If you have computer access, you will find several sites that provide current drug information on the Internet. In addition, there are numerous nursing drug handbooks that provide essential basic information, including drug use, actions, dosages, side and adverse effects, contraindications, interactions, and nursing implications. It is a good idea to have your own handbook for ready access. If you cannot find information about a drug, call a pharmacist to answer your questions.

CHAPTER 2

HOW DO DRUGS WORK?

$\mathcal{F}$or drugs to be useful, they must be absorbed, reach the site of action, and cause some physiologic effect. To avoid adverse effects from prolonged exposure or accumulation, there must also be mechanisms that metabolize or excrete drugs or their byproducts. This chapter addresses the movement of drugs within the body and the ways that they act.

PHARMACOKINETICS

Pharmacokinetics refers to the movement of drug molecules in the body. Pharmacokinetics includes absorption, distribution, metabolism, and excretion of drugs.

Absorption

Absorption can be defined simply as the movement of a drug into the bloodstream from its site of administration. Although some drugs such as antacids and topical ointments act at their sites of administration, most drugs act at some distant site. Some drugs are more readily absorbed than others. Factors that affect drug absorption are fat and water solubility, ionization, pH, concentration or dosage, and route of administration. Once drugs are absorbed, they are transported by body fluids for *distribution* to the site of action.

Routes of Administration

The most common routes of drug administration are classified as enteral and parenteral. *Enteral* drugs are given orally or through a gastrointestinal tube (G-tube or N/G tube). *Parenteral* routes include intravenous (IV), intramuscular (IM), subcutaneous (SC), and intradermal (ID). The percutaneous route is used for drugs that can be absorbed through the skin or mucous membranes. *Percutaneous* routes include *sublingual* (under the tongue), *buccal* (in the cheek), *inhalation* (through the lungs), and *transdermal* (through the skin). Table 2–1 summarizes the barriers to absorption, advantages, and disadvantages of each route.

TABLE 2–1

Routes of Drug Administration

Route	Advantages	Disadvantages
Oral	Easy, convenient, no special skills required, usually least expensive, painless, safest; absorption can be prevented if necessary by gastric lavage, induced vomiting, or activated charcoal.	Variable absorption, some drugs inactivated by gastric acids or liver enzymes, may be irritating to gastrointestinal tract, requires patient cooperation.
Intravenous	Rapid onset of action, more control over amount of drug delivered to the bloodstream, can be given in larger volumes of fluid, less local damage caused by irritating drugs.	Most expensive route, requires special training, effects not readily reversed, risk of fluid volume excess. General complications of IV therapy: infection, embolism.
Intramuscular	Can be used for poorly soluble drugs and for drugs that are intended to be absorbed over time.	Pain, inconvenience, requires special skill.
Subcutaneous	Can be used for poorly soluble drugs and for drugs. intended for absorption over time.	Pain, inconvenience, requires special skill.
Percutaneous	No special skills required; painless; rapid effects with sublingual, buccal, and inhalation routes; transdermal route allows slow absorption over time.	Local irritation, especially with transdermal drugs.

Distribution

Distribution refers to the transportation of a drug to the site of action by body fluids. Factors that influence the rate and extent of drug distribution include:

- Physical and chemical characteristics of the drug such as pH and solubility
- Circulation to the intended site of action
- Plasma protein binding: some drug molecules attach to plasma proteins; if extensively bound to protein, the drug cannot exert effects
- Affinity for fatty tissue: drugs that are attracted to fat tissue are stored there and released slowly over time
- Barriers: limit the passage of drugs and other substances into the brain and the placenta; this is a protective mechanism but must be overcome to treat brain disorders

Metabolism

Metabolism refers to the chemical reactions that alter foreign substances, including drugs, in the body. In relation to drugs, metabolism changes drugs into forms that are inactive or more readily excreted. The liver is the primary site of drug metabolism. Some drugs, such as central nervous system depressants, stimulate the liver to produce increased drug-metabolizing enzymes.

Increased drug-metabolizing enzymes also contribute to the development of *tolerance*, a condition in which increasing amounts of the drug are needed to achieve the same effect. It can also result in rapid metabolism of other drugs, requiring adjustments in their dosages.

When drugs are absorbed into the bloodstream through the intestinal blood vessels, the blood passes through the liver, where a certain amount of the drug may be inactivated. This is referred to as the *first-pass effect*. When a large amount of the drug is inactivated in this way, a parenteral or percutaneous route may be necessary.

Excretion

The elimination of a drug from the body is called *excretion*. The kidneys are the primary organs of drug excretion. Other routes include the gastrointestinal tract, lungs, breast milk, and to a small extent, saliva and sweat.

PHARMACODYNAMICS

Pharmacodynamics describes the interactions of drugs with cells and other body structures or components to produce characteristic effects. The best understood mechanisms of action include interactions with receptors on cells, physical actions, chemical actions, and altered metabolic pathways.

Receptor Theory of Drug Action

The receptor theory of drug action is based on the ability of drugs to attach to specialized regions of cells called *receptors*. You may find it helpful to think of this as a lock-and-key arrangement. The drug is a key and the receptor is the lock. Only certain keys will open specific locks. Once the lock is opened (the drug binds with the receptor), the drug is able to influence the cell in some way.

Defining terminology helps to explain the receptor theory:

- *Affinity* describes a drug's ability to bind to a given receptor. To illustrate, when histamine is released in allergic attacks, it binds with receptors in the capillary walls, causing increased permeability. Fluid leaves the capillary, so the patient with allergies has a "runny nose." You would say that histamine has affinity for these cells. An antihistamine also has affinity for the same receptors. By occupying the receptor sites on the capillary walls, the antihistamine blocks the action of histamine.
- *Efficacy* describes the ability of a drug to produce an effect as a result of binding with a receptor.
- An *agonist* is a drug that produces a pharmacologic effect when it binds with a receptor. An agonist has both affinity and efficacy.
- An *antagonist* is a drug that combines with receptors without producing a pharmacologic effect or a drug that occupies receptor sites so that other drugs and chemicals cannot bind there. As noted earlier, antihistamines block tissue receptors so that histamine cannot bind with that tissue. Antagonists are sometimes referred to as "blockers" because they block the receptor sites.

Physical Actions

Physical drug actions do not involve direct effects on body tissues. For example, osmotic diuretics increase osmotic pressure in the blood, which causes the kidneys to increase urine excretion.

Chemical Actions

An example of a chemical action is the neutralization of gastric acid by an antacid. This represents chemical activity with no direct cellular effects.

Altered Metabolic Pathways

Some drugs, including some anticancer drugs and anti-infectives, are able to interrupt the metabolic processes that maintain cell life. The drugs can destroy cancer cells or pathogens by interfering with metabolism.

Drug Uses

Although drugs have many specific uses, those uses can be classified in terms of the following applications:

- Stimulate, regulate, or suppress physiologic processes (e.g., vasopressors, antihypertensives, anti-inflammatories)
- Supplement or substitute for some essential substance that is deficient (e.g., vitamins, insulin, thyroid hormones)
- Destroy pathogens or abnormal cells (e.g., antimicrobials, antineoplastics/anticancer agents)
- Protect vulnerable tissues (e.g., skin protectants, cytoprotectives)

Factors that Affect Drug Dosages and Actions

Many factors affect the way a person responds to a drug and explain why dosages must be individualized. Biophysiologic factors include body weight, age, gender, genetics, biologic rhythms, medical conditions, and the development of tolerance or cumulation. Psychological factors such as emotional state and beliefs about a drug can also affect the patient's response to the drug.

Body Weight. Drugs are absorbed and distributed in body tissues. To achieve therapeutic effects, a drug must be present in adequate concentration. Therefore, heavier people generally require larger doses of drugs than smaller people. Consider a situation in which you have two postoperative patients who had abdominal surgery yesterday. One weighs 250 lbs, the other 90 lbs. Ten milligrams of morphine may have no effect when given to the 250 lb person, but could effectively relieve pain in a 90 lb person. On the other hand, the 250 lb person might require 30 mg for pain relief—a dose that could excessively sedate the 90 lb patient.

Adult dosages are usually based on a recommended dosage range. Pediatric dosages, however, are often based on the patient's body weight to ensure appropriate, but not excessive, drug therapy.

Age. In general, the very young and the very old are at greater risk of harm from drugs. Young children have immature liver and kidney function, so they may not metabolize or excrete the drugs efficiently. Some elderly people also have reduced liver and kidney function, especially under conditions of severe illness. Therefore, dosages are often proportionately smaller for these patients.

Other special problems with the elderly person are as follows:

- Polypharmacy: taking multiple drugs for multiple medical conditions; interactions among drugs can enhance or diminish individual drug actions
- Limited financial resources: expensive drugs may be unaffordable; the patient may run out of medication and be unable to get refills immediately
- Hearing impairment: the patient may not understand verbal instructions
- Vision impairment: the patient may have difficulty reading drug labels or directions
- Cognitive impairment: though not characteristic of most older people, may make self-medication unsafe

Gender. Male and female patients may respond differently to some drugs. This may be related, in part, to the higher proportion of fat in females, and the effects of female hormonal cycles, or other less-understood mechanisms. In the past, females have not always been well-represented in drug studies, so gender differences were not detected. This problem is receiving attention in many newer drug studies.

Another important consideration in drug therapy is the risk of harm to a developing embryo when pregnant women take drugs. Drugs that cause abnormal embryonic or fetal development are said to be *teratogenic.*

Genetics. Genetics may affect the actions of drugs in a variety of ways. For example, the presence or absence of specific drug-metabolizing enzymes is genetically based. People who lack a particular enzyme are unable to metabolize certain drugs. Therefore, serum levels of those drugs can quickly reach toxic levels.

Genetics account for differences in drug responses based on race. For example, in the treatment of hypertension, white patients respond better to beta-adrenergic blockers than do African-American patients. African-Americans respond better to diuretics.

Biologic Rhythms. Patient responses to some drugs vary with biorhythmic cycles. For example, drugs given to promote sleep work better at the patient's usual sleep time than at other times.

Medical Conditions. Pathologic states can affect drug absorption, distribution, metabolism, and excretion. Following are some examples of these situations:

- People with **inadequate gastric acid** (including those taking drugs to inhibit acid production) may not absorb drugs that require an acid medium to dissolve.
- **Diarrhea** may cause oral drugs to pass through the gastrointestinal tract too quickly to be absorbed.
- Enteric-coated drugs may be eliminated intact through an **ileostomy.**
- **Arterial insufficiency** may prevent distribution of a drug to affected tissues.
- **Liver failure** impairs the ability to metabolize drugs.
- With **renal insufficiency**, the patient may not eliminate drugs normally when under physiologic stress.
- **Renal failure** prevents the elimination of drugs so they accumulate in the body.

Tolerance. *Tolerance* is reduced responsiveness to a drug. It can be congenital, due to genetic factors mentioned earlier, or acquired, due to stimulation of liver enzymes or other physiologic variations. Tolerance is manifested by reduced response to usual dosage levels. This may occur with analgesics, where the patient requires increasing dosages of a drug to achieve the same therapeutic effects. Either the dosage will have to be increased or a different drug used.

In addition, it is possible to have cross-tolerance. *Cross-tolerance* occurs when the patient develops tolerance to one drug that causes tolerance to a second, similar drug without previous exposure to the second drug.

Cumulation. *Cumulation* is increased concentration of a drug in the body because of inability to metabolize or excrete the drug rapidly enough. Cumulation can result in toxic drug effects. You must be especially alert for cumulation in elderly people who take drugs over a long period of time.

Drug Interactions. When two or more drugs are present in the body at the same time, there is a chance of *drug interactions*. Drug interactions can alter the effects of any of the drugs present. They include:

- **Synergism** (working together): this term indicates that the drugs will have combined effects greater than either agent would have alone. Synergism may permit lower doses of each agent to be used, which achieves the goal with less risk of adverse effects from either drug. For example, hypertension can be controlled with low or moderate doses of two agents rather than a high dose of a single agent. Synergism can also result in toxicity of one or both of the drugs.
- **Potentiation** is the term used when the action of one drug is enhanced by the action of another drug.
- **Antagonism** (working against): this term indicates that the interacting drugs will have fewer effects than if either were given alone.

Psychological Factors. In addition to the many biophysiologic factors just listed, the patient's emotional state and expectations can influence drug effects as well. To illustrate, if the patient in pain lacks confidence that a given drug will be effective, it may indeed not work well for that person. On the other hand, belief that an agent will bring relief seems to enhance that effect. A term used to describe the positive drug effects contributed by psychological factors is the *placebo effect*.

A *placebo* is an agent such as normal saline or "sugar pills" that has no pharmacologic activity. In the past, placebos were sometimes given to patients who were believed to be exaggerating their needs for drugs. The fact that these patients often showed a positive response to the placebo was interpreted as evidence that the need was not "real." We now understand that the perceived positive effects were most likely due to the placebo effect and did not mean the patient was "faking it." There is no appropriate place for the clinical use of placebos except in research studies in which the patient is informed that a placebo might be given.

⚠ IMPLICATIONS OF PREGNANCY AND LACTATION

Teratogenesis

One basic fact to remember is that any drug given to a pregnant woman is likely to be distributed to her fetus as well. Although many drugs may be harmless to the fetus, most drugs have not really been tested for their effects on human fetuses. Therefore, with drug use during pregnancy, the benefits must be weighed against the potential risks. The types of risks to the fetus depend on the stage of development. As noted earlier, drugs that are harmful to the embryo or fetus are called *teratogens*. From conception through the second week, teratogens in adequate concentrations cause embryonic death. From the third through the eighth week, teratogens can cause structural abnormalities. For the remainder of the gestation period, teratogen exposure is most likely to cause functional impairments such as behavioral abnormalities or learning problems.

These cautions do not mean that no drugs should be given. Chronic problems such as diabetes or hypertension must be carefully managed during pregnancy. Severe infections must be treated. However, indiscriminate use of drugs is not advised. When drugs are needed, the physician selects the drug thought to be most effective with the least risk to the patient and her fetus. Table 2–2 lists drugs known to be teratogenic.

TABLE 2–2

Known Teratogens*

ACE† Inhibitors
All ACE inhibitors are teratogens

Anticancer Drugs/Immunosuppressants
Aminopterin
Busulfan
Cyclophosphamide
Methotrexate

Antiseizure Drugs
Carbamazepine
Phenytoin
Trimethadione
Valproic Acid

Vitamin A Derivatives
Etretinate
Isotretinoin
Vitamin A (>18,000 IU/day)

Other Drugs
Alcohol (high doses)
Cocaine (high doses)
Lithium
Tetracycline
Thalidomide
Warfarin

Sex Hormones
Estrogens
Progestins
Androgens

---

*The absence of a drug from this table does not mean that the drug is not a teratogen; it only means that teratogenicity has not been proved. For most proven teratogens, the risk of a congential anomaly is only 10%.

†ACE = angiotensin-converting enzyme.

Reprinted with permission from Lehne, R. A. (1998). *Pharmacology for Nursing Care*, 3rd ed. Philadelphia: W. B. Saunders, p. 82.

⚠ Maternal Complications

In addition to fetal injury, drugs can cause complications for the mother during pregnancy. Examples are

- Prostaglandins such as misoprostol (Cytotec), which is used to treat peptic ulcer disease, stimulate uterine contractions and can cause abortion.
- Tetracycline (an anti-infective) is more likely to cause liver damage if taken during pregnancy.
- Heparin (an anticoagulant) tends to contribute to demineralization of bones if taken during pregnancy.
- Aspirin (an antiplatelet agent) can contribute to severe bleeding during and after delivery.

⚠ Lactation

Most drugs taken by a lactating woman are secreted in breast milk. Usually the concentration of the drug is too low to have a pharmacologic effect on the breastfeeding infant. However, some drugs are specifically contraindicated during breastfeeding (Table 2–3).

TABLE 2–3

Drugs that Are Contraindicated During Lactation

Controlled Substances
Amphetamines
Cocaine
Heroin
Marijuana
Phenycyclidine

Anticancer Drugs/Immunosuppressants
Cyclophosphamide
Cyclosporine
Doxorubicin

Others
Bromocriptine
Ergotamine
Lithium
Methotrexate
Nicotine

Reprinted with permission from Lehne, R. A. (1998). *Pharmacology for Nursing Care*, 3rd ed. Philadelphia: W. B. Saunders, p. 83.

⚠ NURSING IMPLICATIONS

Before giving ANY drug to a pregnant woman, be sure to determine whether it is safe during pregnancy. Drug reference sources assign drugs to categories (A, B, C, D, X) in terms of their potential for harm during pregnancy. Category A is safest, and category X is most dangerous (Table 2–4). If questionable, discuss it with the physician or nurse practitioner. Teach pregnant women not to take any drugs without discussing them with their caregiver.

When women have taken dependence-producing drugs during pregnancy, the infant may be born drug-dependent. The mother may not tell you of her dependence out of fear.

Once the infant is deprived of the drug through the mother's blood, drug withdrawal begins and is manifested by extreme irritability, vomiting, and a shrill cry. Decreasing doses of the drug must be given to the infant to wean him or her from the drug.

Advise lactating women not to take drugs without medical approval. When drugs are needed, the concentration in breast milk can be minimized by giving the drug immediately after breastfeeding.

TABLE 2–4

Pregnancy Safety Categories

Category	Category Description
A	*Remote Risk of Fetal Harm:* Controlled studies in women have been done and have failed to demonstrate a risk of fetal harm during the first trimester, and there is no evidence of risk in later trimesters.
B	*Slightly More Risk Than A:* Animal studies show no fetal risk, but controlled studies have not been done in women or Animal studies do show a risk of fetal harm, but controlled studies have failed to demonstrate a risk during the first trimester, and there is no evidence of risk in later trimesters.
C	*Greater Risk Than B:* Animal studies show a risk of fetal harm, but no controlled studies have been done in women or No studies have been done in women or animals.
D	*Proven Risk of Fetal Harm:* Studies in women show proof of fetal damage, but the potential benefits of use during pregnancy may be acceptable despite the risks (e.g., treatment of life-threatening disease for which safer drugs are ineffective). A statement on risk will appear in the "WARNINGS" section of drug labeling.
X	*Proven Risk of Fetal Harm:* Studies in women or animals show definite risk of fetal abnormality or Adverse reaction reports indicate evidence of fetal risk. The risks clearly outweigh any possible benefit. A statement on risk will appear in the "CONTRAINDICATIONS" section of drug labeling.

WHY DO NURSES NEED PHARMACOLOGY?

*D*rug therapy is an important component of medical care today. Indeed, it is rare to find a hospitalized patient who is not receiving drug therapy. In traditional patient care settings, the nurse is the person who administers and documents the drugs ordered by the prescriber. In that role, the nurse is responsible for giving the drug exactly as prescribed. However, nursing responsibilities do not stop there. As a licensed nurse, you are expected to understand the drugs you give and to protect the patient from harm.

These responsibilities require in-depth knowledge of drugs, which is the focus of this textbook. You will be introduced to major classifications of drugs with limited specific examples called *prototypes*. Broad classifications provide the background to understand how drugs in that class work and what effects you can expect. However, you must always look up new drugs to identify information specific to that drug. Even within a classification, there are often different indications, dosages, adverse effects, and contraindications for various individual drugs.

THE NURSING PROCESS AND DRUG THERAPY

Assessment

The assessment includes information about the patient and the prescribed drug. On admission, a complete health history should be taken. Ongoing assessments are needed to determine the patient's continued need for drug therapy and to evaluate the response to drug therapy.

Health History

During the health history, document the following:

- Age
- Diagnosed health problems and current reason for seeking care
- All drugs being taken (including prescription and nonprescription drugs): name, dosage, route, schedule, and frequency of administration of each drug

- Any symptoms that might be related to drug therapy
- Use of any herbal or other "natural" products for medicinal purposes
- Use of caffeine, tobacco, alcohol, street drugs
- Patient's understanding of the purpose of the drugs

The review of systems may elicit significant data related to drug effects. Throughout the health history, assess the patient's vocabulary, emotional state, and cognitive state. This will help you develop appropriate teaching plans.

Physical Examination

A systematic physical examination enables you to evaluate the therapeutic effects of drug therapy and to detect possible adverse drug effects. For example:

- Vital signs: slow pulse may reflect digitalis toxicity, slow respirations may result from central nervous system depressants, low blood pressure may be associated with vasodilators
- Weight: increase may be associated with corticosteroids, decrease may be associated with fluid loss caused by diuretics
- Skin: a rash and urticaria (hives) are associated with allergic reactions
- Head: headache may be caused by vasodilators
- Eyes: cholinergic drugs constrict the pupil, anticholinergics dilate them
- Ears: tinnitus (ringing in the ears) can be caused by aspirin toxicity
- Mouth: dry mouth is associated with anticholinergics like atropine
- Thorax: wheezing is one symptom of anaphylaxis, the most serious, life-threatening allergic response
- Heart: abnormal heart rhythms can be caused by stimulants or depressants
- Abdomen: increased bowel sounds may be related to laxatives
- Musculoskeletal: muscle weakness may be due to hypokalemia caused by diuretics

Nursing Diagnoses

Your assessment in relation to drug therapy can support many nursing diagnoses. A few examples are:

- **Noncompliance** with drug therapy related to intolerable side effects, poor understanding of need, financial limitations
- **Ineffective individual management of therapeutic regimen** related to lack of understanding of drug therapy, inability to pay for drugs
- **Constipation** related to side effects of anticholinergic drug therapy
- **Risk for injury** related to sedating side effects of drug therapy

Interventions

Nursing responsibilities in drug therapy include drug administration; monitoring, recording, evaluating, and reporting responses; managing side and adverse effects; patient education; care of patients with drug dependency; and, for some advanced practice nurses, prescribing drugs.

Drug Administration

Nursing responsibilities in drug administration requires that you do five things correctly. These are commonly referred to as *The Five Rights*. They are:

1. Right **drug**
2. Right **dose**
3. Right **time**
4. Right **route**
5. Right **patient**

Right Drug. To select the right drug, you must first correctly interpret the drug order (see Chapter 53). Always read a drug label three times: when you select the container, when you remove the dose from the container, and when you replace the container. When you have unit-dose drugs, leave the drug packaged until you are ready to administer it. That way it can readily be identified.

Right Dose. The dose is included in the medical order. Look up the drug to be sure the dose is within the usual range. See what the dosage is in the available form of the drug. It may be necessary to convert the ordered dosage from one system of measurement to another. You may also need to calculate the amount of the drug to give (e.g., tablets, milliliters). Chapter 53 explains these procedures. Any time you are uncertain of your calculations, ask a more experienced nurse or the pharmacist to confirm your figures.

Be suspicious if you calculate more than 2 tablets or capsules or more than 3 milliliters (mL) of an intramuscular drug. For example, ask yourself if it is sensible to give 25 tablets orally or 15 mL intramuscularly.

Right Time. The timing of drug doses is important to maintain therapeutic blood levels consistently. Maintaining a therapeutic blood level means the amount of drug in the blood is adequate to produce therapeutic effects without toxicity. The drug order will indicate the number of times the drug is to be given in a day. For example, it may be ordered QID (four times a day) or q 8 h (every 8 hours). Most agencies have standard administration times. It is generally acceptable to give drugs within ½ hour before to ½ hour after the scheduled time.

Right Route. The drug order will also indicate the route by which the drug should be given, most often oral, intramuscular, intravenous, or topical. Many drugs are available in multiple preparations, so you must be sure to select the correct preparation for the ordered route. Once you have chosen the correct drug form for the intended route, you must know how to administer it correctly. Important factors to remember are the following:

- Follow oral drugs with a minimum of 100 mL of fluid to help the drug reach the stomach and to facilitate absorption.
- For injections
  - Select the smallest syringe that will hold the volume of drug to be given.
  - Determine the most appropriate needle length and gauge for the type of drug being given, the administration site, and the patient's size.
- For intravenous infusions
  - Be sure which, if any, drugs you are permitted to give intravenously.
  - Determine whether the drug is given IV push or IV piggyback.
  - Determine whether IV drugs are compatible with the fluid being infused.
  - Determine the rate of infusion and monitor carefully.
- For topical medications
  - Be sure you have the correct preparation; e.g., ophthalmic for the eyes, otic for the ears.

Right Patient. Prior to giving each medication, you must always identify the patient. Ask the patient's name and check the wrist identification band against the medication record. Many long-term care facilities have photographs of residents on the medication record to help with positive identification. Especially in long-term care settings, do not assume that patients are always in the right room or even the right bed. Also, confused patients may not correct you if you call them by another person's name.

Right Documentation. Some nurses consider Right Documentation to be a "sixth right." Right documentation includes prompt and accurate recording of all drugs as soon as they are given as well as noting assessment findings related to therapeutic and adverse effects of drugs.

Management of Drug Side and Adverse Effects

Managing side and adverse drug effects is an important part of the nurse's role. For example, a nursing diagnosis presented earlier was **Constipation** related to side effects of anticholinergic drug therapy. Nursing interventions would include monitoring bowel elimination, encouraging fluid and fiber intake, and possibly giving prescribed stool softeners. Another nursing diagnosis was **Risk for injury** related to sedating side effects of drug therapy. In this situation, you would keep the bed in low position, instruct the patient to call for help to get up, and provide a call button.

Patient Education

An important aspect of nursing care and drug therapy is patient education. The challenge is to provide vital information about the drugs without overwhelming the patient. For hospitalized patients, the amount of information depends on the patient's condition. To a fairly recent postoperative patient, you might say, "This is your pain medication. It should relieve your pain within 15 to 20 minutes. It will make you drowsy, so call for help if you need to get up." That is probably all the patient needs to know at that point.

If you are sending a patient home on insulin, however, think how much he or she needs to know for safe self-medication: type(s) of insulin, correct number of units, schedule, injection technique, and symptoms and treatment of low blood glucose. For this situation, teaching should begin as soon as the need is identified so that the patient can have opportunities to practice in your presence.

An important problem with drug therapy is *noncompliance* or *nonadherence* with the prescribed therapy. Patients may fail to take the drug as ordered. It is important to determine why patients do not take their medications correctly. Possible factors include the following:

- Lack of understanding of the importance of the drug
- Intolerable side effects
- Inability to afford the drug
- Difficulty with self-administration

If you can determine the reason, you may be able to find a solution. However, remember that the patient always

has the right to refuse to take medication. Be sure to document patient teaching and any concerns identified.

Evaluation

Immediately after you give a drug, it should be documented. Never chart a drug before giving it. Since no drug has only one effect, you must routinely assess the patient for the desired drug effect as well as any side or adverse effects. Record your observations and bring them to the attention of the physician.

LEGAL CONSIDERATIONS

Your role in relation to drug therapy is defined by your state board of nursing, and you must not exceed your limitations. In addition, your employing agency may have additional policies that you must know and follow. Your legal responsibilities are as follows:

- You must administer drugs safely and accurately (Five Rights).
- You must be knowledgeable about the drugs you give.
- You must question orders that appear to be incorrect, such as excessive doses.
- You must refuse to give a drug that you believe to be unsafe.
- You must recognize serious and common adverse effects of drugs that you administer.
- You must follow legal requirements and agency procedures for administering and accounting for controlled substances

The bottom line is: **You are accountable for your actions as a licensed nurse.** Following physician's orders is no defense when the drug order is inappropriate.

Participation in Drug Studies

You may become involved in drug studies that are testing new drugs or comparing multiple drug effects. Your role may be to give the drug, but your responsibility does not stop there. In some studies, you will not know if you are giving a drug or a placebo. As a nurse, you must know that the patient has given informed consent, and you must understand the drug being studied and the study protocol. You should notify the researcher of any problems noted.

REVIEW QUESTIONS: UNIT 1

Match the term on the left with the definition on the right:

1. _____ drugs

2. _____ pharmacokinet-
ics

3. _____ pharmacology

4. _____ pharmacody-
namics

5. _____ absorption

6. _____ distribution

7. _____ metabolism

8. _____ excretion

9. _____ affinity

10. _____ efficacy

11. _____ agonist

12. _____ antagonist

A. A drug that produces a pharmacologic effect when it binds with a receptor

B. Study of chemicals that act on living tissue

C. Drug's ability to bind to a given receptor

D. Chemical used in the prevention or treatment of disease

E. Movement of a drug into the bloodstream

F. Movement of drug molecules in the body

G. Drug that combines with a receptor without producing a pharmaco-logic effect

H. Transportation of a drug to the site of action

I. Elimination of a drug from the body

J. Chemical reactions that alter foreign substances

K. Ability of a drug to produce an effect as a result of binding with a receptor

L. Interactions of drugs with cells and other body structures to produce characteristic effects.

Match the type of name with the example:

13. _____ cephalexin

14. _____ Keflex

15. _____ 7-(D-q-amino-α-phenylacea-mido)-3-methyl-3-cephem-4-carboxylic acid, monohydrate

A. Trade name

B. Generic name

C. Chemical name

State in which Schedule each controlled substance is listed:

16. pentobarbital (Nemb-utal) _____

17. heroin _____

18. buprenorphine _____

19. diazepam (Valium) _____

20. paregoric _____

List five factors that affect drug distribution in the body:

21.

22.

23.

24.

25.

26. List the Five Rights:

27. A drug is given orally. After absorption, most of the drug is inactivated as the blood passes through the liver, so there is no therapeutic effect. This is called:

A. tolerance.

B. first-pass effect.

C. antagonism.

D. pharmacodynamics.

28. The ability of drugs to attach to specialized regions of cells is the basis of which theory of drug action?

A. Chemical action

B. Physical action

C. Altered metabolic pathways

D. Receptor theory of drug action

29. Drugs that cause abnormal embryonic or fetal development are said to be:

    A. teratogenic.

    B. synergistic.

    C. antagonistic.

    D. efficacious.

30. Which statement is true regarding your responsibilities for drug therapy?

    A. You are not liable for mistakes as long as you follow doctor's orders.

    B. You are accountable for your actions as a licensed nurse.

    C. You cannot be expected to recognize adverse drug effects.

    D. You cannot refuse to carry out a legal order.

DRUGS USED RELATED TO PHYSIOLOGIC RESPONSES TO ILLNESS

OBJECTIVES

1. Identify classifications of drugs used to treat the following physiologic responses to illness: inflammation, infection, immune responses, fluid and electrolyte disorders, and pain.

2. Describe the general actions, side and adverse effects, interactions, and contraindications of drugs employed to treat physiologic responses to illness.

3. Identify nursing considerations for drugs used to treat physiologic responses to illness.

CHAPTER 4

ANTI-INFLAMMATORY AGENTS

*I*nflammation is a generalized response to tissue damage. It is said to be *localized* when it is confined to a specific region of the body. When the whole body responds, it is called *systemic inflammation*.

LOCALIZED INFLAMMATION

Localized inflammation begins with tissue trauma that may be caused by invasion of pathogens, mechanical injury, exposure to harmful substances, or ischemia. In response to tissue damage, mast cells release chemical mediators, including complement, histamine, leukotrienes, prostaglandins, and others. Chemical mediators act on target tissues, causing three important effects:

1. Blood vessels dilate, bringing increased blood to the affected tissue.

2. Capillary permeability increases so that extra fluid shifts into the affected tissue.

3. White blood cells, especially neutrophils and monocytes, are attracted to the area, a process called *chemotaxis*.

The outcome of this process is that white blood cells move into the tissue and destroy the pathogens. Macrophages clean up cellular debris, and tissue healing begins.

The sequence of events just described explains the classic signs and symptoms of inflammation. Increased blood flow causes the tissue to become red and warm, and fluid shifting into the area causes swelling. Prostaglandins and other chemical mediators stimulate pain receptors.

SYSTEMIC INFLAMMATION

When inflammation extends beyond a single area of the body, systemic defenses come into play. The bone marrow increases production of white blood cells. That is why patients with infections have elevated white blood cell counts (leukocytosis). Foreign substances trigger white blood cells to produce endogenous pyrogens. Pyrogens act on the hypothalamus to reset the body's thermostat, which activates mechanisms that cause the body temperature to rise (fever).

In some situations, such as anaphylaxis, generalized vasodilation and increased capillary permeability cause a precipitous drop in blood pressure.

INFLAMMATORY DISORDERS

A wide variety of conditions can cause inflammation. Examples are:

- Local tissue trauma: surgical incision, thermal burn, chemical burn, abrasion, muscle strains, deterioration of joint linings
- Tissue ischemia: myocardial infarction, pulmonary embolism
- Immune responses: acute rhinitis, dermatitis, rheumatoid arthritis
- Infection: pneumonia, otitis media, appendicitis

ANTI-INFLAMMATORY AGENTS

Anti-inflammatory agents fall into two categories: steroidal and nonsteroidal. The steroidal anti-inflammatory drugs are corticosteroids produced by the adrenal cortex. These naturally occurring hormones, which are used pharmacologically, are discussed in Chapter 43. Therefore, this chapter will focus on the nonsteroidal anti-inflammatory agents, which are commonly referred to as NSAIDs.

Nonsteroidal anti-inflammatory drugs are classified as prostaglandin synthetase inhibitors (PSIs) or nonprostaglandin synthetase inhibitors (non-PSIs).

Prostaglandin Synthetase Inhibitors

Prostaglandin synthetase inhibitors include carboxylic acids and enolic acids. Examples of carboxylic acids are salicylic, acetic, propionic, and anthranilic acids. The prototype you will probably recognize is aspirin (acetylsalicylic acid). Enolic acids include oxicams and pyrazolones.

Actions and Uses

Prostaglandin synthetase inhibitors prevent the synthesis and release of prostaglandins. They are useful in a variety of situations in which there is inflammation, pain, or fever. This could include acute infectious conditions as well as chronic inflammatory conditions such as osteoarthritis.

Side and Adverse Effects

Adverse effects of PSIs most commonly occur in the gastrointestinal tract, kidneys, and blood cells. Central nervous system effects are less common.

- Gastrointestinal effects: heartburn, nausea, vomiting, ulceration and bleeding, and abdominal pain
- Kidneys: renal impairment, retention of sodium and water, hyperkalemia
- Blood cells: decreased platelet aggregation (clumping), decreased white blood cells
- Central nervous system effects: tinnitus, vertigo, altered vision, confusion, drowsiness, dizziness, and headache

In addition, some people are allergic to PSIs. Manifestations of allergy are itching, rash, wheezing, and edema.

Interactions and Contraindications

Even though PSIs are available as over-the-counter drugs, you must always assess any potential interactions with other drugs the patient is taking because PSIs interact with many other drugs. Some important examples are diuretics and antihypertensives, which may be counteracted by PSIs. If given with anticoagulants, PSIs increase the risk of bleeding. Gastrointestinal adverse effects are enhanced by alcohol.

Nursing Actions

Assess for gastrointestinal symptoms, edema, decreased urine output, and easy bruising or bleeding. Be aware that older people taking PSIs are at greater risk for adverse effects, especially confusion. Evaluate local pain, swelling, redness, and warmth. With long-term therapy, monitor complete blood cell counts for decreased platelets and white blood cells. Patient teaching is especially important because these drugs are widely used and can be obtained without a prescription.

Patient Teaching
• Take PSIs 15 to 30 minutes before meals and with 8 ounces of water.
• If gastrointestinal upset occurs, you can take the drug with a little food or milk.
• Do not exceed the recommended dosage.
• Alcohol and caffeine tend to increase gastrointestinal distress with these drugs.

Salicylic Acid Prototype: Acetylsalicylic Acid (Aspirin)

Actions and Uses

Aspirin has anti-inflammatory, antipyretic, and analgesic effects. It is used to treat various symptoms, including headache, fever, and joint and muscle pain. Because of its antiplatelet effects, small daily doses are used to prevent thrombosis responsible for myocardial infarction and stroke.

Side and Adverse Effects

Aspirin has the general PSI adverse effects (gastrointestinal distress, renal damage, bleeding) already discussed. In addition, with prolonged or excessive use, there is a risk of salicylate poisoning (called salicylism). Symptoms of salicylism are tinnitus (ringing in the ears), headache, sweating, nausea and vomiting, and hyperventilation. In older people, the only symptom may be confusion. Allergic reactions occur most often in people who have asthma or nasal polyps.

Interactions and Contraindications

Aspirin interacts with many other drugs. For example, excretion of aspirin is enhanced by antacids and urine alkalinizers. Aspirin enhances the effects of insulin, oral hypoglycemics, and anticoagulants. It also increases the risk of toxicity from methotrexate and zidovudine. Be sure to assess all drugs the patient is taking for potential interactions.

General contraindications to aspirin therapy are bleeding disorders, anticoagulant therapy, history of asthma or nasal polyps, and the third trimester of pregnancy. If aspirin is given to young children or adolescents for viral infections, there is a risk of Reye's syndrome. Reye's syndrome is an often fatal syndrome that affects the central nervous system, kidneys, and liver.

Nursing Actions

Same as general PSI implications.

Patient Teaching

- Same as general PSI implications.

Acetic Acid Derivative Prototype: Indomethacin (Indocin)

Indomethacin (Indocin) is similar to aspirin in action, adverse effects, interactions, and contraindications. It is, however, 20 to 30 times more potent than aspirin. One unique action is that indomethacin causes the ductus arteriosus to close. Therefore, it is not given during the last trimester of pregnancy, when it could cause the ductus to close prematurely. The drug may be given to premature infants to induce closure of the ductus. It should be noted that some older people experience depression when on indomethacin.

Other acetic acid derivatives are sulindac (Clinoril), tolmetin sodium (Tolmetin), and diclofenac sodium (Voltaren).

Propionic Acid Derivative Prototype: Ibuprofen (Motrin, Advil, et al.)

Ibuprofen (Motrin) is similar to aspirin in action, adverse effects, interactions, and contraindications. In addition to assessing for gastrointestinal bleeding, renal function must be monitored with long-term therapy. Many patients who are allergic to aspirin are also allergic to ibuprofen. This and other propionic acid derivatives can cause photosensitivity, so patients should protect their skin from direct sunlight.

Another propionic acid derivative is ketoprofen (Orudis).

Prototypes of other PSI inhibitors are presented in Table 4–1.

TABLE 4–1

Miscellaneous Prostaglandin Synthetase Inhibitors

Type	Examples	Specific Considerations
Arylacetic acid derivatives	naproxen (Naprosyn) naproxen sodium (Anaprox) fenoprofen calcium (Fenoprofen)	Naproxen and naproxen sodium should not be given concurrently. Be alert for fluid retention with sodium preparation.
Anthranilic acid derivatives	mefenamic acid (Ponstel) meclofenamate sodium (Meclomen)	Both have significant adverse gastrointestinal effects. Mefenamic acid can cause agranulocytosis. Meclofenamate sodium has especially high incidence of colitis and diarrhea; also can cause renal and liver damage with long-term therapy.
Phenylalkanoic acid derivatives	flurbiprofen (Ansaid)	Similar to other PSIs
Oxicams	piroxicam (Feldene)	In addition to other PSI effects, can cause drowsiness and reduced hemoglobin and hematocrit.
Pyrrolacetic acid derivatives	ketorolac tromethamine (Toradol)	Only injectable NSAID. In addition to other PSI effects, is nephrotoxic with long-term use and causes drowsiness.

Non-Prostaglandin Synthetase Inhibitors (Non-PSIs)

Acetaminophen (Tylenol, et al.) is an example of a non-PSI. It is often used with inflammatory conditions, but it actually does not reduce inflammation. It is effective as an antipyretic and analgesic, so it is commonly used to treat mild pain and fever. It is discussed in greater detail in Chapter 8.

Gold Salts

One other type of drug that is used specifically for rheumatoid arthritis is gold salts. The prototype is gold sodium thiomalate (Myochrysine).

Actions and Uses

This drug seems to suppress the immune response in joint tissues, thereby decreasing inflammation and slowing the disease progression.

Side and Adverse Effects

Gold salts are very toxic. They can cause dermatitis, pruritus, skin pigmentation, stomatitis, renal toxicity, and bone marrow suppression. Some people are allergic to this drug.

Interactions and Contraindications

Do not give gold salts with other drugs that can suppress bone marrow. Use is contraindicated with diabetes mellitus, renal or hepatic dysfunction, enterocolitis, congestive heart failure, hypertension, and blood dyscrasias.

Nursing Implications

Gold sodium thiomalate is given intramuscularly on a weekly basis until a specific total dose has been given. For the injection, the patient should lie down and remain recumbent for at least 10 minutes. Toxic or anaphylactic reactions are treated with dimercaprol (BAL).

ANTI-INFECTIVES

*A*t the turn of the 20th century, infectious diseases were among the leading causes of death in the United States. With the advent of anti-infective agents and widespread use of immunizations by the 1950s, however, it was thought that eradication of infection was within our reach. There was a relatively brief period of dramatic decline in infectious disease deaths before new pathogens (agents capable of causing disease) and resistant strains of old pathogens began to emerge. Medical science was once again confronted with the task of developing drugs capable of destroying pathogens. It is now recognized that it will be an ongoing battle to stay one step ahead of the adaptive organisms that cause infectious disease.

Anti-infectives and *antimicrobials* are interchangeable terms used to describe pharmacologic agents employed to destroy microorganisms. Anti-infectives include antibacterial, antifungal, antiviral, antiparasitic, and miscellaneous other agents that are effective against specific types of pathogens. Anti-infectives that are effective against a broad range of organisms are said to be *broad-spectrum* drugs, whereas those that are effective against only a few organisms are said to be *narrow-spectrum* drugs.

MECHANISMS OF ACTION

Anti-infectives may be *bacteriostatic,* meaning they suppress the growth of bacteria, or *bactericidal,* meaning they kill actively growing bacteria. This is an important characteristic the physician must consider in selecting a specific drug. Patients with normal immune systems can usually resist infection and may be effectively treated with bacteriostatic drugs. The drugs hold the organisms in check and natural body defenses defeat them. Patients who lack normal immune response, however, may require bactericidal drugs to actually destroy the invading pathogens.

Anti-infectives exert their effects through a variety of mechanisms, including the following:

- Damage to cell walls either directly or by inhibiting cell wall synthesis
- Alteration of metabolic processes or structures required to maintain cell metabolism
- Interference with reproduction of organisms

RESISTANCE: NATURAL AND ACQUIRED

A major problem in the treatment of infection is the ability of microorganisms to resist destruction by drugs. The appearance of pathogens that are resistant to previously effective anti-infectives reflects the adaptability of the organisms. Organisms can resist drugs by natural or acquired resistance. Natural resistance is conferred by protective mechanisms such as a slime layer that is not readily penetrated or the production of enzymes that break down chemicals, including anti-infectives. To illustrate natural resistance, some pathogens produce penicillinase, an enzyme that breaks down penicillin. Organisms that produce penicillinase cannot be effectively treated with that drug; that is, the organisms are resistant to penicillin.

Acquired resistance can occur when genetic mutations produce a protective mechanism, or when resistant organisms transfer genes that confer resistance on nonresistant organisms. One other way that resistance is acquired is through "survival of the fittest." In any colony of organisms, some are stronger (more resistant) than others. Over time, the weakest die off and the strongest (most resistant) survive.

Factors that contribute to the development of resistant strains of microorganisms include the inappropriate use of anti-infectives and the indiscriminate use of broad-spectrum agents. An example of inappropriate use is prescribing antibacterial agents for the common cold, which is caused by a virus and for which there is no known effective drug. Remember that we all have pathogenic organisms on and in our bodies. Normally our natural defenses, including nonpathogenic organisms, control their multiplication so they do not cause illness. However, whenever these pathogens are unnecessarily exposed to anti-infectives that do not eradicate them, they begin to develop resistance.

Another situation that promotes resistance is failure to complete a course of anti-infective therapy. Typically, the patient is given a prescription for a week or 10 days. After a few days, the patient begins to feel better and becomes lax about taking the drug on time or stops taking it completely. This allows the blood level to fall so that pathogens are exposed to a low concentration of the drug—another situation that encourages the development of resistance.

Examples of dangerous pathogens that have developed significant antimicrobial resistance are MRSA (methicillin-resistant *Staphylococcus aureus*) and VRE (vancomycin-resistant *Enterococcus*).

PREVENTING RESISTANCE TO ANTI-INFECTIVES

The development of resistant strains of pathogens can be reduced by limiting the use of anti-infectives to appropriate circumstances, using the most effective drug for a given infection, using combinations of drugs, and scheduling doses to maintain therapeutic blood levels.

Anti-infectives have been so widely used in our society that people have come to expect them whenever they have any kind of infection. Since the widespread use of anti-infectives contributes to the development of resistant strains of microorganisms, these drugs should be used only when there is a serious infection known to be sensitive to available drugs. Most healthy people recover from common infections without anti-infective drugs.

Furthermore, it is important that the most appropriate drug be selected. The best choice is based on the results of culture and sensitivity (C & S) tests that identify the infecting organism and the drugs that are effective against it. With serious infections, the physician may order a C & S, then begin an anti-infective pending results of the test. When a C & S is ordered, collect specimens for culture before giving the first dose of an anti-infective. Once results are known, a decision is made whether to continue the first anti-infective or begin a different one. The drug with the narrowest possible spectrum of effectiveness should be used, avoiding indiscriminate use of the most powerful and broad-spectrum drugs. Some anti-infectives are very toxic and should be reserved for the most serious infections.

Using combinations of anti-infectives is one strategy that is sometimes helpful in curbing the development of resistance. An example of this approach is the use of two or more drugs in the treatment of tuberculosis. The organism that causes tuberculosis is highly adaptive and quickly develops resistance to single drugs.

To maintain a therapeutic blood level, anti-infectives are often scheduled at even intervals, such as every 6 or 8 hours rather that TID or QID. The consistent blood level more effectively kills pathogens and is less likely to foster resistance.

SIDE AND ADVERSE EFFECTS

Side and adverse effects common to many anti-infectives are presented here. Any time you give an anti-infective, these are effects to be aware of, but always look up the specific effects of each drug as well.

Allergic Reactions

The allergic response is caused by a process called *sensitization*. When people are exposed to antigens (in this case, drugs), plasma cells produce substances called immunoglobulin E (IgE) antibodies. IgE antibodies attach to mast cells in the gastrointestinal tract, the skin, and the respiratory tract. When the person is exposed to that same drug at a later time, it binds with the IgE antibodies that are attached to the mast cells. Mast cells respond by releasing chemicals, including histamine and leukotrienes. These chemicals trigger reactions that are commonly associated with allergies. Mild responses could be rash, diarrhea, rhinorrhea (runny nose), and sneezing. Intense itching and skin eruptions can be attributed to the allergic effects of some drugs.

A much more serious response is anaphylaxis. Anaphylactic reactions typically begin shortly after exposure to the drug to which the patient has become sensitized. Constriction of bronchi interferes with gas exchange and the patient struggles to breathe. Wheezing can be heard on auscultation of the lungs. As blood vessels dilate, blood pressure falls and circulation to the brain becomes inadequate. The heart rate increases in an attempt to compensate for the falling blood pressure. The patient feels dizzy, then may lose consciousness. The shift of fluid into body tissues causes massive edema. These dramatic effects can cause the patient to go rapidly into shock. Death can occur from respiratory and circulatory failure. Because the consequences of an allergic drug reaction can be fatal, you must always assess known drug allergies before giving anti-infective agents.

It is possible to have a delayed allergic reaction commonly called "serum sickness." It may occur weeks or months after exposure to a drug and is characterized by fever, vasculitis (inflammation of small blood vessels), enlarged lymph nodes, swollen joints, urticaria (hives), and bronchospasm.

An important concept to understand is *cross-sensitivity*. Many drugs share common chemical structures. Therefore, it is possible for a patient to be sensitized to one drug after being exposed to another drug with similar chemical structure. For example, glyburide is one of several sulfonylureas used to treat diabetes. The sulfonylureas can sensitize patients to sulfonamide anti-infectives. So, when the patient who has taken a sulfonylurea receives an initial dose of a sulfonamide, an unexpected allergic reaction can occur. This type of sensitization explains how allergic reactions can occur the first time a person is given a drug.

Mild allergic reactions can be treated with antihistamines and corticosteroids. Anaphylaxis is also treated with epinephrine, which counteracts bronchial constriction and vasodilation.

Superinfection

Not all microorganisms are harmful. Nonpathogenic bacteria that reside on the skin and in the gastrointestinal, genitourinary, and respiratory tracts help suppress the growth of pathogens. If these nonpathogenic organisms are eliminated by anti-infectives, pathogens may flourish and cause secondary infections. Such infections are called *superinfections*. They are often caused by drug-resistant gram-negative organisms or by fungi and may be more difficult to treat than the original infection.

Examples of superinfections commonly associated with anti-infective therapy are stomatitis (inflamed oral tissues with white patches, "black furry tongue"), diarrhea, and vaginal candidiasis (yeast infection). An especially serious superinfection is pseudomembranous colitis, caused by *Clostridium difficile*, and manifested by abdominal pain and bloody diarrhea. The patient may also develop signs of new or worsening local or systemic infections.

Superinfections are treated by discontinuing the first anti-infective and prescribing drugs effective against the organisms responsible for the new infection.

Direct Toxicity

Anti-infectives are potentially harmful to various body tissues, most often the kidneys, liver, gastrointestinal tract, nerves, and blood vessels.

Nephrotoxicity

Since most anti-infectives are eliminated through the kidneys, renal tissue is exposed to potentially high concentrations of these drugs. Drugs that can damage renal tissue are said to *nephrotoxic*. To reduce the risk of kidney damage, patients on anti-infectives are encouraged to maintain a high fluid intake unless contraindicated. This dilutes the concentration of the drug in the urine and decreases the potential for harm. Patients on nephrotoxic drugs should be monitored for decreasing urine output and elevated blood urea nitrogen and creatinine.

Neurotoxicity

Examples of toxic effects of drugs on nerve tissue are peripheral neuropathy, ototoxicity, and optic neuritis. Peripheral neuropathy refers to effects on the peripheral nerves and is often evident by numbness and tingling or burning sensations in the extremities. Ototoxicity refers to effects on the vestibulocochlear nerve, simply called the eighth cranial nerve. Symptoms of ototoxicity are tinnitus (ringing in the ears), hearing loss, and problems with balance. Optic neuritis refers to inflammation of the optic nerve and may be manifested by blurred vision.

Gastrointestinal Distress

Oral anti-infectives are often irritating to the gastrointestinal tract and may cause nausea, vomiting, and diarrhea.

Hepatotoxicity

Anti-infectives are transported throughout the body in the bloodstream, circulating through the liver. In addition, some anti-infectives are metabolized by the liver. This contact with hepatic tissue can result in direct tissue damage, called *hepatotoxicity*. The best way to assess hepatic damage when patients receive hepatotoxic drugs is by laboratory measurement of liver enzymes. Increasing enzymes can indicate liver damage and may require discontinuing the drug. One other sign of liver dysfunction is jaundice, a golden color of the sclera, skin, and urine.

Hematologic Effects

Some anti-infectives can affect blood components by suppressing blood cell production by the bone marrow or damaging circulating cells. A deficiency of red blood cells (RBCs) is called *anemia*. Signs and symptoms of anemia include fatigue, tachycardia, and pallor. A deficiency of white blood cells (WBCs) is called *leukopenia*. Leukopenia should be suspected in the patient who seems to have poor resistance to infection. Evidence of a deficiency of platelets, called *thrombocytopenia*, includes easy bruising and bleeding. In most situations, hematologic effects of anti-infectives are reversed when the drug is discontinued. However, some drugs pose a risk of severe and permanent bone marrow suppression. Therefore, patients on drugs that affect the bone marrow or blood cells must be monitored carefully with periodic blood tests. This is especially true with long-term therapy.

Photosensitivity

People with *photosensitivity* are excessively susceptible to the effects of sunlight. They may develop sunburn during relatively short periods of exposure. In severe cases, the affected areas of the skin become red and swollen, then darkly pigmented. Peeling, and sometimes scarring, follow. Light-skinned people are more likely than those with dark skin to develop photosensitivity.

NURSING ACTIONS

Before giving an anti-infective, check the chart for documented allergies and ask the patient about any known allergies. Never administer a drug to patient if there is reason to believe he or she might be allergic to it. Sometimes patients think that any adverse effect is an allergic reaction. Therefore, when patients indicate allergies, note the signs and symptoms that they experienced. Be sure the physician is aware of this information.

Always consider the possibility of allergic drug reactions at any time in the course of drug therapy. If patients are given parenteral anti-infectives in outpatient settings, have them remain at the site and under observation for at least 30 minutes before leaving. This allows prompt treatment of any serious reactions, which usually occur soon after administration.

When patients are taking nephrotoxic drugs, monitor urine output, blood urea nitrogen (BUN), and creatinine as indicators of kidney function. Check liver enzyme reports for increases consistent with hepatotoxicity. Assess the color of the sclera and skin for jaundice.

Parenteral anti-infectives should not be mixed with other drugs. Carefully follow directions for reconstituting and administering drugs. Most oral drugs should be given on an empty stomach. Check your drug handbook for specifics. Laws regarding the role of the vocational or practical nurse in administering IV drugs varies from state to state. You must know what is permitted in the state where you practice.

Assess for evidence that the drug is effectively eliminating the infection. Monitor the patient's temperature and white blood cell count for a return to normal. With local infections, assess wounds for decreasing redness, swelling, warmth, and pain.

Patient Teaching

- When taking anti-infectives, immediately notify your physician of rash, diarrhea, sneezing, difficulty breathing, dizziness, change in your skin color, or symptoms of new infections.
- Advise all health care providers of any drug allergies you have.
- If you are allergic to any drug, wear a medical alert tag stating the drug name. This would alert health providers if you require treatment in an emergency and cannot speak for yourself.
- Be sure to take this drug as scheduled and to complete the entire course of therapy.
- Avoid excessive sunlight while on drugs that cause photosensitivity. If you must be outside, wear long sleeves and pants and a brimmed hat. Put sunscreen on exposed skin.
- Take at least 2000 mL of fluids each day, unless advised otherwise by your physician

---

SPECIFIC ANTI-INFECTIVE DRUGS

There are hundreds of individual anti-infectives, and you must familiarize yourself with them when you encounter them in clinical situations. However, for efficiency, this book will introduce you to the major classifications of these drugs and offer limited examples. An understanding of major classifications will equip you with basic information common to most drugs within that classification. The classifications

are organized under antibacterial, antiviral, antifungal, antiparasitic, antiprotozoal, and miscellaneous drugs.

Antibacterial Drugs

Penicillins

Penicillin was discovered by Alexander Fleming in 1928 but was not available for clinical use until 1939. Imagine life before that time with no means to combat infectious diseases. Infants succumbed to deadly childhood infections, women died from sepsis following childbirth, and soldiers and laborers were lost to infected injuries—common situations then that are rare today. Indeed, the discovery of the medical applications for anti-infective agents changed the world forever.

Actions. The rigid cell walls of bacteria encase contents that have very high osmotic pressure. Penicillins work by weakening the bacterial cell wall. Without the protective barrier, water is drawn into the cell, causing it to rupture and die. Therefore, the penicillins are bactericidal. Penicillins are effective only against bacteria that are actively growing and multiplying. These drugs are excreted by the kidneys.

Side and Adverse Effects. Penicillins are among our safest antibacterials. Nevertheless, like all drugs, there are side and adverse effects. Effects common to most penicillins are noted here. Table 5–1 lists other effects of specific agents.

- Allergic response: An estimated 1–10% of people who are given penicillins have allergic reactions. Reactions can range from a rash to anaphylaxis. There are approximately 300 deaths each year in the United States from penicillin-allergic reactions.
- Superinfection: colitis
- Gastrointestinal effects: nausea, vomiting
- Neurotoxicity (with high blood levels): confusion, seizures, hallucinations
- Local tissue effects: pain at intramuscular injection site, thrombophlebitis at intravenous infusion site
- Nephrotoxicity: with high parenteral doses

Interactions and Contraindications. The risk of bleeding is increased if anticoagulants are given with high-dose penicillins. The effectiveness of oral contraceptives may be diminished during penicillin therapy, so patients should employ alternate means of birth control while under treatment. The effects of penicillins are increased if given with probenecid (Benemid) because probenecid interferes with penicillin excretion.

Penicillins are contraindicated with known allergy to penicillins or cephalosporins. They are used with extreme caution in patients with renal or gastrointestinal disease, bleeding disorders, and a history of asthma. Check your drug handbook for additional specific information about individual drugs.

TABLE 5–1

Penicillin Prototypes

Type	Specific Considerations
Natural penicillins: most effective against gram-positive *Cocci*	
Penicillin G benthazine (Bicillin, Permapen)	Penicillins that contain potassium or sodium can contribute significant amounts of electrolytes. Rapid IV infusion of potassium forms can cause hyperkalemia and cardiac dysrhythmias, especially with renal impairment. With potassium forms, monitor for hyperkalemia: cardiac dysrhythmias including bradycardia, muscle weakness, and tingling of the hands, feet, and tongue.
Penicillin G potassium (Pentids, Pfizerpen)	
Penicillin G procaine (Crysticillin, A. S. Wycillin)	
Penicillin G sodium (Na Pen G)	
Penicillin V potassium (Pen-Vee K, V-Cillin K, Veetids)	Sodium forms can cause fluid volume excess and heart failure; monitor for fluid volume excess: increased blood pressure, bounding pulse.
	Assess urine output before giving potassium or sodium penicillin preparations.
	Penicillin V decreases absorption of oral contraceptives. Advise patients who are taking oral contraceptives to use alternative means of birth control while taking penicillin V.
Extended spectrum: effective against some gram-negative organisms including *Pseudomonas aeruginosa* (Often given with an aminoglycoside)	
Carbenicillin (Geocillin)	Carbenicillin is an oral drug; should not be taken with meals.
Mezlocillin (Mezlin)	Ticarcillin contains much sodium, so it can cause fluid volume excess and heart failure. With ticarcillin, monitor for signs and symptoms of heart failure: increased blood pressure and pulse, dyspnea, decreased urine output.
Piperacillin (Pipracil)	
Piperacillin tazobactam (Zosyn)*	
Ticarcillin (Ticar)	Ticarcillin, mezlocillin and piperacillin interfere with platelet function, which can cause bleeding. Assess for easy bruising and unexplained or excessive bleeding.
Ticarcillin and clavulanate potassium (Timentin)*	
	Mezlocillin and piperacillin doses must be reduced in patients with renal dysfunction. None of these drugs should be mixed in the same IV solution with aminoglycosides. Some oral extended-spectrum drugs should be given on an empty stomach; others with meals. Check drug handbook for specifics. Monitor intake and output and blood studies for elevated BUN and creatinine. Some should be given on an empty stomach; others with meals. Check drug handbook. Monitor intake and output and blood studies for increasing BUN and creatinine.
Broad-spectrum: effective against some gram-positive *Cocci* and some gram-negative bacteria	
Amoxicillin (Amoxil, Polymox, Trimox, Wymox)	Tend to cause diarrhea. Amoxicillin is preferred for oral therapy because it causes less diarrhea than others.
Amoxicillin clavulanate (Augmentin)*	Ampicillin may cause rash in addition to diarrhea.
Ampicillin (Omnipen, Polycillin, Principen)	
Ampicillin sulbactam (Unasyn)*	Bacampicillin is a form of ampicillin but produces higher blood levels than regular ampicillin. Tell patient to report diarrhea. Record frequency of stools.
Bacampicillin (Spectrobid)	
	Inspect skin for rash.
	Amoxicillin, amoxicillin-clavulanate, bacampicillin may be taken with meals; others should be taken on empty stomach with full glass of water.

(Continued on p. 26)

Penicillinase-resistant: effective against penicillinase-producing *Staphylococcus aureus*

Oxacillin (Prostaphlin, Bactocill)

Cloxacillin (Cloxapen, Tegopen)

Dicloxacillin (Dynapen, Pathocil)

Methicillin (Staphcillin)

Oxacillin, cloxacillin, and dicloxacillin are available for PO use and can be given with meals. Others are usually given parenterally.

Methicillin can cause an inflammatory process in the kidney that may progress to renal failure; monitor renal function (urine output, BUN, creatinine).

---

*Sulbactam, clavulanic acid, and tazobactam are agents that inhibit penicillinase. When combined with various penicillins, it makes them more effective against penicillinase-resistant organisms.

Cephalosporins

The cephalosporins and the penicillins both have a beta-lactam ring as part of their chemical structures. Therefore, you will often see them referred to as beta-lactams. This common structure explains why there are many similarities in the actions and adverse effects of the cephalosporins and penicillins.

Actions. Cephalosporins are bactericidal. Like the penicillins, cephalosporins weaken the bacterial cell wall that protects the vital structures of the organism. As the wall deteriorates, water enters the cell, causing it to swell, rupture, and die. Cephalosporins are most effective against organisms that are actively growing and reproducing. Most cephalosporins are excreted through the kidneys.

Cephalosporins are classified as first-, second-, third-, and fourth-generation. Each generation is defined by the range of organisms against which it is effective (Table 5–2).

Side and Adverse Effects. The most serious adverse effect of cephalosporins is anaphylaxis. Because of the common beta-lactam structure, people who are allergic to penicillins may also be allergic to cephalosporins. This is an example of cross-sensitivity, which was described earlier. A person who has been sensitized to penicillin may have an allergic reaction with the first exposure to cephalosporin. Therefore, before giving a cephalosporin, always inquire about any previous reactions to penicillins. Cephalosporins are contraindicated in the person who has had an anaphylactic reaction to penicillin.

Other adverse effects are as follows:

- Local tissue effects: inflammation and pain at injection and infusion sites
- Gastrointestinal effects: nausea and vomiting (mostly with high-dose oral forms)
- Superinfection: can cause pseudomembranous colitis, which is severe, bloody diarrhea caused by *Clostridium difficile*. Treatment includes stopping the cephalosporin and treating the *Clostridium* infection.

- Nephrotoxicity: acute interstitial nephritis (AIN), possibly progressing to renal failure. Most likely with high doses. Signs: blood, protein, and white blood cells in urine; decreased urine output; increased blood urine nitrogen and creatinine.
- Neurotoxicity: confusion, seizures, muscle twitching. Most likely with renal dysfunction and with high intravenous doses.
- Hematologic effects: some cephalosporins destroy intestinal bacteria that produce vitamin K, which is needed to activate prothrombin. Without adequate prothrombin, the patient's blood does not clot normally and abnormal bleeding can occur.

Interactions and Contraindications. The effects of cephalosporins are increased by loop diuretics such as furosemide (Lasix), aminoglycoside antibacterials, and probenecid. They are decreased by tetracyclines.

Some cephalosporins interact with alcohol to cause nausea, vomiting, abdominal pain, headache, chest pain, hypotension, and palpitations. This is called a disulfiram-like reaction because it is similar to the effects of combining alcohol and disulfiram (Antabuse). Disulfiram is a drug used to treat alcoholism. Alcohol consumed up to 72 hours after taking some cephalosporins can trigger this response.

Contraindications include allergy to cephalosporins or penicillins. They are used cautiously with renal or hepatic dysfunction, bleeding disorders, and gastrointestinal disorders. Other contraindications and precautions during pregnancy and lactation vary with the individual drug.

Nursing Actions. Assess history of allergies before administering. If previous allergic response to cephalosporins or penicillins is suspected, withhold the drug and notify the physician. Administer doses at evenly spaced intervals to maintain therapeutic blood levels. With intravenous administration, infuse slowly at first to assess for allergic response. Have emergency equipment and drugs available.

Patient Teaching

- Take this medication on the prescribed schedule with doses evenly spaced.
- Complete the entire course of therapy.
- Notify your physician if you have rash, itching, difficulty breathing, swelling, dizziness, or diarrhea.
- Do not drink alcohol until at least 72 hours after completing the course of therapy.
- Contact your physician if your symptoms of infection do not improve within several days.
- Drink at least 2000 mL of fluid daily unless your physician advises otherwise. This is about eight 8-ounce glasses of fluid.

TABLE 5–2

Cephalosporins: Four Generations

Generation and Activity	Specific Prototypes
First Most effective against gram-positive organisms; moderately effective against some gram-negatives	cefadroxil (Duricef, Ultracef) cefazolin (Ancef, Kefzol) cephalexin (Keftab, Keflet) cephalothin (Keflin, Seffin)
Second Effective against more gram-negatives than first generation	cefaclor (Ceclor) cefamandole (Mandol) cefmetazole (Zefazone) cefonicid (Monocid) cefotetan (Cefotan) cefoxitin (Mefoxin) cefpodoxime (Vantin) cefprozil (Cefzil) cefuroxime (Ceftin, Kefurox, Zinacef) loracarbef (Lorabid)
Third More gram-negative, and less gram-positive effectiveness. Better action against *Pseudomonas aeruginosa*. Cross blood-brain barrier.	cefdinir (Omnicef) cefixime (Suprax) cefoperazone (Cefobid) cefotaxime (Claforan) ceftazidime (Fortaz, Tazicef, Tazidime) ceftibuten (Cedax) ceftizoxime (Cefizox) ceftriaxone (Rocephin)
Fourth Effective against both gram-positives and gram-negatives. Cross blood-brain barrier.	cefepime (Maxipime)

Other Beta-Lactams

In addition to penicillins and cephalosporins, carbapenems and monobactams are beta-lactams. All have the beta-lactam ring in common and act in similar fashion. Table 5–3 summarizes specific applications for the carbapenems and monobactams. Side and adverse effects are similar to those of the other beta-lactams.

TABLE 5–3

Miscellaneous Beta-Lactams

Beta-Lactams	Specific Considerations
Carbapenems imipenem/cilastatin (Primaxin)	Imipenem has the broadest range of effectiveness of all antibacterial drugs. Cilastatin is added because it inhibits an enzyme that breaks down imipenem. Dosage should be reduced with renal impairment. Be aware that the IM preparation contains lidocaine (a local anesthetic), so **assess for allergies** to lidocaine before administering.
meropenem (Merrem)	Meropenem is similar to imipenem: it has a broad spectrum of effectiveness, but it is more expensive.
Monobactam aztreonam (Azactam)	Aztreonam is effective against many drug-resistant gram-negative organisms, but not against gram-positive or anaerobic organisms.

Aminoglycosides

Actions and Uses. The aminoglycosides penetrate bacterial cell membranes and attach to organelles that synthesize proteins. By interfering with protein synthesis, they prevent reproduction of the organism. Aminoglycosides are most often used for gram-negative infections when other, less toxic, drugs fail.

Side and Adverse Effects. Side effects of aminoglycosides include nausea, diarrhea, anorexia, headache, and increased salivation. Intramuscular injections are painful and intravenous infusions can cause thrombophlebitis. The most serious adverse effects are ototoxicity and nephrotoxicity. Aminoglycosides also have a neuromuscular blocking effect that may be manifested by muscle weakness, difficulty breathing, and respiratory arrest. Other manifestations of neurotoxicity are headache, dizziness, lethargy, tremors, and visual disturbances.

Interactions and Contraindications. The risk of toxicity increases if aminoglycosides are given in combination with other ototoxic or nephrotoxic drugs. The neuromuscular blocking effects are enhanced by other neuromuscular blockers, which include drugs used during surgical procedures to cause paralysis.

Oral aminoglycosides are contraindicated with bowel obstruction, pregnancy, and lactation. They are used only with caution in people with Parkinson's disease or myasthenia gravis—both neuromuscular disorders that may be worsened by a blocking agent.

Nursing Actions. Assess for symptoms of ototoxicity (tinnitus, dizziness, hearing loss) and neuromuscular blockade (muscle weakness, shallow breathing). Monitor for signs of nephrotoxicity: increasing serum BUN and creatinine, proteinuria, and decreasing urine output. Assess for muscle weakness and difficulty breathing, which may reflect neuromuscular blockade. Intramuscular injections are less painful in the gluteus maximus than in the lateral thigh. Inject slowly. Blood samples may be drawn to assess serum drug levels at peak and lowest (trough) points in the day.

Patient Teaching
• Notify your physician if you have "ringing" in your ears, dizziness, muscle weakness, or difficulty breathing.
• Drink at least eight 8-ounce glasses of fluids each day (unless contraindicated).

Selected aminoglycosides are summarized in Table 5–4.

TABLE 5–4

Aminoglycosides

Drug	Specific Considerations
amikacin (Amikin)	Among aminoglycosides, has lowest incidence of resistance and broadest spectrum of action against gram-negative bacilli. Dosage based on ideal body weight.
gentamicin (Garamycin)	Less expensive than other aminoglycosides, but more organisms are resistant. Organisms that resist tobramycin often have cross-resistance to gentamicin as well. Do not mix in same solution with penicillin.
kanamycin (Kantrex)	Many pathogens are resistant. Oral form not absorbed; given to reduce bacterial flora before bowel surgery.
neomycin (Mycifradin)	Most toxic aminoglycoside if given parenterally. Oral form not absorbed; used to reduce bacterial flora before bowel surgery. Topical preparation used for infections of the skin, eye, and ear.
paromomycin (Humatin)	Given orally for intestinal amebiasis and tapeworm. May cause nausea, cramping, and diarrhea.
streptomycin (Streptomycin)	First aminoglycoside drug. Not widely used now except for treatment of some uncommon infections such as plague, tularemia, glanders, and brucellosis. Used in some tuberculosis regimens.
tobramycin (Nebcin)	Organisms that resist gentamicin often have cross-resistance to tobramycin as well. Do not mix in same solution with penicillin.

Tetracyclines

Actions and Uses. Tetracyclines, like aminoglycosides, pass through the cell walls of pathogens, attach to ribosomes, and interfere with protein synthesis. Unable to manufacture protein, the cell cannot maintain structural integrity or reproduce, and eventually dies.

Tetracyclines are broad-spectrum drugs, effective against an array of gram-positive and gram-negative organisms as well as rickettsiae, mycoplasmas, and some protozoa and spirochetes. Some specific uses for the tetracyclines include treatment of chlamydial infections and acne and prevention of "traveler's diarrhea." They are used to treat syphilis and gonorrhea in patients who are allergic to penicillin.

Many tetracyclines are excreted in the urine; however, doxycycline and minocycline are secreted into the intestine in the bile and eliminated in the feces.

Side and Adverse Effects. Adverse effects of tetracyclines include the following:

- Gastrointestinal effects: nausea, vomiting, epigastric pain, diarrhea
- Effects of bones and teeth: yellow-brown discoloration in developing teeth; suppression of growth of long bones in premature infants
- Superinfection: severe diarrhea associated with *Clostridium difficile*; candidal (yeast) infections of the mouth, vagina, and bowel
- Hepatotoxicity: most likely in pregnant women
- Nephrotoxicity: especially with pre-existing renal dysfunction
- Photosensitivity: exaggerated sunburn
- Local tissue effects: pain and irritation at site of injection or infusion
- Pseudotumor cerebri: (rare) elevated intracranial pressure

Interactions and Contraindications. Absorption of tetracyclines may be impaired by dairy products, antacids, iron, cholestyramine, and colestipol. Their effects can also be decreased by carbamazepine and phenytoin. Tetracyclines may interfere with oral contraceptives. Tetracyclines are contraindicated after the fourth month of pregnancy and in children younger than 8 years because of the risk of discolored teeth. Only doxycycline and minocycline should be given to patients with renal dysfunction; other tetracyclines may precipitate renal failure.

Nursing Actions. Assess for adverse effects as listed. Maintain prescribed rate of administration of intravenous doses; follow manufacturer directions. Rapid infusion may be harmful. Schedule oral doses at least 2 hours apart from antacids or iron preparations. Give oral drugs with nondairy liquids.

Patient Teaching

- If you have diarrhea or develop a rash or itching in your mouth or genitals, notify your physician.
- Do not take tetracycline within 2 hours of consuming dairy products, antacids, or iron preparations.
- If the drug irritates your stomach, you can take it with food (other than dairy products).
- If you use oral contraceptives, you will need to use an alternate form of birth control while on tetracycline.
- When outdoors, protect your skin from sun exposure.
- Drink at least eight 8-ounce glasses of fluids every day (unless contraindicated).

TABLE 5–5
Prototypes: Tetracyclines

Prototype	Specific Considerations
tetracycline hydrochloride (Achromycin, et al.)	Available as generic or under many trade names.
doxycycline (Vibramycin)	Unlike other tetracyclines, is safe with renal impairment.
demeclocycline (Declomycin)	Greatest risk of photosensitivity, so caution patient to protect skin from direct sunlight. In addition to antibacterial uses, is used to produce diuresis associated with SIADH (syndrome of inappropriate antidiuretic hormone).
minocycline (Minocin)	May cause vertigo and drowsiness. Possibly severe photosensitivity.

Macrolides

Actions and Uses. The macrolides, like tetracycline, penetrate the bacterial cell wall, attach to ribosomes, and inhibit protein synthesis, which eventually leads to cell death. Macrolides are effective against gram-positive organisms and gram-negative *Cocci* that often cause respiratory and skin infections.

Side and Adverse Effects. The most common adverse effects of macrolides are nausea, vomiting, and diarrhea. Some patients have reported headache. Hepatotoxicity has occurred on rare occasions. Like other anti-infectives, there is a risk of allergic responses and superinfections, most importantly severe diarrhea associated with *Clostridium difficile*. Other adverse effects specific to individual drugs are noted in Table 5–6.

Interactions and Contraindications. See Table 5–6 for interactions. Macrolides are contraindicated in people who are allergic to penicillins or cephalosporins because of possible cross-sensitivity.

Nursing Actions. General nursing measures include monitoring for adverse effects.

Patient Teaching

- Notify your physician if you have severe and/or bloody diarrhea.
- Drink at least eight 8-ounce glasses of water each day while taking this drug.

TABLE 5–6
Macrolides

Prototype	Specific Considerations
erythromycin (E-Mycin, Ery-Tab, Ilosone, Erythrocin, et al.)	Specific adverse effects: hepatotoxicity, cardiotoxicity, hearing loss, pancreatitis Interactions: • decreased effects of chloramphenicol and clindamycin • increased effects of carbamazepine, cyclosporine, felodipine, lovastatin, simvastatin, and warfarin • increased risk of hepatotoxicity if given with other hepatotoxic drugs • increased risk of cardiotoxicity if given with cisapride, terfenadine Can be given without regard to meals

(Continued on p. 30)

(Concluded from p. 29)

Prototype	Specific Considerations
azithromycin (Zithromax)	Specific adverse effects: dizziness, nephrotoxicity (acute interstitial nephritis) Interactions: • increased effects of carbamazepine, cyclosporine, theophylline, and warfarin • effects of azithromycin decreased if given with aluminum or magnesium antacids Give on empty stomach, 1 hour AC or 2 hours PC. Do not give within 2 hours of antacids.
clarithromycin (Biaxin)	Specific adverse effects: abnormal taste, hepatotoxicity, nephrotoxicity (acute interstitial nephritis) Interactions: • increased effects of astemizole, carbamazepine, cisapride, digoxin, terfenadine, theophylline, and warfarin • decreased effects of zidovudine • rifampin decreases concentration of clarithromycin Do not refrigerate, shake well before pouring, can be given without regard to meals
dirithromycin (Dynabac)	Specific adverse effects: weakness and nonspecific pain, heartburn, flatulence, insomnia, rash, urticaria (hives), pruritus (itching) Interactions: none significant Should be given with food or within 1 hour after eating

Sulfonamides

In 1935, the sulfonamides became available as the first clinically useful, safe antibacterial drugs.

Actions and Uses. Bacteria must synthesize their own folic acid to manufacture proteins. Sulfonamides interfere with the synthesis of folic acid, thereby suppressing bacterial growth. This is an example of bacteriostatic action. Sulfonamides have a broad spectrum of activity; however, many organisms have developed resistance over the many years that sulfonamides have been in use. These drugs continue to be important in the treatment of urinary tract infections. A combination of sulfonamide with trimethoprim (Bactrim, Septra) is widely used for a variety of infections.

Side and Adverse Effects

• Hypersensitivity reactions: mild allergic reactions to the sulfonamides are fairly common. A serious hypersensitivity response is the Stevens-Johnson syndrome, a potentially fatal reaction with lesions of the skin and mucous membranes. People who are allergic to oral sulfonylureas, thiazide diuretics, or loop diuretics may have cross-sensitivity to sulfonamide antibacterials.

• Hematologic effects: sulfonamides can suppress the production of red blood cells, white blood cells, and platelets. Hemolytic anemia (breakdown of red blood cells) may occur in people with a genetic predisposition.

• Kernicterus: sulfonamides can facilitate the passage of bilirubin across the blood-brain barrier in newborn infants. Bilirubin is toxic to brain tissue and can cause a disorder called kernicterus. There is a risk of neurologic damage and even death.

• Renal damage: older sulfonamides tend to form crystals in the urine. These crystals can obstruct kidney tubules, possibly causing severe kidney damage.

• Gastrointestinal effects: nausea, vomiting, and diarrhea.

Interactions and Contraindications. Sulfonamides increase the effects of oral hypoglycemics, phenytoin, and warfarin. They are contraindicated in pregnant women near term, breastfeeding mothers, and infants under 2 months of age.

Nursing Actions. Assess for allergy to any sulfonamide, oral hypoglycemic agent, loop diuretic, or thiazide diuretic. If an allergy is reported, withhold the drug and notify the physician. Inspect skin and mucous membranes for lesions. Monitor for fatigue, easy bruising or bleeding, and continued signs of infections. Monitor urine output. Encourage enough fluids to maintain a urine output of at least 1500 mL/day to reduce crystal formation and kidney damage.

Patient Teaching
• Drink at least eight 8-ounce glasses of fluid each day (unless contraindicated). • Protect your skin from sun exposure when outside. • If you develop a skin rash, stop taking this drug and notify your physician. • Notify your physician if you have unexplained or prolonged bleeding or easy bruising.

TABLE 5–7

Prototypes: Sulfonamides

Prototype	Specific Considerations
sulfamethoxazole (Gantanol)	Significant risk of crystalluria, so high fluid intake is especially important.
sulfasalazine (Azulfidine)	Poor oral absorption; remains in the bowel. Does not harm normal bacteria in colon. Has anti-inflammatory and antibacterial actions. Used to treat inflammatory bowel disease, rheumatoid arthritis. Give after meals. Hepatotoxic.
sulfisoxazole (Gantrisin)	Lower risk of crystalluria than most other sulfonamides.
sulfamethoxazole-trimethoprim (Bactrim, Septra, et al.)	Combination drug. Broad-spectrum. Can be nephrotoxic, so encourage additional fluids unless contraindicated.
Topicals mafenide (Sulfamylon) silver sulfadiazine (Silvadene)	Both are applied to burn wounds to prevent bacterial infections. Mafenide: stings when applied; is absorbed through the wound surface, which can lead to metabolic acidosis. Silver sulfadiazine: painless; is absorbed, but does not disturb acid-base balance.

Miscellaneous Antibacterials

In addition to the many drugs included in the above classifications, there are several other anti-infectives that merit mention. For efficiency, these are presented in table format, in Table 5–8.

TABLE 5–8

Miscellaneous Anti-infectives

Anti-infective	Uses and Adverse Effects	Nursing Considerations
chloramphenicol (Chloromycetin)	Broad-spectrum antibacterial. Rarely first choice because of toxicity. Adverse effects: <ul><li>Suppression of red and white blood cells and platelets</li><li>Gastrointestinal distress: nausea, vomiting, diarrhea</li><li>Neurotoxicity: optic neuritis, peripheral neuritis, depression</li><li>"Gray syndrome" in infants and children under age 2: abdominal distention, circulatory and respiratory failure, death. Reversible if drug stopped at onset of symptoms.</li><li>Superinfections</li></ul>	Monitor blood cell counts for bone marrow suppression. Assess for signs of agranulocytosis: sore throat, fever, fatigue, bleeding. Contraindicated with hepatic or renal impairment, in children under age 2, and in women nearing full term of pregnancy or breastfeeding. Risk of bone marrow depression is increased if given with anticonvulsants or other bone marrow depressants. Effects of oral hypoglycemics, warfarin, phenytoin, and phenobarbital may be increased, putting patient at risk for effects of overdose.

(Continued on p. 32)

(Concluded from p. 31)

Anti-infective	Uses and Adverse Effects	Nursing Considerations
vancomycin (Vancocin)	Effective against a variety of gram-positive pathogens, including methicillin-resistant *Staphylococcus aureus* (MRSA) and *Clostridium difficile*. Adverse effects: • Ototoxicity: permanent hearing loss possible • Nephrotoxicity • "Red man syndrome": rash on neck, face, chest, and arms; related to rapid IV infusion • Unpleasant taste in mouth, nausea, vomiting • Local tissue effects: thrombophlebitis and pain at infusion site	Risk of ototoxicity and nephrotoxicity increases if given with other drugs that can be ototoxic or nephrotoxic. Tell patient to report change in hearing or ringing in the ears. Monitor urine output, serum BUN, and serum creatinine. If patient develops rash during IV infusion, discontinue the infusion. Give future doses at a slower rate. Encourage oral hygiene. Antiemetics PRN. Assess infusion site for signs of infiltration; if present, restart at different site.

Fluoroquinolones
  ciprofloxacin (Cipro)
  ofloxacin (Floxin)
  norfloxacin (Noroxin)
  lomefloxacin (Maxiquin)
  sparfloxacin (Zagam)
  trovafloxacin (Trovan)
	Broad-spectrum antibacterials. Effective by PO route.
	Adverse effects:
	• Gastrointestinal effects: nausea, vomiting, diarrhea, abdominal pain
	• Central nervous system effects: dizziness, restlessness, confusion, headache
	• Musculoskeletal effects: (rare) rupture of tendons
		Contraindicated in children age 18 or younger and during ⚠ pregnancy or breastfeeding.
		Increases effects of warfarin and theophylline.
		If taking warfarin, monitor prothrombin time and assess for bleeding. If taking theophylline, monitor serum level; assess for cardiac dysrhythmias.
		Absorption decreased by milk, aluminum or magnesium antacids, iron, zinc, and sucralfate so do not give with these agents.
		Discontinue at first sign of musculoskeletal pain.

Antitubercular Drugs

Tuberculosis is a bacterial infection caused by *Mycobacterium tuberculosis*. It is transmitted by airborne droplets. Tuberculosis usually affects the lungs but can involve the kidneys, meninges, bone, adrenal glands, and gastrointestinal tract. It was a leading cause of death at the turn of the 20th century, but had declined dramatically with the advent of anti-infective agents. From 1986 to 1995, the incidence steadily increased and then began to level off. A major concern in the treatment of tuberculosis is the adaptability of the causative organism. *Mycobacterium tuberculosis* readily develops resistance to drugs, especially when it is exposed to a single drug. The key to managing tuberculosis seems to be using various combinations of drugs, which discourages the development of resistant strains. Because of the unique treatment programs required, antitubercular regimens are addressed separately in this chapter.

General nursing considerations with antitubercular drugs are as follows.

- Nursing Actions
  - Monitor for improvement: decreased sputum, cough, fever, night sweats, and fatigue.
  - Patients who cannot take their medications independently may come into a clinic for their medications.

- Patient Teaching
  - It is important to complete the entire course of therapy even after symptoms improve. If you do not complete the treatment, you will become reinfected and the disease may be much harder to treat.
  - Keep appointments for periodic blood studies to be sure you are not developing any problems related to your drugs.
  - Do not take other drugs without consulting your physician.

Primary Drugs

Primary, or first-line, drugs used to treat tuberculosis include isoniazid (INH), rifampin (Rifadin), ethambutol, pyrazinamide, and streptomycin. Combinations of these drugs are usually employed initially. If the patient does not respond, second-line drugs are prescribed.

Isoniazid (INH, Laniazid)

Actions and Uses. Isoniazid is a bactericidal agent that disrupts bacterial cell walls. It is the drug of choice in preventing tuberculosis in high-risk individuals and is used in combination with other drugs to treat active tuberculosis.

Side and Adverse Effects. More common side effects of isoniazid include peripheral neuritis, nausea, vomiting, dry mouth, dizziness, and hyperglycemia. Isoniazid inhibits the effects of pyridoxine (vitamin B_6) on the nervous system. Pyridoxine deficiency causes peripheral neuritis, manifested by numbness or tingling in the extremities. The symptoms are managed by giving vitamin B_6 supplements. Serious adverse effects are uncommon but can include neurotoxicity and hepatotoxicity.

Interactions and Contraindications. Alcohol decreases the effects of isoniazid by stimulating metabolism of the drug. It also increases the risk of hepatotoxicity, as does the concurrent use of other hepatotoxic agents. The effects of isoniazid on the nervous system are enhanced by disulfiram, so the patient may have behavior changes and impaired coordination. Also, sympathomimetics combined with isoniazid can cause a serious increase in blood pressure. This drug is contraindicated with liver disease.

Nursing Actions. Monitor for rash and fever, which suggest an allergic response to isoniazid. Check blood studies for elevated liver enzymes.

Patient Teaching

- Report abnormal sensations, gastrointestinal distress, or jaundice (yellow skin color).
- Avoid alcohol while taking isoniazid.
- Do not take laxatives or antacids at the same time you take isoniazid.
- Over-the-counter cold remedies can cause your blood pressure to rise dangerously.

Rifampin (Rifadin)

Actions and Uses. Rifampin exerts a bactericidal effect by interfering with protein synthesis and reproduction. In addition to tuberculosis, it is used to treat *Neisseria* meningitis and MRSA (methicillin-resistant *Staphylococcus aureus*).

Side and Adverse Effects. Rifampin imparts a reddish color to body fluids. This is not cause for concern. In addition to gastrointestinal distress and allergy, rifampin may cause:

- Neurologic effects: headache, visual disturbances, confusion, drowsiness
- Hepatotoxicity
- Hematologic effects: suppressed production of red blood cells, white blood cells, and platelets

Interactions and Contraindications. The risk of hepatotoxicity increases if other hepatotoxic drugs, including alcohol, are taken. Rifampin can decrease the effects of a variety of drugs including oral contraceptives, warfarin, oral hypoglycemics, digoxin, verapamil, and theophylline. The only specific contraindication is allergy, but rifampin is used cautiously with liver disease or alcoholism.

Nursing Actions. Same as isoniazid.

Patient Teaching

- Your urine will appear red while on this medication; this is normal and is not harmful.
- If you wear soft contact lens, rifampin can discolor them.
- It is best to take this drug 1 hour before or 2 hours after meals with 8 ounces of water. However, if it upsets your stomach, you can take it with food.
- Oral contraceptives may not be reliable when you are taking rifampin.

Ethambutol (Myambutol)

Actions and Uses. Ethambutol is a bacteriostatic agent that interferes with bacterial reproduction. It is used to treat tuberculosis and atypical mycobacterial infections.

Side and Adverse Effects. Ethambutol can cause gastrointestinal distress, headache, dizziness, joint pain, and dermatitis. More serious adverse effects are:

- Neurologic effects: optic neuritis (usually with long-term use, high dosage); peripheral neuritis
- Hematologic effects: suppression of platelet production
- Allergic reactions: anaphylaxis (rare)

Interactions and Contraindications. Neurologic effects are enhanced by other neurotoxic drugs. Ethambutol is contraindicated with optic neuritis.

Nursing Actions and Patient Teaching. General nursing care has been outlined. In addition, advise the patient of specific adverse effects to be reported.

Pyrazinamide (Pyrazinamide)

Actions and Uses. Pyrazinamide is used to treat tuberculosis. The exact mechanism of action is not known.

Side and Adverse Effects. Pyrazinamide often causes muscle and joint pain. The primary adverse effects are hepatotoxicity and decreased platelet production. Photosensitivity develops in some patients.

Interactions and Contraindications. Pyrazinamide can decrease the effects of other drugs, including several used in the treatment of gout. The most important contraindication is liver disease.

Nursing Actions. In addition to the general considerations presented earlier, teach the patient the specifics of this drug as outlined in Patient Teaching.

Patient Teaching
• Report unexplained bleeding or easy bruising. • The drug can be taken with food to prevent gastrointestinal distress. • If you find that you sunburn easily, protect your skin from direct exposure when outside.

Streptomycin (Streptomycin)

Streptomycin is an aminoglycoside that can be used in combination with other antitubercular drugs. Aminoglycosides are discussed in detail earlier in this chapter.

Second-Line Drugs

If the patient fails to respond to first-line drugs, additional antitubercular drugs are selected. These drugs are outlined in Table 5–9.

TABLE 5–9

Second-Line Antitubercular Drugs

Drug	Specific Considerations
paraaminosalicylic acid (PAS)	PAS raises the blood level of isoniazid. Causes significant gastrointestinal distress: diarrhea, abdominal pain, vomiting. Tolerated by children better than adults. Protect tablets from light, heat, and moisture.
capreomycin (Capastat)	Nephrotoxic: monitor urine output, BUN, creatinine. Contraindicated with renal disease. Ototoxic: assess hearing and balance. Only given per IM route.
ethionamide (Trecator-SC)	Gastrointestinal distress is common. Hepatotoxic and neurotoxic. Assess for peripheral neuritis and confusion.
cycloserine (Seromycin)	Neurologic effects are common; may include confusion, anxiety, hallucination, seizures, psychosis. Hepatotoxic.

Courses of Therapy

Examples of the many courses of antitubercular treatment are as follows:

- INH, rifampin, pyrazinamide, and streptomycin or ethambutol for 2 months, followed by INH and rifampin alone for an additional 4 months
- INH and rifampin with or without streptomycin for 4 to 6 months
- INH, rifampin, and pyrazinamide for 2 months, followed by INH and rifampin for an additional 4 months

Antiviral Drugs for Non-Human Immunodeficiency Virus (Non-HIV) Infections

Viruses are infectious agents that consist of genetic material encased in a protective coat. They lack the biochemical processes needed for replication (reproduction). Therefore, viruses invade host cells and use the biochemical mechanisms of the host cells to support replication. As the virus replicates, it can promptly destroy the host cell, alter the reproduction of the host cell, or remain dormant for a long period of time. People who harbor dormant viruses may be carriers. That means they are able to transmit the infection even though they manifest no symptoms of the disease.

From a medical perspective, the challenge in treating viral infections is to destroy the virus without destroying the host cells. Viral replication can be prevented only by interrupting biochemical mechanisms, which, in this case, will also prevent replication of host cells. For that reason, there are relatively few antiviral agents in use as compared with antibacterial agents. In the last decade, however, several effective and safe drugs have been developed. These drugs generally have narrow ranges of effectiveness. Several antiviral agents are discussed in detail. Others are summarized in Table 5–10.

Amantadine (Symmetrel)

Actions and Uses. Amantadine has long been used in the treatment of Parkinson's disease but is now recognized for its ability to suppress growth of some strains of the type A influenza virus. The exact mechanism of action is unclear. To be most effective in treating active influenza A infection, therapy with amantadine should be started within 48 hours of the onset of symptoms. If started promptly, amantadine can significantly reduce the severity and duration of the infection. When used to prevent influenza A infection, amantadine is given for 5 to 6 weeks during epidemics.

Side and Adverse Effects. Adverse effects tend to be mild with amantadine. However, it can cause the following:

- Neurologic effects: most often nervousness, insomnia, and difficulty concentrating; depression, hallucinations, and seizures occur less often
- Cardiovascular effects: orthostatic hypotension and (rarely) congestive heart failure
- Teratogenesis: crosses the placental barrier; harmful to embryos in laboratory animals; risks to fetus must be considered during pregnancy

Interactions and Contraindications. Teach patients, especially the frail and elderly, to seek medical attention as soon as influenza symptoms develop (fever, chills, cough, muscle aches, sore throat, gastrointestinal disturbances). Amantadine intensifies the effects of anticholinergic drugs. There are no specific contraindications, although it is used only with caution in people with histories of congestive heart failure, orthostatic hypotension, and liver or renal disease.

Nursing Actions. Assess for fluid retention: edema, dyspnea, decreased urine output. Assess mental-emotional status. Monitor blood pressure with position changes to detect orthostatic hypotension.

Patient Teaching

- Complete the full course of therapy, even if you are feeling better.
- Change positions slowly, avoid prolonged standing and hot baths or showers.
- Report changes in your mental or emotional state.

Rimantadine (Flumadine)

Rimantadine closely resembles amantadine in action, uses, and side effects. However, rimantadine has a much lower incidence of neurologic side effects.

Acyclovir (Zovirax)

Actions and Uses. Acyclovir is the first choice in the treatment of herpes simplex and varicella-zoster virus infections. It suppresses the synthesis of viral DNA. Resistance is most likely in patients with suppressed immune responses.

Side and Adverse Effects. When given intravenously, acyclovir may cause inflammation at the infusion site. Nephrotoxicity can be caused by acyclovir being deposited in the kidney tubules. This can be minimized by providing extra fluids during and for 2 hours after the infusion of acyclovir. The most common side effects of oral therapy are nausea, vomiting, diarrhea, headache, and dizziness. More serious adverse effects are uncommon. Topical acyclovir stings when applied to lesions.

Interactions and Contraindications. The risk of nephrotoxicity increases if given with other nephrotoxic drugs. The effects of acyclovir may be enhanced by probenecid. Other than known allergy, there are no contraindications to acyclovir.

Nursing Actions. Monitor for increased blood urea nitrogen and creatinine, which suggest nephrotoxicity. Be aware that intravenous infusions should run slowly, at least over 1 hour. Inspect the infusion site for redness or swelling. Dosages should be reduced for patients with renal impairment.

Patient Teaching

- Do not crush or break capsules.
- You can take this drug with or without food.
- When receiving intravenous acyclovir, report pain at the site of infusion.
- Apply topical acyclovir with a gloved finger.
- Acyclovir does NOT cure herpes simplex infections; it only decreases symptoms.
- To prevent infecting sexual partners, avoid sexual contact when lesions are present.

Ganciclovir (Cytovene, Vitrasert)

Actions and Uses. Ganciclovir interferes with synthesis of viral DNA and replication. Because of its toxicity, it is reserved for the treatment of cytomegalovirus (CMV) in patients with acquired immunodeficiency syndrome (AIDS) and for prevention of CMV in people who have had transplants. It can be given intravenously, orally, or via an implanted insert. Vitrasert is the form of the drug that is implanted in the eye for treatment of CMV retinitis (inflammation of the retina of the eye). The implant dispenses the drug over 5 to 8 months, then can be replaced.

Side and Adverse Effects. Side effects include nausea, rash, fever, confusion, and liver dysfunction. The most serious adverse effect of ganciclovir is bone marrow suppression with resulting deficiencies in white blood cells and platelets. Visual disturbances and retinal detachment have occurred. There is a risk of sterility in males. Ganciclovir may be teratogenic.

Interactions and Contraindications. The risk of bone marrow suppression is increased if ganciclovir is given with zidovudine (AZT) or other drugs that suppress the bone marrow. Ganciclovir is contraindicated in people with normal immune function.

Nursing Actions. Monitor blood counts throughout the course of therapy. Withhold the drug and notify the physician if the neutrophil count falls below 500 mm^3 or the platelet count falls below 25,000/mm^3. Assess for signs and symptoms of infection: fever, sore throat. Monitor rate of intravenous administration to flow over at least 1 hour.

Patient Teaching

- Report any signs of infection, easy bruising, or bleeding.
- Follow-up blood studies are critical because the drug can affect your blood cells.
- This drug can cause sterility in males.
- This drug can be harmful to a fetus; females should avoid pregnancy during and for 3 months after therapy.
- Drink at least eight 8-ounce glasses of fluids each day (unless contraindicated).

TABLE 5–10

Miscellaneous Antiviral Drugs for Non-Human Immunodeficiency Virus Infections

Drug	Specific Considerations
famciclovir (Famvir)	Used to treat acute herpes zoster (the virus that causes chickenpox and "shingles"). Action and side adverse effects similar to acyclovir. With renal impairment, space doses 12–24 hours apart. Can be taken alone or with meals.
valacyclovir (Valtrex)	Used to treat herpes zoster in patients with normal immune function. Effects similar to acyclovir, except it can cause very serious hematologic and renal effects in people with impaired immune function. Reduced dosage with renal impairment.
cidofovir (Vistide)	Used to treat CMV retinitis in patients with AIDS. Administered IV weekly or every other week. Most important adverse effect is renal damage. To reduce harm to kidneys, oral probenecid and additional IV fluids are given with each infusion. Can also suppress production of white blood cells, so neutrophil count must be monitored.
foscarnet (Foscavir)	Effective against all herpes viruses, but is more expensive and has more adverse effects: nephrotoxicity, hypocalcemia, hypokalemia, hypomagnesemia, hypophosphatemia or hyperphosphatemia, gastrointestinal distress, anemia, and headache. IV pump must be used to control flow rate because too rapid rate contributes to adverse effects. Reduced dose with renal impairment.
ribavirin (Virazole)	Used only for severe respiratory syncytial virus (RSV) in limited situations. Very expensive. Administered by oral inhalation using an oxygen hood for 12–18 hours a day from 3–7 days. Low toxicity, but can cause respiratory problems in selected patients, especially those on mechanical ventilation. Contraindicated during pregnancy. **Pregnancy Category X.**
rimantadine (Flumadine)	Similar to amantadine in uses, actions, and effects. Central nervous system side effects less common than with amantadine.
interferon alfa alfa-2a (Roferon-A) alfa-2b (Intron A) alfa-n3 (Alferon N)	Used to treat various viral infections including hepatitis B and C. Also used in cancer treatment. Adverse effects: fever, chills, fatigue, muscle aches, headache, anorexia, diarrhea, abdominal pain, dizziness, and cough. With high doses: bone marrow suppression, neurotoxicity, hair loss, cardiotoxicity, and thyroid dysfunction.
ophthalmic agents trifluridine (Viroptic) vidarabine (Vira-A) idoxuridine (Herplex Liquifilm)	Trifluridine and vidarabine are used for eye infections caused by herpes simplex virus (HSV) types 1 and 2; idoxuridine only for HSV type 1 eye infections. Common side effects include a stinging sensation, photophobia, and edema of the eyelids. Systemic absorption minimal.

Antiviral Drugs For Human Immunodeficiency Virus Infections

The human immunodeficiency virus (HIV) destroys CD4 T lymphocytes, leaving the patient at risk for overwhelming infections and certain types of cancer. HIV is classified as a *retrovirus*. For replication, retroviruses require an enzyme called RNA-dependent DNA polymerase (simply called reverse transcriptase) to convert RNA to DNA.

Although no current drug is capable of killing HIV, several have been found that suppress the replication of the virus, enabling patients to live longer. The three types of anti-HIV drugs in use at this time are nucleoside reverse transcriptase inhibitors, non-nuclide reverse transcriptase inhibitors, and protease inhibitors. With all of these drugs, a positive therapeutic response is indicated by rising CD4 T cell counts and declining plasma HIV RNA.

A prototype for each type of anti-HIV drug is presented here with other examples summarized in Table 5–11.

Nucleoside Reverse Transcriptase Inhibitors

Nucleoside reverse transcriptase inhibitors (NRTIs) include zidovudine (Retrovir), didanosine (ddI), zalcitabine (ddC), stavudine (d4T), and lamivudine (3TC). Zidovudine will be used as the prototype NRTI.

Zidovudine (Retrovir)

Actions and Uses. By inhibiting reverse transcriptase, zidovudine interferes with viral DNA synthesis, thereby suppressing replication of HIV. The drug is used in combination with other anti-HIV drugs to decrease the development of resistance. Zidovudine can be administered orally or intravenously.

Side and Adverse Effects. The most serious adverse effects of zidovudine are hematologic: suppression of red and white blood cells. Gastrointestinal effects include anorexia, nausea, vomiting, abdominal pain, and diarrhea. Symptoms of neurotoxicity include confusion, headache, anxiety, insomnia, and seizures. There may be damage to muscle fibers, referred to as *myopathy*.

Interactions and Contraindications. Probenecid raises the serum level of zidovudine, thereby increasing the risk of toxicity. The blood level is decreased by clarithromycin. Toxic effects of zidovudine are enhanced by other drugs with similar effects. For example, ganciclovir increases the risk of adverse hematologic effects.

Zidovudine is contraindicated only in patients who have had serious allergic reactions to it. However, it is used cautiously in people with renal or hepatic disorders and those with bone marrow suppression.

Nursing Actions. Monitor blood studies for declining red or white blood cell counts and for increasing liver enzymes, blood urea nitrogen, or creatinine. Assess for fatigue and pallor, which suggest anemia, and signs of infection including fever. Intravenous zidovudine is given over 1 hour; it is not mixed with blood products or protein solutions.

Patient Teaching

- Zidovudine does not cure HIV; it only slows the progress of the infection. Therefore, you must take precautions not to transmit it to others.
- It is very important to take this drug exactly as prescribed with doses evenly spaced to maintain blood levels.
- Do not take any other medications without consulting your physician.
- You must have blood studies done every 2 weeks to be sure your blood cells remain normal.
- Notify your physician if you have any new symptoms.

Non-Nucleoside Reverse Transcriptase Inhibitors

Non-nucleoside reverse transcriptase inhibitors (NNRTIs) directly interfere with growth of the DNA strand, thereby preventing replication of the virus. The two NNRTIs in use at this time are nevirapine (Viramune) and delavirdine (Rescriptor). Nevirapine is presented as the prototype.

Nevirapine (Viramune)

Side and Adverse Effects. The only serious adverse effect of nevirapine is rash. The rash is mild in most people but can be extensive (Stevens-Johnson syndrome), with blisters, oral lesions, conjunctivitis, and muscle and joint pain.

Interactions and Contraindications. Nevirapine increases the metabolism of many other drugs, including oral contraceptives and protease inhibitors, which decreases the serum levels of these drugs. The serum level of nevirapine may be decreased by rifampin and rifabutin.

Nursing Actions. Monitor CD4 T cell counts and plasma HIV RNA for decreases, which would indicate positive response to the drug. Be aware of drug interactions and anticipate the need for some dosage adjustments.

Patient Teaching	**Patient Teaching**
• This drug does not cure HIV, so you must still take precautions to avoid transmitting the infection to others. • Notify your physician immediately if you develop a rash. • Complete the full course of treatment. • Take doses at evenly spaced intervals to maintain even blood levels.	• Always take saquinavir with food. • Do not take saquinavir with grapefruit juice. • Take the drug exactly as prescribed with doses evenly spaced. • Report an increase in thirst, appetite, and/or urine output, which may indicate diabetes. • Do not take other drugs without consulting your physician. • Saquinavir does not cure HIV, so you must still take precautions to prevent transmission of the infection to others.

Protease Inhibitors

The replication of HIV requires the synthesis of enzymes and structural proteins that are produced as a chain-like structure. Protease is an enzyme that breaks the chain into individual units. This frees the enzymes and proteins for the developing virion (virus particle) to use. Without protease, the enzymes and proteins are useless and the virion is unable to mature and become infectious.

Saquinavir (Invirase)

Action and Uses. Protease inhibitors, including saquinavir, prevent protease from breaking the chain of enzymes and proteins. The HIV virion remains immature. Treatment of HIV is the only approved use for saquinavir.

Side and Adverse Effects. Adverse effects are rare but may include headache, nausea, diarrhea, abdominal pain, and possibly diabetes.

Interactions and Contraindications. Saquinavir decreases the metabolism of some other drugs, allowing them to accumulate and possibly reach toxic levels. Some drugs, including rifampin, can accelerate the metabolism of saquinavir so that it falls below therapeutic levels. Others drugs slow saquinavir metabolism, causing the blood level to rise. Interestingly, grapefruit juice also slows saquinavir metabolism.

Nursing Actions. Monitor results of CD4 T cell count and plasma HIV RNA studies. Anticipate the effects of specific drug interactions; dosage adjustments may be necessary.

TABLE 5–11

Additional Antiviral Drugs for Human Immunodeficiency Virus (HIV) Infections

Classifications and Examples	Specific Considerations
Nucleoside Reverse Transcriptase Inhibitors	
didanosine (Videx)	Route: oral; food interferes with absorption so best taken 1 hour before or 2 hours after meals. Adverse effects: Risk of potentially fatal pancreatitis. Less risk of bone marrow suppression than with zidovudine. Can cause chills and fever, rash, peripheral neuropathy (numbness and tingling), and diarrhea. Dosage based on body weight; reduced with renal impairment. Tablets should be chewed or crushed and dissolved in at least 1 ounce of water. Powders are mixed with 4 ounces of water and dissolved before drinking.
zalcitabine (Hivid)	Route: oral. Adverse effects: potentially severe and irreversible peripheral neuropathy, pancreatitis, and ulcerations of the oral mucosa. Risk of pancreatitis increases with alcohol and with IV pentamidine. Tell patient to report any numbness, tingling, or pain in extremities promptly.
stavudine (Zerit)	Route: oral; not affected by meals. Adverse effects: pancreatitis, peripheral neuropathy.
lamivudine (Epivir)	Route: oral; can be given with food. Adverse effects: no major adverse effects; transient insomnia and headache.
Non-Nucleoside Reverse Transcriptase Inhibitors	
delavirdine (Rescriptor)	Similar to nevirapine. Adverse effects: serious rash, headache, fatigue, gastrointestinal distress, elevated liver enzymes. Can raise blood levels of other drugs taken concurrently. Absorption of delavirdine impaired by antacids and didanosine, so these drugs should be given at least 1 hour apart.

Protease Inhibitors

indinavir (Crixivan)	Route: oral; take on empty stomach or with light, low-fat meal. Adverse effects: kidney stones, diabetes, gastrointestinal distress, headache, dizziness, blurred vision, rash, weakness, metallic taste, and thrombocytopenia (low platelet count). Indinavir can impair metabolism of other drugs, leading to toxic effects of those drugs. Give 1 hour apart from didanosine.
ritonavir (Norvir)	Route: oral; food improves absorption with capsules. Solution can be dissolved in chocolate milk, Ensure, or Advera to improve taste. Adverse effects (most are transient): nausea, diarrhea, vomiting, muscle weakness, altered taste, numbness or tingling. May cause diabetes. Decreases metabolism of some drugs, leading to toxicity of those drugs; increases metabolism of other drugs, leading to decline in blood level of those drugs.
nelfinavir (Viracept)	Route: oral; absorption increased by food. Adverse effects: diarrhea; may cause diabetes.

Antifungal Drugs

Fungi are capable of causing diseases, including histoplasmosis, coccidioidomycosis, ringworm, athlete's foot, and thrush. Fungal infections can be superficial or systemic. Superficial infections are more common, but systemic infections are more dangerous.

Systemic Antifungal Drugs

Drugs used to treat systemic fungal infections include amphotericin B (Fungizone Intravenous), ketoconazole (Nizoral), itraconazole (Sporanox), fluconazole (Diflucan), and flucytosine (Ancobon). Amphotericin B and ketoconazole will be discussed in detail. Key features of others are summarized in Table 5–12.

Amphotericin B

Actions and Uses. Amphotericin B increases the permeability of the fungal cell wall, which can lead to destruction of the cell. This drug is reserved for the most serious systemic fungal infections. Treatment may require as long as 4 months for eradication of the infection. Amphotericin B is almost always administered intravenously for systemic infections.

Side and Adverse Effects. Amphotericin B is very toxic. Adverse effects include the following:

- Reactions to intravenous infusion: chills, fever, nausea, and headache
- Local tissue toxicity: phlebitis at infusion site
- Nephrotoxicity: renal damage almost always occurs; not always reversible.

- Electrolyte imbalance: hypokalemia (low serum potassium) associated with renal damage
- Hematologic effects: bone marrow depression
- Neurologic effects: delirium
- Respiratory effects: wheezing, hypoxia
- Cardiovascular effects: hypotension or hypertension
- Other uncommon effects: dysrhythmias, anaphylaxis, liver failure, rash, diabetes insipidus

Interactions and Contraindications. Other nephrotoxic drugs increase the risk of renal damage with amphotericin B. Flucytosine enhances amphotericin B; therefore, a combination of the two may be used. This can achieve therapeutic effects with a lower dose of amphotericin B, which poses less risk of toxicity. Amphotericin B is contraindicated in patients with known allergy to it or to sulfites. It is used only with caution with renal impairment.

Nursing Actions. Before intravenous amphotericin is given, administer diphenhydramine (Benadryl), aspirin or acetaminophen, and meperidine (Demerol) as ordered to reduce adverse reactions. Monitor vital signs during administration. Assess every 15 minutes during the first ½ hour, then every 30 minutes for the next 4 hours. Inspect the infusion site for redness or swelling. Measure intake and output. Check results of blood urea nitrogen and creatinine tests. Assess for signs and symptoms of hypokalemia: cardiac dysrhythmias, muscle weakness. Note that nursing research has found that wrapping the extremities in towels or blankets to conserve warmth decreases the chills and shaking associated with intravenous administration.

Patient Teaching

- Let me know if you feel like you are having a chill while receiving this drug.
- We will be monitoring your vital signs and urine output frequently.

Ketoconazole (Nizoral)

Ketoconazole is a safer alternative to amphotericin B in the treatment of less serious systemic fungal infections.

Actions and Uses. Ketoconazole, like amphotericin B, disrupts the fungal cell membrane. It is effective against many fungi including *Candida albicans,* which causes "yeast" infections. Therapy may extend over several months.

Side and Adverse Effects. The most common adverse effects of ketoconazole are nausea and vomiting, which can usually be managed by giving the drug with food. Other side effects include rash, fever, chills, constipation or diarrhea, headache, and photophobia. Hepatotoxicity is the most serious adverse effect. By inhibiting testosterone synthesis in males, ketoconazole can cause gynecomastia (breast enlargement), decreased libido, and reversible sterility. Females may have menstrual irregularities associated with decreased synthesis of hormones.

Interactions and Contraindications. Ketoconazole absorption requires an acid environment; therefore, it should not be given within 2 hours of antacids or drugs that decrease gastric acid secretion. Other hepatotoxic agents, including alcohol, increase the risk of liver damage. Ketoconazole can increase or decrease the serum level of several other drugs. The only specific contraindication is allergy to ketoconazole, but it is used cautiously with liver disease.

Nursing Actions. Monitor liver enzymes.

Patient Teaching

- Notify your physician if you have unusual fatigue, dark urine, or pale stools.
- Nausea and vomiting can usually be controlled by taking this drug with food.
- It is important to complete the course of therapy and to take the drug exactly as prescribed.
- Do not take antacids or drugs that reduce gastric acid secretion within 2 hours of taking this drug.
- Do not take any other drugs without consulting your physician.

TABLE 5–12
Systemic Antifungal Drugs

Drug	Specific Consideration
itraconazole (Sporanox)	Route: oral; absorption enhanced by food. Used for a variety of infections including blastomycosis, histoplasmosis, aspergillosis, and onychomycosis. Adverse effects: gastrointestinal distress, rash, headache, abdominal pain, edema. Rarely: hepatitis.
fluconazole (Diflucan)	Route: oral. Adverse effects (less than ketoconazole): gastrointestinal distress, diarrhea, headache. Rare: liver necrosis, Stevens-Johnson syndrome, anaphylaxis.
flucytosine (Ancobon)	Most often used with amphotericin B to treat infections caused by *Candida* or *Cryptococcus neoformans*. Adverse effects: bone marrow depression, hepatotoxicity. When given with amphotericin B, monitor renal function closely.

Antifungal Drugs for Superficial Infections

Superficial fungal infections may affect the skin, hair, and nails. They are caused by *Candida* species or dermatophytes. Sites of candidal infections are the vulvovaginal area, the mouth, and the bowel. Oral candidiasis is called "thrush." Dermatophytic infections are commonly called "ringworm" and include tinea pedis (athlete's foot), tinea corporis (ringworm of the body), tinea cruris (ringworm of the groin), and tinea capitis (ringworm of the scalp).

TABLE 5–13
Antifungal Drugs for Superficial Infections

Drugs	Specific Considerations
Azoles clotrimazole (FemCare, Gyne-Lotrimin, Mycelex-7, Mycelex-G) ketoconazole (Nizoral) fluconazole (Diflucan), et al.	Used to treat dermatophytic and candidal infections. Various preparations: lotions, creams, powders, vaginal suppositories. Adverse effects: topical preparations can cause stinging, itching, and edema. Fluconazole is used for oral therapy.
griseofulvin (Fulvicin)	Used to treat dermatophytic infections. Route: oral. Adverse effects: transient headache, rash, insomnia, gastrointestinal distress. Contraindicated with porphyria and liver disease due to increased risk of hepatotoxicity. Can decrease effects of warfarin.
Polyene Antibiotics amphotericin B (Fungizone) nystatin (Mycostatin)	For superficial candidal infections, only the topical preparation of amphotericin B is used. Topical or oral nystatin may be used. Adverse effects: topicals can cause skin irritation. Oral nystatin can cause gastrointestinal distress.

Antiparasitics

Human parasitic infections can include the following:

- Helminths: nematodes (roundworms), cestodes (tapeworms), and trematodes (flukes) can infest the intestines, liver, lymphatic system, and blood vessels.
- Protozoa
  — *Plasmodium:* causes malaria
  — *Entamoeba histolytica:* causes amebiasis
  — *Giardia lamblia:* causes giardiasis
  — *Leishmania:* causes leishmaniasis
  — *Toxoplasma gondii:* causes toxoplasmosis
  — *Trichomonas vaginalis:* causes trichomoniasis
  — *Trypanosoma:* causes trypanosomiasis (sleeping sickness, Chagas' disease)

Anthelmintics

Some of the drugs used to treat specific helminth infestations and related nursing considerations are summarized in Table 5–14.

TABLE 5–14		
Anthelmintics		
Antiparasitic Drug	Use	Specific Considerations
mebendazole (Vermox)	Giant roundworm, pinworm, hookworm, whipworm, pork roundworm	Poorly absorbed, so has minimal side/adverse effects. Not recommended during pregnancy.
thiabendazole (Mintezol)	Threadworm	High incidence of adverse effects: nausea, vomiting, diarrhea, dizziness, drowsiness, hepatotoxicity. Contraindicated with liver disease.
diethylcarbamazine (Hetrazan)	Filariae	Adverse effects: headache, weakness, nausea, vomiting, dizziness. Secondary to death of parasites, patient may become acutely ill. Pretreatment with glucocorticoids reduces adverse effects.
pyrantel (Antiminth)	Giant roundworm, hookworm, pinworm	Poorly absorbed, so has minimal systemic effects (dizziness, insomnia, headache). Patient may have nausea, vomiting, cramping, and diarrhea.
praziquantel (Biltricide)	Tapeworms: pork, fish, beef Flukes: intestinal, blood, lung	Adverse effects: drowsiness, transient headache and abdominal discomfort.

Antiprotozoal Drugs

Antimalarial Agents

Malaria is an infectious disease caused by a protozoan, *Plasmodium*, that is transmitted by mosquitoes. Antimalarial drugs can be used to treat an acute malarial attack, prevent a relapse, or prevent an initial infection. Acute attacks are best treated with a 3-day course of chloroquine (Aralen). With chloroquine-resistant strains, tetracycline, clindamycin, or pyrimethamine with sulfadoxine may be used in combination with chloroquine. Primaquine is used to prevent a relapse. Depending on the malarial strain to which a person is likely to be exposed, chloroquine or mefloquine may be used for prevention. Chloroquine is the prototype for the antimalarials.

Chloroquine (Aralen). Chloroquine may destroy *Plasmodium* by causing toxic metabolic substances to accumulate in the parasite. Serious adverse effects are uncommon, but the patient may have headache, visual disturbances, itching, and gastrointestinal distress. Taking the drug with food minimizes the gastrointestinal effects. When the drug is being taken for prevention, the patient should begin the drug 1 week before anticipated exposure and continue the drug for 4 weeks after leaving the area of potential exposure.

Primaquine. The most important adverse effect of primaquine is hemolysis, which tends to occur in people whose red blood cells lack an enzyme referred to as G-6-PD. This deficiency is an inherited trait found most often among dark-skinned whites and blacks. Before primaquine is administered, screening for this characteristic is recommended.

Mefloquine (Lariam). Mefloquine is the drug of choice for preventive treatment when exposure to chloroquine-resistant strains is expected. Mild nausea and dizziness may occur at low doses. Higher doses used to treat acute attacks can cause gastrointestinal distress, nightmares, headache, and visual disturbances. Neurotoxicity can occur, with confusion and psychosis. Mefloquine is contraindicated with psychiatric disorders or epilepsy.

Miscellaneous Antiprotozoal Drugs. A variety of drugs are employed to treat protozoal infections other than malaria (Table 5–15).

TABLE 5–15

Miscellaneous Antiprotozoal Drugs

Drug	Protozoal Infection
iodoquinol (Yodoxin)	Asymptomatic intestinal amebiasis
metronidazole (Flagyl)	Symptomatic intestinal amebiasis, *Trichomonas vaginalis* infection, giardiasis
trimethoprim plus sulfamethoxazole (Bactrim, Septra)	*Pneumocystis carinii* pneumonia
pentamidine (Pentam 300)	*Pneumocystis carinii* infection
atovaquone (Mepron)	*Pneumocystis carinii* pneumonia
melarsoprol (Arsobol) eflornithine (Ornidyl) suramin (Germanin)	African trypanosomiasis (sleeping sickness)
nifurtimox (Lampit)	American trypanosomiasis (Chagas' disease)
pyrimethamine (Daraprim)	Toxoplasmosis
sodium stibogluconate (Pentostam)	Leishmaniasis

CHAPTER 6

IMMUNIZING AGENTS

*I*mmunity protects us from infectious diseases. A person is said to be immune to a particular pathogen if he has antibodies that prevent him from being infected when exposed to that pathogen. There are two types of immunity: natural and acquired. Natural immunity is manifested by nonspecific responses to any foreign protein. The inflammatory response is an example of natural immunity. The response is essentially the same regardless of the invader.

Acquired immunity, on the other hand, develops after exposure to the foreign protein. Antibodies specific to that protein are manufactured and protect the patient if there is subsequent exposure. This mechanism can be activated by vaccinating people to render them immune to various infections.

Vaccines are the materials administered to stimulate antibody production. They are described as *killed vaccines* or *live vaccines,* depending on the state of the organisms used. Killed vaccines contain whole dead microbes or components isolated from microbes. Live (attenuated) vaccines contain live organisms that have been weakened. In people with normal immune function, live vaccines stimulate antibody production but do not cause disease.

Another term used in relation to vaccinations is *toxoid.* A toxoid is made of a bacterial toxin that has been altered so it is nontoxic. When the toxoid is administered, a patient develops antibodies against the toxin but not against the microbe itself.

IMMUNIZATION

Immunization, the process of becoming immune to a specific microbe or toxin, can be passive or active. *Passive immunity* results when a person is given preformed antibodies or sensitized lymphoid cells. *Active immunity* develops when people are given vaccines or toxoids that cause them to develop antibodies. The term *vaccination* is used only to describe treatment with vaccines or toxoids.

TARGET DISEASES

Vaccination is recommended during childhood for the following diseases: diphtheria, tetanus, pertussis, measles, mumps, rubella, invasive *Haemophilus influenzae* type b, hepatitis B, poliomyelitis, and varicella. The vaccines for diphtheria, tetanus, and pertussis are combined into one, commonly referred to as DTP. Measles, mumps, and rubella vaccines are combined and referred to as MMR.

The vaccine for varicella is given in a single injection. Vaccinations for the rest of these conditions require a series of doses over a period of months or years. It is important to complete the series to ensure immunity. Although various factors may affect individual schedules, a common childhood immunization schedule is presented in Table 6–1.

TABLE 6–1

Typical Childhood Immunization Schedule

Age	Hepatitis B	Oral Polio	Diphtheria, Tetanus, Pertussis, (DTP)	*Haemophilus* B Conjugate	Measles, Mumps, Rubella (MMR)	Varicella
Birth to 2 Months	X					
2 Months		X	X	X		
1–4 Months	X					
4 Months		X	X	X		
6 Months			X	X		
6–18 Months	X					
12–15 Months				X	X	
12–18 Months		X				X
15–18 Months			X			
4–6 Years		X	X		X or	
11–12 Years					X	
14–16 Years			Tetanus and diphtheria booster			

Recommended Childhood Immunization Schedule: United States, 1997. From Lehne, R. A. (1998). *Pharmacology for Nursing Care.* Philadelphia: W. B. Saunders, p. 741.

GENERAL CONTRAINDICATIONS

General contraindications to vaccination include the following:

- Previous anaphylactic reaction to a vaccine
- Previous anaphylactic reaction to any component of a vaccine
- Moderate or severe illness with or without fever
- Pregnancy

Children with immunosuppression should not be given *live* vaccines. Lacking normal immune responses, they can develop active infections from the live viruses. Other contraindications are included in Table 6–2.

ADVERSE EFFECTS OF SPECIFIC VACCINES AND TOXOIDS

Most people tolerate vaccinations with only minimal adverse effects. Mild fever and local reactions are common. Local reactions include soreness, redness, and swelling at the injection site. Other adverse effects are noted in Table 6–2.

TABLE 6–2

Vaccines and Toxoids: Adverse Effects and Contraindications

Preparation	Mild Side Effects	Serious Adverse Effects	Additional Specific Contraindications
Measles, mumps, and rubella virus vaccine	Local reactions; rash; fever; swollen glands in cheeks and neck and under the jaw; pain, stiffness, and swelling in joints	Anaphylaxis, thrombocytopenia	Pregnancy ⚠️ Children with a history of thrombocytopenia, thrombocytopenic purpura, or anaphylactic reactions to gelatin, eggs, or neomycin ⚠️
Diphtheria and tetanus toxoids and pertussis vaccine, whole-cell or acellular*	Local reactions, fever, fretfulness, drowsiness, anorexia, persistent crying	Acute encephalopathy, convulsions, shock-like state	Encephalopathy within 7 days of prior vaccination
Haemophilus influenzae type b conjugate vaccine	Local reactions, fever, crying, diarrhea, vomiting	None	
Poliovirus vaccine (IPV and OPV)	Local reactions (only from IPV)	Rare: Vaccine-assisted paralytic poliomyelitis (only from OPV)	
Varicella virus vaccine	Local reactions, fever, mild varicella-like rash (local or generalized)	None	Pregnancy ⚠️ Some cancers: leukemia, lymphoma Allergy to neomycin, gelatin Patient should not take aspirin for 6 weeks due to risk for Reye's syndrome Patient can transmit virus to others; should avoid contact with pregnant women, newborns, susceptible people ⚠️
Hepatitis B vaccine	Local discomfort, fever	Anaphylaxis	Anaphylactic reaction to baker's yeast

*Acellular DTP causes fever and milder effects than whole-cell DTP.

Adapted with permission from Lehne, R. A. (1998). *Pharmacology for Nursing Care*, 3rd ed. Philadelphia: W. B. Saunders, p. 740.

NURSING IMPLICATIONS

Nursing Actions

- Prior to administering a vaccine or toxoid, assess for contraindications.
- Obtain signed consent form per agency policy.
- Record the following in the patient's permanent record: date of vaccination; route and site; vaccine type, manufacturer, lot number, and expiration date; and name, address, and title of person administering the vaccine.
- Provide written information about immunizations and reportable reactions.

Patient Teaching

- It is essential to complete the series of immunizations to protect you or your child from illness.
- Children commonly have mild fever and ⚠️ redness, soreness, and swelling at the injection site.
- Side effects of vaccinations can be treated with acetaminophen or a nonsteroidal anti-inflammatory agent other than aspirin.
- Notify your health care provider if side effects last over 72 hours.

FLUIDS AND ELECTROLYTES

PHYSIOLOGY OF FLUID BALANCE

About 60% of the adult human body is water. Fluid inside the blood vessels is known as intravascular fluid (IVF) and fluid outside the blood vessels is extravascular fluid (EVF). Fluid within cells is called intracellular fluid (ICF); outside cells it is called extracellular fluid (ECF). Interstitial fluid (ISF) is the fluid in the spaces between cells, tissue, and organs.

The regulation of the volume and composition of body water is essential because all metabolic reactions occur in body water. The body maintains water balance by keeping the amount of water taken in daily equal to the amount of water lost. If the amount of water gained exceeds the amount of water lost, water excess, or overhydration, occurs. This is known as hypervolemia. If the amount of water lost exceeds the amount gained, fluid volume deficit, or dehydration, occurs. This is known as hypovolemia.

FLUID IMBALANCE

Hypervolemia

The primary symptom of hypervolemia is edema occurring in three general body areas: circulatory edema, pulmonary edema, and peripheral edema.

The symptoms of circulatory edema include fast, bounding pulse; hypertension; distended neck veins; and increased body weight. An enlarged heart may be noted on radiograph.

The symptoms of pulmonary edema may include abnormal breath sounds (especially rales, which are bubbling or popping sounds), dyspnea, and altered respiratory rate. Arterial blood gases may also be abnormal.

Periorbital edema (around the eyes) may be the first sign of peripheral edema, especially when the patient has been lying down. Position-related dependent edema (in any part of the body lower than the heart) may occur in feet and ankles or sacrococcygeal area. Ascites is the accumulation of fluid in the abdomen and may or may not be position-related.

Nursing actions related to hypervolemia include the following:

- Careful monitoring of intake and output, especially if the patient has an intravenous line
- Monitoring blood pressure and pulse as often as necessary
- Daily weights, at the same time of day, in the same type of clothes, on the same scale
- Assessment for peripheral edema
- Checking for distended neck veins
- Assessment of lung sounds
- Measurement of abdominal girth daily, at the same place, in the same position.

Hypovolemia

The primary sign of hypovolemia is dehydration. Symptoms may include dry skin and mucous membranes; poor skin turgor; decreased perspiration, tears, and saliva; and decreased urine output.

Nursing care of a patient with hypovolemia includes administration of fluids, either orally or intravenously, and, in some cases of extreme fluid volume loss, use of plasma volume expanders. Nursing actions include careful monitoring of intake and output, frequent blood pressure and pulse checks, and assessment of skin turgor.

PHYSIOLOGY OF ELECTROLYTE BALANCE

Chemical composition of the fluid compartments varies from compartment to compartment. The primary electrolytes in the ECF are sodium (Na^+) and chloride (Cl^-), whereas potassium (K^+) is the major electrolyte of the ICF. Calcium (Ca^{++}), phosphorus (P), and magnesium (Mg^{++}) are other important electrolytes.

Potassium

Potassium is necessary to the body for the conduction of nerve impulses, production of muscle contractions, and regulation of the cardiac pacemaker. All muscles, both voluntary and involuntary, require potassium for normal functioning. Potassium is also essential in the maintenance of acid-base balance and is an essential component of gastric secretion, kidney function, tissue synthesis, and carbohydrate metabolism. Potassium-rich foods include citrus fruits, bananas, milk, tomatoes, potatoes, bran, and chocolate. Normal serum potassium level is 3.5 to 5.0 mEq/L.

Hyperkalemia

Renal failure is the most common cause of excessive serum potassium. Other causes include burns, trauma, infections, potassium supplements, and potassium-sparing diuretics. Signs and symptoms of hyperkalemia include voluntary muscle weakness, weak, irregular pulse, cardiac arrhythmias, respiratory paralysis, and cardiac arrest.

The drug most commonly used to treat hyperkalemia is sodium polystyrene (Kayexalate). As the trade name indicates, this drug makes the "K exit," so that the body releases excess potassium through the gastrointestinal tract. Sodium polystyrene can be given either orally or rectally by enema. Nursing actions include careful monitoring of serum potassium levels and assessment for hypokalemia.

Hypokalemia

Hypokalemia is a deficiency of potassium, most often caused by excessive potassium loss rather than lack of dietary potassium. This loss is related to the use of potassium-wasting diuretics and steroids, excessive vomiting and diarrhea, crash diets, ingestion of large amounts of licorice, and prolonged misuse of laxatives. Burn patients may also exhibit hypokalemia.

It is important to recognize the early symptoms of hypokalemia to prevent serious, life-threatening consequences. Early (mild) symptoms include anorexia, lethargy, mental confusion, nausea, muscle weakness, and hypotension. Late (severe) symptoms are muscle tetany, neuropathy, paralytic ileus, and cardiac arrhythmias. Mild hypokalemia can usually be corrected by consumption of potassium-rich foods or addition of a potassium supplement to the treatment plan. Severe hypokalemia may be corrected by oral potassium supplements but usually requires initial treatment with intravenous potassium chloride (KCl). The chloride is required to correct the decreased serum chloride that frequently accompanies potassium deficiency. Adverse effects from oral potassium preparations are primarily gastrointestinal and may include gastrointestinal bleeding and ulceration. Parenteral KCl will cause pain at the injection site. Nursing actions include monitoring of serum potassium levels and assessment for hyperkalemia. Careful inspection of the intravenous site must be done, as infiltration of KCl can lead to tissue necrosis and sloughing. Intravenous potassium must always be diluted and administered slowly (over an hour). Rapid infusion may cause fatal cardiac arrhythmias.

Sodium

Sodium is essential in the maintenance of the body's fluid balance. It is primarily involved in the control of water distribution and fluid and electrolyte balance. Sodium, chloride, and bicarbonate also assist in the regulation of acid-base balance. Chloride closely complements the physiologic action of sodium. Normal sodium concentration is maintained through dietary intake of salt (NaCl) and fish, meats, and other foods flavored, preserved, or seasoned with salt. Normal serum sodium level is 135 to 145 mEq/L. Normal serum chloride level is 95 to 108 mEq/L.

Hypernatremia

Hypernatremia is an excess of serum sodium. Its most common cause is poor renal excretion due to kidney disease. Inadequate water intake and dehydration and the use of sodium supplements may also cause hypernatremia. Symptoms include red, flushed skin, dry, sticky mucous membranes, increased thirst, oliguria or anuria, and fever. Hypernatremia may lead to hypertension, edema, tachycardia, weakness, convulsions, and possibly coma. Treatment includes increased fluid intake and sodium-restricted diet. The intravenous administration of dextrose may be necessary to help promote renal excretion of sodium. Nursing actions include monitoring serum sodium levels and assessment for hyponatremia.

Hyponatremia

Low serum sodium is caused by some of the same conditions that cause hypokalemia (see earlier discussion). Other causes for hyponatremia are excessive perspiration, especially in hot weather, kidney disease, and impairment of the adrenal glands. Children are particularly vulnerable to hyponatremia from vomiting and diarrhea. Signs and symptoms include lethargy, tachycardia, hypotension, stomach cramps, vomiting, diarrhea, and convulsions. Mild hyponatremia is usually treated with salt tablets. Normal saline or Ringer's lactate solutions intravenously may be necessary to correct more severe symptoms. Nursing actions include monitoring serum sodium levels and assessment for hypernatremia. Intravenous sites must be checked for the occurrence of venous phlebitis.

Calcium

Calcium is necessary for the production of bones, teeth, and nerve and muscle tissue, and in the process of blood clotting. Vitamin D helps the body utilize calcium. Calcium and Vitamin D–rich foods include dairy products (milk, cheeses, yogurt, ice cream) and dark green leafy vegetables. Sunshine is also an excellent source of vitamin D because it changes a substance in the skin to a vitamin D precursor. Phosphorus, in combination with calcium, oxygen, and hydrogen, forms the substance of bones. Phosphorus also plays an important role in cell metabolism. It is obtained from milk products, cereals, meats, and fish. Its use is controlled by vitamin D and calcium.

Calcium is regulated by parathormone, the hormone produced by the parathyroid glands (see Chapter 42). When serum calcium levels are low, parathormone promotes release of calcium from bones. When serum calcium levels are high, calcitonin, from the thyroid gland, inhibits release of calcium from bones (see Chapter 42). A third hormone (hydroxycholecalciferol) is produced from vitamin D to regulate calcium absorption by the intestine. Normal serum calcium level is 4.4 to 5.2 mEq/L.

Hypercalcemia

Hypercalcemia is primarily seen in overdoses of calcium supplements, although disorders of the endocrine system may affect calcium levels. Symptoms of hypercalcemia include anorexia, nausea, muscle weakness, dehydration, and irregular pulse rate or rhythm. Treatment is stopping calcium supplements or treating the specific endocrine disorder. Nursing actions include monitoring intake and output, as kidney stones may develop from hypercalcemia. Encourage an intake of 2000 to 3000 mL per day unless contraindicated by another medical condition. Patient teaching includes the following: physical activity helps prevent kidney stones; report decreased output; check pulse daily for irregularities or changes in rate (hypercalcemia may cause serious cardiac arrhythmias); take calcium supplements only as prescribed (overdose may lead to coma or death).

Hypocalcemia

Hypocalcemia is caused by thyroidectomy (the parathyroid glands are embedded in the posterior capsule of the thyroid gland), renal failure, cardiac arrest, rickets, osteomalacia, and pregnancy. Postmenopausal women may be more vulnerable to hypocalcemia due to osteoporosis.

Symptoms of hypocalcemia may vary from person to person. These may include numbness and tingling of fingers and toes and abdominal cramping, or may involve muscle tetany and convulsions. Calcium is necessary for normal muscle response from the nervous system. The cluster of symptoms that constitute tetany usually begins with numbness and tingling of the lips, progressing to the extremities. If the hypocalcemia is not treated, cardiac arrhythmias, tremors, severe muscle spasms, and convulsions will occur. Treatments include a calcium-rich diet and oral or parenteral supplements as indicated. Before administration of a calcium supplement, assess for neuromuscular irritability by checking for Chvostek's sign (see under Nursing Actions).

Magnesium

Magnesium is used by the body for transmission of nerve impulses and for complete metabolism of carbohydrates. Magnesium is obtained in sufficient quantities from a normal diet that includes meats, dairy products, whole-grain cereals, fruits (especially bananas), and green leafy vegetables. Normal serum magnesium level is 1.8 to 3.0 mEq/L.

Hypermagnesemia

Elevated serum magnesium levels are most often seen in cases of overdoses of magnesium supplements but are also common in renal failure. Abuse of magnesium-based laxatives and antacids may also produce hypermagnesemia. Symptoms include decreased deep tendon reflexes, lethargy, hypotension, flushing and diaphoresis, decreased respirations (< 12/minute), bradycardia, and cardiac arrhythmias.

Hypomagnesemia

Decreased serum magnesium is most commonly seen in patients with renal failure and eclampsia of pregnancy. Symptoms include muscle weakness, tremors, hyperactive reflexes, personality changes, and convulsions. Initial treatment is parenteral magnesium, usually magnesium sulfate ($MgSO_4$), followed by maintenance on oral magnesium supplements if necessary. Magnesium can also be added to total parenteral nutrition mixtures to enhance carbohydrate metabolism. Oral preparations include magnesium sulfate, magnesium gluconate, magnesium lactate, and magnesium oxide.

FLUID AND ELECTROLYTE NURSING ACTIONS

Monitor serum electrolyte levels. Assess fluid volume status (i.e. edema, skin turgor, mucous membranes, pulses, and blood pressure). Carefully monitor intake and output. Take daily weights as indicated. Perform close assessment of the intravenous site for infiltration, venous phlebitis, pain, tissue necrosis, or sloughing. Assess for adequate urine output in patients receiving intravenous potassium replacements (>30 mL/hour). Assess for signs and symptoms of electrolyte imbalances. Intramuscular and intravenous calcium solutions should be warmed to body temperature to decrease the risk of inflammation. To check for Chvostek's sign, tap the cheek near the ear (where the facial nerve is located); if the nose, mouth, and eye twitch on the side tapped, the sign is present. Report findings to the physician immediately. For patients taking oral calcium supplements, monitor for indigestion, constipation, or gastrointestinal hemorrhage (check stool for color changes). Prior to administration of parenteral magnesium, check deep tendon reflexes, respiratory rate, and urine output (should be > 30 mL/hour).

C H A P T E R 8

ANALGESICS

An analgesic is a drug that relieves pain. Analgesics can be classified as opioids or nonopioids. Table 8–1 shows the classifications of drugs used as analgesics.

TABLE 8–1

Types of Analgesics by Classification

Type	Example
Opioids	
Opioid agonists	codeine
	methadone (Dolophine)
	hydromorphone (Dilaudid)
	meperidine (Demerol)
	morphine
	fentanyl (Duragesic, Sublimaze)
Opioid agonist-antagonists	buprenorphine (Buprenex)
	nalbuphine (Nubain)
	butorphanol (Stadol)
	pentazocine (Talwin)
Non-Opioids	
Nonsteroidal anti-inflammatory drugs (NSAIDs)	
Nonprostaglandin synthetase inhibitors (non-PSIs)	acetaminophen (Tylenol, et al.)
Prostaglandin synthetase inhibitors (PSIs)	aspirin
	naproxen (Naprosyn)
	naproxen sodium (Anaprox)
	fenoprofen calcium (Fenoprofen)
	mefenamic acid (Ponstel)
	meclofenamate sodium (Meclomen)
	flurbiprofen (Ansaid)
	piroxicam (Feldene)
	ketorolac tromethamine (Toradol)

OPIOID ANALGESICS

An *opioid* is "any drug, natural or synthetic, that has actions similar to those of morphine" (Lehne, 1998, p. 229). The term *opioid* is preferred to "narcotic" because it is more specific. The term *narcotic* has been used to describe a wide variety of drugs, including illegal "street drugs." Note that opioid is broader than *opiate,* which refers only to opium compounds such as morphine or codeine.

The two types of opioids used for analgesia are opioid agonists and opioid agonist-antagonists. Opioid agonists include codeine, methadone (Dolophine), hydromorphone (Dilaudid), meperidine (Demerol), morphine, and fentanyl (Duragesic, Sublimaze). Opioid agonists-antagonists include buprenorphine (Buprenex), nalbuphine (Nubain), butorphanol (Stadol), and pentazocine (Talwin).

Action and Uses

Opioids act on receptors in the central nervous system to raise the pain threshold, reducing the perception of pain, and to reduce the emotional response to pain. As analgesics, they are most often used to treat moderate to severe acute pain and chronic cancer pain. Other uses are in the treatment of cough and diarrhea, and for preoperative sedation.

Side and Adverse Effects

The two types of opioids have slightly different side and adverse effects. In addition to pain relief, both cause sedation. The opioid agonists also can cause respiratory depression, euphoria, and physical dependence. Infants and the elderly are at greatest risk for respiratory depression. Intracranial pressure may increase because respiratory depression results in increased carbon dioxide in the blood, which dilates cerebral blood vessels. Nausea and vomiting may occur, but this effect usually diminishes with repeated doses. Constriction of the pupil (miosis) is a classic response to opioids. The classic signs of opioid toxicity are coma, respiratory depression, and pinpoint pupils. All of these effects are related to the actions of the drug on the central nervous system.

Opioids also have some effects on receptors outside the central nervous system. The effects on the digestive tract include decreased gastrointestinal motility and decreased gastric, biliary, and pancreatic secretions. Morphine sulfate can cause spasms of the bile duct. Opioids can decrease urine production by stimulating the release of antidiuretic hormone (ADH), can cause urinary retention or urgency, and

49

can reduce the perception of a full bladder. Cardiovascular effects include vasodilation in response to histamine release, orthostatic hypotension, and bradycardia.

With prolonged or high-dose use, the patient may develop tolerance or physical dependency. After gradual withdrawal, it is rare for a patient to seek continued use of opioids.

Interactions and Contraindications

If given with other central nervous system depressants (including alcohol), the risk of hypotension, sedation, and respiratory depression increases. Fatal reactions have occurred in patients taking monoamine oxidase (MAO) inhibitors who receive opioids. Concurrent use of anticholinergics greatly increases the incidence of constipation and urinary retention. With elderly patients, who often take multiple drugs, it is especially important to be aware of interactions that can cause hypotension, constipation, and urinary retention.

Opioids are contraindicated after biliary tract surgery. They are used only with extreme caution in patients with central nervous system depression, head injuries, shock, seizures, untreated myxedema (severe hypothyroidism), and respiratory depression. If given during the early stage of labor, opioids can slow the patient's progress. They can also cause the neonate to have respiratory depression.

Some drugs are pure opioid antagonists. These drugs block the effects of opioids, so are used to reverse opioid effects in the event of overdose. They include naloxone (Narcan), naltrexone, and nalmefene.

Nursing Actions

Do not wait until pain is severe before medicating with analgesics. Assess pain location, type, and severity; pulse, blood pressure, and respiratory rate; and mental status before administration. You can ask patients to rate their pain on a scale of 1 to 10 with 10 being the worst pain imaginable. The patient's rating can then be used to measure the effectiveness of interventions. If the respiratory rate is 12

or less, withhold the opioid and notify the registered nurse or the physician. Assist the patient to assume a recumbent position before giving parenteral opioids. This reduces symptoms of orthostatic hypotension and nausea. Take safety precautions such as raising side rails, and provide a call bell. After administration, reassess pain and vital signs. Monitor urine output and palpate for bladder distention. Assess stool frequency and characteristics for constipation. Patients with chronic pain who are treated with opioids over a long period of time should be placed on a program to promote regular bowel elimination. This may include increased fluids and exercise as well as stool softeners.

Remember that analgesics are only one of many means of pain management. Other measures such as relaxation exercises, massage, and imagery may be used with, or sometimes in place of, analgesics.

Patient Teaching
• This drug will help you feel better; I will check on you soon to be sure you are more comfortable. • You will probably feel drowsy. • To prevent dizziness or falls, change positions slowly and ask for help to get up. • Let me know if you have difficulty emptying your bladder. • There is little reason to fear addiction when opioid analgesics are used for short-term management of pain. • With long-term therapy, your physician may advise stool softeners to prevent constipation.

Prototypes

The information just presented is true of opioid analgesics in general. Table 8–2 lists various opioids and considerations specific to those drugs.

TABLE 8–2

Specific Opioid Analgesics

Drug	Side and Adverse Effects	Special Considerations
morphine sulfate (Astramorph, Duramorph, MS Contin, et al.)	Causes more smooth muscle spasm than other opioids, making it inappropriate with biliary colic.	Especially useful for pain of acute myocardial infarction, and for dyspnea caused by pulmonary edema. Most effective with constant, dull pain. Routes: PO, IM, IV, SC, and epidural and intrathecal. Larger doses are needed for PO than other routes because of first pass effect.
meperidine (Demerol)	Patients with renal disease may develop seizures and a sense of anxiety because of accumulation of drug metabolites.	Preferred over morphine during labor because it does not slow labor and causes less neonatal respiratory depression. Routes include PO (tablets and syrup), IM, IV, and SC.
methadone (Dolophine)	Orthostatic hypotension, sedation. Nausea, vomiting, dizziness more common in ambulatory patients.	In addition to analgesic use, is used to treat people addicted to opioids. People can function normally while taking methadone to treat addiction. Routes: PO (tablets and liquid), IM, SC. Dilute PO syrup in water. IM preferred over SC; SC painful and irritating.
fentanyl parenteral: Sublimaze transdermal: Duragesic transmucosal: Fentanyl Oralet	Sublimaze, which is used as part of surgical anesthesia, can cause muscle rigidity. Parenteral form, patches, and lozenges all have same adverse effects as other opioids.	Routes: IM, IV, transdermal (patch), transmucosal (lozenge). Used Duragesic patches should be flushed down the toilet. Patches may be changed at 48- or 72-hour intervals. Even though lozenge looks like a lollipop, it provides a significant drug dosage and must be treated with the same caution as any other opioid.
codeine phosphate, codeine sulfate	Less abuse potential than morphine.	Usually given orally for mild to moderate pain. Combinations with aspirin or acetaminophen are available and provide more pain relief than either given alone. Especially effective as antitussive (relieves cough). Routes: PO, SC, IM.
propoxyphene (Darvon)	Large doses can cause toxicity with psychosis; can be fatal. Therefore, not usually given to people thought to be suicidal.	Often combined with nonopioids for improved analgesic effect. Route: PO.
tramadol (Ultram)	Serious adverse effects rare. Can cause headache and dry mouth in addition to constipation, sedation, and respiratory depression. Not a controlled substance; low abuse potential.	Absolutely contraindicated with MAO inhibitors. Route: PO.
pentazocine (Talwin) nalbuphine (Nubain) butorphanol (Stadol)	Less respiratory depression and euphoria than morphine. Low blood levels can cause psychotomimetic reactions (anxiety, nightmares, hallucinations). Pentazocine and butorphanol increase cardiac workload, so not recommended after acute myocardial infarction.	Blocks effects of agonist opioids, so should not be given to opioid dependent people: will trigger opioid withdrawal reaction. Pentazocine routes: PO, IV, IM, SC Nalbuphine routes: IV, IM, SC. Butorphanol routes: IM, IV, nasal spray.

NONOPIOID ANALGESICS

Nonopioid drugs used for analgesic actions include a variety of drugs that are classified as nonsteroidal anti-inflammatory agents (NSAIDs). NSAIDs are further classified as prostaglandin synthetase inhibitors (PSIs) and nonprostaglandin synthetase inhibitors (non-PSIs). Most commonly used NSAIDs are PSIs. Acetaminophen is a non-PSI.

Nonsteroidal Anti-Inflammatory Drugs: Prostaglandin Synthetase Inhibitors

Nonsteroidal anti-inflammatory drugs are covered in Chapter 4. Prostaglandin synthetase inhibitors (PSIs) have analgesic, antipyretic, and anti-inflammatory effects. They are briefly reviewed here in relation to analgesic effects. Examples of PSIs are aspirin, indomethacin (Indocin), ibuprofen (Motrin), ketoprofen (Orudis), naproxen (Naprosyn), and ketorolac tromethamine (Toradol). Table 4–1 provides a more complete list.

Action and Uses

Prostaglandins are substances produced by body tissues in response to various stimuli. When inflammation occurs, prostaglandins potentiate (make greater) the effects of natural chemicals that cause pain and edema. By inhibiting the formation of prostaglandins, NSAIDs reduce pain and edema.

Aspirin also has an antiplatelet effect, which reduces blood clotting.

Side and Adverse Effects

Aspirin and most other PSIs can cause abdominal pain and cramping, heartburn, and allergic responses. Serious gastric bleeding may occur. In addition to gastrointestinal bleeding, large doses of aspirin can cause salicylism, a toxic state. It is manifested first by nausea, vomiting, changes in vision and hearing, drowsiness, confusion, and hyperventilation. Later, the patient may develop seizures and mental changes progressing to coma and to death if not successfully treated. NSAIDs can cause fluid retention, which may interfere with the management of hypertension.

Interactions and Contraindications

Gastrointestinal irritation is increased if PSIs are taken with alcohol. Antacids and other alkalinizing drugs promote excretion of aspirin, reducing its effectiveness. The risk of bleeding is enhanced if given with anticoagulants, thrombolytics, or platelet inhibitors. Because there are numerous other drug interactions, you must look up each drug before giving it to see if the patient is at risk for adverse effects of these interactions.

Prostaglandin synthetase inhibitors are generally contraindicated with gastrointestinal bleeding or ulceration, history of allergic reactions, impaired liver function, and any bleeding disorders. Aspirin should not be given with chickenpox or flu in children or teenagers because of the risk of potentially fatal Reye's syndrome. The elderly patient who may use PSIs long-term is at greater risk for toxicity if liver function is impaired.

Nursing Actions

Assess for allergies before giving any NSAID. Assess pain before and after drug administration. Determine the potential for drug interactions. Assess for signs of bleeding: easy bruising, minor injuries that bleed excessively, black or maroon stools.

Patient Teaching

- You should not exceed the recommended dosage of these drugs because they can be harmful in excessive amounts.
- Treat fever in children and teenagers with acetaminophen rather than aspirin.
- Report any abdominal pain or signs of bleeding to the physician.
- Check expiration dates of over-the-counter drugs.
- If you are allergic to aspirin, always read labels of over-the-counter drugs, since many contain aspirin.
- If you have high blood pressure, ask your physician which pain reliever is best for you, because some nonprescription drugs can raise blood pressure.

Nonprostaglandin Synthetase Inhibitor: Acetaminophen

Actions and Uses

Acetaminophen is a widely used over-the-counter drug for fever and pain. It is preferred over aspirin for the treatment of febrile illness in children because it does not cause Reye's syndrome. Reye's syndrome is a potentially fatal condition with neurologic and hepatic symptoms that has been associated with viral diseases treated with aspirin. Unlike aspirin, acetaminophen does not cause gastrointestinal bleeding, nausea, and vomiting. However, it lacks the anti-inflammatory actions of aspirin and other PSIs. Therefore, it may relieve pain associated with inflammation, but will not act on the underlying problem.

Side and Adverse Effects

Acetaminophen has a relatively low incidence of serious side effects. With acetaminophen overdose, toxic metabolites accumulate in the liver, causing potentially fatal liver necrosis. Early signs of toxicity are anorexia, nausea, diaphoresis, and weakness. Late signs include vomiting, tenderness in the right upper abdominal quadrant, and elevated liver enzymes.

Interactions and Contraindications

The risk of liver toxicity increases if acetaminophen is taken with drugs that stimulate the production of certain liver enzymes. This includes alcohol and cimetidine. Of course, the risk also increases if taken with other hepatotoxic drugs. The antidote for toxicity is acetylcysteine.

Acetaminophen is contraindicated with known hypersensitivity and is used cautiously with liver damage.

Nursing Actions

Assess pain before and after administering acetaminophen.

Patient Teaching
• Acetaminophen is safe when taken as directed, but can be toxic if taken in excess or with alcohol.

REVIEW QUESTIONS: UNIT 2

1. List three to four nursing actions related to hypervolemia.

2. Kayexalate is the most commonly used drug to treat which of the following conditions?
   A. Hyperkalemia
   B. Hyponatremia
   C. Hypokalemia
   D. Hypercalcemia

3. Patients receiving parenteral potassium or magnesium must have adequate urine output. Minimum urine output should be at least:
   A. 10 mL/hour.
   B. 30 mL/hour.
   C. 100 mL/hour.
   D. 200 mL/hour.

4. A calcium- and phosphorus-rich diet has been prescribed for your patient to help prevent hypocalcemia. What foods would you recommend?

5. Patients taking diuretics are at risk for hyponatremia. What are the symptoms of hyponatremia?

6. The two categories of anti-inflammatory agents are _____ and _____.

7. Which system is most often affected by adverse effects of PSIs?
   A. Gastrointestinal
   B. Central nervous
   C. Cardiovascular
   D. Endocrine

8. Teaching for the patient who is taking aspirin should include which of the following?
   A. There are no dosage limits.
   B. You can take aspirin with alcohol
   C. Always take aspirin after meals.
   D. Report "ringing in the ears."

9. Aspirin should not be used to treat viral infections in children because it can cause:
   A. kidney failure.
   B. gastric ulcers.
   C. Reye's syndrome.
   D. confusion.

10. The actions of acetaminophen are similar to those of aspirin except that acetaminophen is NOT:
    A. anti-inflammatory.
    B. analgesic.
    C. antipyretic.
    D. antimicrobial.

11. Gold salts are used to treat:
    A. osteoarthritis.
    B. Alzheimer's disease.
    C. rheumatoid arthritis.
    D. lupus erythematosus.

Match the term on the left with the definition on the right:

12. _____ bacteriostatic

13. _____ broad spectrum

14. _____ bactericidal

15. _____ narrow spectrum

A. Effective against few organisms

B. Kills bacteria

C. Inhibits bacterial growth

D. Effective against many organisms

16. Which action would promote the development of drug-resistant pathogens?

    A. Liberal use of antimicrobials

    B. Using combinations of antimicrobial agents

    C. Spacing doses evenly over 24 hours

    D. Basing drug choice on culture and sensitivity results

17. Histamine and leukotriene are released by:

    A. antibodies.

    B. antigens.

    C. goblet cells.

    D. mast cells.

18. The most serious type of allergic reaction is:

    A. anaphylaxis.

    B. rhinorrhea.

    C. diarrhea.

    D. urticaria.

19. Mrs. Jones had an allergic reaction to penicillin. She indicated she had never taken penicillin before. What could explain her sensitization?

    A. Idiosyncratic response

    B. Cross-sensitivity

    C. Hypersensitive immune system

    D. It is impossible to have an allergic reaction with the first exposure to a drug.

20. A secondary infection caused by elimination of normal flora by an antimicrobial is called:

    A. opportunistic infection.

    B. superinfection.

    C. tertiary infection.

    D. fulminating infection.

21. When giving a nephrotoxic drug, you should monitor:

    A. bowel sounds.

    B. skin color.

    C. liver enzymes.

    D. urine output.

22. When a drug causes photosensitivity, advise the patient to:

    A. avoid exposure to sunlight.

    B. wear sunglasses.

    C. drink extra fluids.

    D. use skin moisturizer.

23. Mrs. Smith is taking Pen-Vee K. In her medication history, you note that she uses birth control pills for contraception and takes an over-the-counter antihistamine for allergies. What teaching will be important?

    A. The antihistamine will interfere with the action of penicillin.

    B. Discontinue birth control pills while taking penicillin.

    C. Use an alternate means of contraception while taking penicillin.

    D. Take penicillin at least 1 hour before taking birth control pills.

24. When preparing to give Mr. Black his first dose of ceftriaxone (Rocephin), you ask if he is allergic to any drugs. He replies that he had an anaphylactic reaction to penicillin in the past. You should:

    A. administer the ceftriaxone and observe him closely.

    B. withhold the ceftriaxone and contact the physician.

    C. tell him ceftriaxone is not a type of penicillin so it will be safe for him.

    D. tell him "This is what the doctor ordered!"

25. The most serious adverse effects of aminoglycosides are:

    A. constipation and abdominal pain.

    B. headache and phlebitis.

    C. weakness and dry mouth.

    D. ototoxicity and nephrotoxicity.

26. Which type of antimicrobial should not be given with dairy products?

    A. Tetracycline

    B. Aminoglycoside

    C. Beta-lactam

    D. Sulfonamide

Match the adverse effect with the antimicrobial:

27. _____ chloramphenicol

28. _____ sulfonamide

29. _____ tetracycline

30. _____ aminoglycoside

A. Neuromuscular blockade

B. Tooth discoloration

C. Crystals in the urine

D. Agranulocytosis

Mr. Harrison had a positive tuberculosis skin test, but no signs of active disease. He is being treated with isoniazid (INH) to prevent the development of active tuberculosis.

31. The physician has ordered pyridoxine (vitamin B_6) for Mr. Harrison. Why?

    A. People with tuberculosis tend to be undernourished and need vitamin supplements.

    B. Vitamin B_6 will decrease neurologic side effects of isoniazid.

    C. Pyridoxine is effective against the organism that causes tuberculosis.

    D. Vitamin B_6 promotes absorption of isoniazid.

32. Patient teaching for Mr. Harrison should include which of the following?

    A. You do not have to take the isoniazid when you are feeling well.

    B. Do not drink alcohol while you are on isoniazid.

    C. Take isoniazid with antacids to decrease stomach upset.

    D. You can expect a reddish color to your urine.

Mr. Harrison's wife is being treated for active tuberculosis. In addition to isoniazid, she is also taking rifampin.

33. The combined effects of isoniazid and rifampin put Mrs. Harrison at greater risk for what condition?

    A. Hepatotoxicity

    B. Nephrotoxicity

    C. Neurotoxicity

    D. Cardiotoxicity

34. Why are multiple drugs recommended to treat active tuberculosis?

    A. Tuberculosis is a very serious infection.

    B. Many different types of bacteria cause tuberculosis.

    C. The *Mycobacterium tuberculosis* quickly becomes resistant to single drugs.

    D. The rationale is not known, but patients generally recover faster when on combinations of drugs.

35. If Mrs. Harrison does not respond to her prescribed drugs, what second-line drug might be prescribed?

    A. Cycloserine

    B. Pyrazinamide

    C. Streptomycin

    D. Ethambutol

36. To be effective in the treatment of influenza A, amantadine (Symmetrel) must be given:

    A. for a minimum of 2 weeks.

    B. before symptoms develop.

    C. 24 hours after exposure to the infection.

    D. within 48 hours of the onset of symptoms.

37. Drugs used to treat HIV infection act by:

    A. killing the virus that causes HIV infection.

    B. improving the patient's immune status.

    C. suppressing replication of the HIV virus.

    D. preventing the virus from entering human cells.

38. The effects of HIV drugs are assessed by monitoring:

    A. body temperature.

    B. CD4 T cell counts.

    C. white blood cell counts.

    D. urine HIV RNA.

39. While receiving an intravenous infusion of amphotericin B, your patient complains of headache, nausea, and chills. You should:

    A. explain that this is expected.

    B. discontinue the infusion.

    C. contact the pharmacist for guidance.

    D. call "code red."

40. The adverse effects of amphotericin B infusion can be reduced by premedicating the patient with:
    A. diphenhydramine, aspirin, and meperidine.
    B. morphine, diazepam, and acetaminophen.
    C. codeine, chlorpromazine, and Maalox.
    D. meperidine, diazepam, and aspirin.

41. What type of immunization is contraindicated for children with immunosuppression?
    A. Killed vaccine
    B. Live vaccine

42. After receiving her immunization, your 5-year-old complains that her arm hurts. You observe slight redness and swelling at the injection site. You should:
    A. give her acetaminophen and tell her it will feel better soon.
    B. take her to the emergency room.
    C. call the physician.
    D. do nothing.

43. Pregnant women should avoid contact with people who have recently been vaccinated for:
    A. mumps.
    B. polio.
    C. varicella.
    D. hepatitis B.

44. Codeine, morphine, and meperidine are examples of:
    A. nonsteroidal anti-inflammatory drugs.
    B. opioid agonists.
    C. opioid agonist-antagonists.
    D. nonopioid analgesics.

45. The two types of opioids can cause:
    A. respiratory depression.
    B. euphoria.
    C. physical dependence.
    D. sedation.

46. The classic signs of opioid toxicity are:
    A. nausea, vomiting, and diarrhea.
    B. respiratory depression, euphoria, and physical dependence.
    C. coma, respiratory depression, and pinpoint pupils.
    D. increased intracranial pressure, coma, and pain relief.

47. Place the patient in a recumbent position to administer parenteral opioids to reduce the risk of:
    A. orthostatic hypotension.
    B. respiratory depression.
    C. increased intraocular pressure.
    D. cardiac depression.

48. Nausea, vomiting, changes in vision and hearing, drowsiness, confusion, and hyperventilation are classic signs of:
    A. opioid overdose.
    B. salicylate toxicity.
    C. orthostatic hypotension.
    D. drug dependency.

SURGICAL CARE

Drugs Used in the Perioperative Period

The nervous system is composed of all nerve tissues: brain, spinal cord, nerves, and ganglia (groups of nerve cell bodies located outside the central nervous system [CNS]). The nervous system is divided into the central nervous system and the peripheral nervous system. The central nervous system, composed of the brain and spinal cord, regulates body functions. The CNS interprets information sent by impulses from the peripheral nervous system and returns instructions through the peripheral nervous system for appropriate cellular actions (drugs affecting the peripheral nervous system and CNS stimulants are discussed in Unit 6). Drugs used in the perioperative period are considered CNS depressants. The broad classifications of these drugs are general anesthetic agents, narcotic analgesics, and sedative-hypnotics. This unit includes discussion of general and local anesthetic agents, sedative-hypnotics, and selected skeletal muscle relaxants used in the perioperative period. Unit 2 covers analgesic drugs.

In the brain, CNS depressant agents inhibit the reticular activating system (includes the senses, balance, motor activity, and level of awareness), the medulla oblongata (cardiac, respiratory, vasomotor centers; centers for coughing, vomiting, sneezing, swallowing, and salivating), and the limbic system (emotions and behavior). General anesthetic agents (inhalation and intravenous) affect the CNS in general with dose-related degrees of depression. Some depressants are more selective and inhibit only certain CNS functions. Examples of selective depressants are antiseizure drugs, which reduce seizure activity when given in amounts that do not interfere with normal psychomotor or psychosensory function (see Chapter 19); narcotic analgesics, which reduce reaction to severe pain without unconsciousness (see Chapter 8); and major tranquilizers, which calm emotionally disturbed patients without inducing sleep (see Unit 17).

OBJECTIVES

1. Identify classifications of, rationales for, and examples of drugs commonly used in the perioperative period.

2. Differentiate between a sedative and a hypnotic agent.

3. Describe the differences between barbiturates and benzodiazepines as sedative-hypnotics.

4. Identify the actions, uses, side effects, contraindications, and interactions of selected sedative-hypnotic drugs.

5. Identify the actions, uses, side effects, contraindications, and interactions of selected skeletal muscle relaxants used in the perioperative period.

6. Define *local anesthesia, general anesthesia*, and *balanced anesthesia.*

7. List routes of administration for local and general anesthesia.

8. Identify the actions, uses, side effects, contraindications, and interactions of selected local and general anesthetic agents.

9. Discuss nursing actions and patient teaching associated with drugs used in the perioperative period.

PREOPERATIVE AGENTS: SEDATIVES-HYPNOTICS

*D*rugs that depress the central nervous system (CNS) to have a calming effect are known as anxiolytics (antianxiety drugs) (see Unit 17) and sedative-hypnotics. Sedatives and anxiolytics reduce nervousness, excitability, and irritability and increase relaxation without causing sleep, but if the dose is increased, they can become hypnotic drugs. Hypnotics cause sleep and have a much more potent effect on the CNS than sedatives. Therapeutic doses of hypnotics given at bedtime may have residual sedative effects the following morning (morning hangover). Because these drugs produce varying dose-dependent degrees of CNS depression, some are also used as anticonvulsants (see Chapter 19) and anesthetic agents (see Chapter 10). The most commonly used groups of sedative-hypnotics are the barbiturates and benzodiazepines.

To understand the significant effects these drugs can have on sleep, it is necessary to understand normal sleep patterns. Sleep is a transient, reversible, periodic state of decreased mental and physical activity during which the person is relatively unresponsive to sensory and environmental stimuli. There are two basic stages of sleep that appear to cycle at about 90-minute intervals in normal adults: nonrapid eye movement (non-REM or NREM) and rapid eye movement (REM). There is an initial period of drowsiness that lasts about 30 minutes (stage I) progressing to deep sleep (stage IV). These stages are characterized by nonrapid eye movements, depressed bodily functions, and nondreaming; this non-REM sleep constitutes about 80% of the sleep cycle and is thought to be necessary for physical restoration. Stage IV is followed by approximately 5 to 20 minutes of rapid eye movements (REM), dreaming, and increased physiologic activity. REM sleep constitutes about 20% of the sleep cycle and is believed to be necessary for mental and emotional restoration. REM sleep deprivation can produce serious psychological problems, including psychosis.

BARBITURATES

Barbiturates were first introduced as sedative-hypnotics in the early 1900s, and, until the advent of the benzodiazepines in the 1960s, were the standard drugs for treating insomnia and producing sedation. Although there have been as many as 2,000 barbiturates developed, only a few are in common clinical use today. This is due to four major problems associated with their use: (1) suppression of REM sleep, (2) induction of drug-metabolizing enzymes in the liver, (3) development of tolerance and cross-tolerance, and (4) high potential for dependence and abuse.

When barbiturates are given in hypnotic doses for insomnia, suppression of REM sleep will occur. When the drug is discontinued, decreased REM sleep is followed by a compensatory increase in REM sleep ("rebound" effect), which appears to be the mind's way to make up for lost dreaming time. This rebound effect may occur even when barbiturates are used for only 3 or 4 days; with longer drug use, REM rebound may be severe and include vivid dreams, nightmares, restlessness, and frequent awakening (this may partially contribute to the dependence and abuse potential because people continue taking the drugs to avoid REM rebound). It may take several weeks for sleep patterns to return to normal following discontinuation of the drug. REM suppression and the rebound effect with its dependence potential does not occur at doses given to treat seizures or epilepsy.

When a drug is known as a *liver enzyme inducer*, it means that it has the capacity to produce larger amounts of drug-metabolizing enzymes. This allows more of the particular drug, as well as other drugs given concurrently, to be metabolized faster during a given period of time. Barbiturates increase the liver's ability to metabolize themselves, several other drugs (e.g., phenytoin, oral anticoagulants, oral contraceptives), and other substances that may be endogenous or administered as drugs (e.g., corticosteroids, sex hormones, vitamin K). Enzyme induction produces tolerance (loss of effectiveness as sedative-hynotics in about 2 weeks of daily use), and cross-tolerance with other CNS depressants and other drugs metabolized by the same enzymes. This enzyme induction effect disappears a few weeks after the barbiturate is discontinued.

Action

Barbiturates are CNS depressants that act primarily on the brainstem in the reticular activating system. They act by inhibiting nerve cell function and by reducing nerve impulse transmission to the cerebral cortex. Barbiturates can also raise the seizure or convulsive threshold. Their CNS depressant effects are dose-related. In low doses, barbiturates act as sedatives, with increasingly higher doses producing a hypnotic effect.

Uses

The clinical uses for barbiturates are subclassified by potency, onset, and duration of action:

Ultrashort-acting:

Onset: < 60 seconds (intravenous route); duration < 2 hours

> Uses: anesthesia induction, anesthetic for short procedures or diagnostic tests, control of convulsions, narcoanalysis (psychoanalysis with use of sedative drugs), reduction of intracranial pressure in neurosurgical patients.

> Drugs: thiopental (Pentothal), methohexital (Brevital), thiamylal (Surital)

Short-acting:

Onset: oral: 15–20 minutes; duration 2–4 hours

> intramuscular: 10–15 minutes; duration 1–4 hours

> intravenous: 1 minute; duration 15 minutes

> Uses: preanesthetic sedation, sedative-hypnotic, control of acute convulsive states from meningitis, poisons, eclampsia of pregnancy, alcohol withdrawal, or tetanus.

> Drugs: pentobarbital (Nembutal), secobarbital (Seconal)

Intermediate-acting:

Onset: oral: 30–60 minutes; duration 6–8 hours

> intramuscular: 20–30 minutes; duration 6–8 hours

> intravenous: 5–10 minutes; duration 3–6 hours

> Uses: sedative-hypnotic, control of convulsive conditions. Butabarbital may be combined with aspirin, acetaminophen, and caffeine to treat migraine headaches.

> Drugs: amobarbital (Amytal), aprobarbital (Alurate), butabarbital (Butisol)

Long-acting:

Onset: oral: 30–60 minutes; duration 10–12 hours

> intramuscular: 20–30 minutes; duration 10–12 hours

> intravenous: 5–10 minutes; duration 4–6 hours

> Uses: convulsive disorders, acute generalized convulsions associated with toxic reactions, eclampsia of pregnancy, meningitis, tetanus, and status epilepticus, as prevention and treatment of neonatal hyperbilirubinemia, narcotic withdrawal, and premenstrual syndrome.

> Drugs: phenobarbital (Luminal), mephobarbital (Mebaral)

Side and Adverse Effects

The primary adverse effect of barbiturates is dose-dependent respiratory depression. Overdose may result in death from respiratory failure. Other CNS effects include drowsiness, lethargy, headache, confusion, dizziness, morning hangover, and paradoxical excitation or restlessness. With long-term use, barbiturates may cause blood dyscrasias such as megaloblastic anemia, thrombocytopenia, leukopenia, agranulocytosis, and folic acid and vitamin D deficiency. Other adverse effects include laryngospasm, bronchospasm, liver damage, exfoliative dermatitis, and ataxia. An additional potentially fatal adverse effect is the occurrence of Stevens-Johnson syndrome, characterized by fever, cough, muscle aches and pains, headache, and the appearance of wheals or blisters on the skin, mucous membranes, and other organs. Allergic or hypersensitivity reactions to barbiturates are not common but can be severe due to the severe edema of mucous membranes of mouth, lips, tongue, face, and viscera. Other potential adverse effects are related to REM suppression and REM rebound, liver enzyme induction, tolerance and cross-tolerance, and dependence and abuse potential.

Interactions and Contraindications

Alcohol, antihistamines, benzodiazepines, opioids, and tranquilizers potentiate the depressant and adverse effects of barbiturates. Monoamine oxidase inhibitors inhibit metabolism of barbiturates, prolonging their effects. Liver enzyme induction decreases the effect of oral anticoagulants, oral contraceptives, theophylline, cortocosteroids, anticonvulsants, and digitoxin. Concurrent use with fluoxetine (Prozac) may produce hypertension, diaphoresis, ataxia, flushing, nausea, dizziness, and anxiety.

Contraindications include severe respiratory disorders, severe liver or kidney disease, and a history of alcohol or other drug abuse. Barbiturates should not be given to laboring women because of the potential for neonatal respiratory depression. Cautious use is advised for geriatric patients and patients with history of depression, psychosis, or suicidal tendencies. **Pregnancy category D.**

Nursing Actions

Assess vital signs and level of consciousness; document as baseline data. Obtain patient history regarding renal or hepatic disease, respiratory disorders, psychiatric disorders, alcohol or drug abuse, and drug and food allergies. Determine patient's use of other prescription and OTC drugs, particularly CNS depressants. Monitor serum renal and liver function tests and complete blood cell count (CBC) for baseline and periodically for long-term therapy. Always maintain (and document) patient safety measures: side rails up, call light within reach, assistance with ambulation. Do not administer intramuscularly unless absolutely necessary (because of pain and possible necrosis at injection site). If an intramuscular route is selected, use a large muscle mass, rotate injection sites, and monitor sites for irritation. Do not mix injectable forms (particularly pentobarbital) with other drugs, as they may form a precipitate in the container. Check intravenous site frequently for infiltration; extravasation of drug may cause tissue necrosis. Prior to administering the drug, assess the patient for the presence of pain (restlessness and paradoxical excitement may occur if pain is present). Assess for effectiveness of other drugs given concurrently with barbiturates (e.g., oral anticoagulants, digitoxin, oral contraceptives). Monitor for and report chronic toxicity symptoms: ataxia, slurred speech, irritability, poor judgment, confusion, insomnia, malaise. Monitor for and report acute toxicity symptoms: profound CNS and respiratory depression, hypoventilation, cyanosis, hypothermia, oliguria, tachycardia, and hypotension. To prevent withdrawal syndrome, avoid abrupt discontinuation of the drug (especially if taken for more than 14 consecutive days or nights). Early symptoms of withdrawal syndrome (8–12 hours after last dose) include anxiety, involuntary muscle tremors, weakness, dizziness, insomnia, orthostatic hypotension, nausea and vomiting, and visual disturbances. More severe symptoms, which may occur 2–8 days later, are delirium, illusions/delusions/hallucinations, paranoia, convulsions, and cardiovascular collapse.

Patient Teaching

- Use nondrug measures to promote relaxation, rest, and sleep (e.g., warm bath, soothing music, no caffeinated drinks after dinner).
- Take medication only as prescribed. Do not double dose if one dose is not effective.
- Report side effects such as morning hangover; drug selection or dose may need to be changed.
- Avoid driving, operating equipment or heavy machinery, and activities requiring mental alertness while taking medication.
- Do not take other CNS drugs, especially CNS depressants such alcohol, tranquilizers, or opioids.
- Check with health care provider before taking any over-the-counter medication (e.g., antihistamines).
- Avoid chronic use (more than 14 consecutive days or nights) if possible.
- Do not abruptly stop taking the drug (may cause rebound REM sleep and insomnia or withdrawal syndrome).
- If on long-term therapy, report fever, sore throat or mouth, malaise, easy bruising or bleeding, petechiae, jaundice, or rash.
- Do not keep drug on bedside table or in a readily accessible place (to avoid accidental overdose).
- Consider alternative methods of contraception in addition to or instead of oral contraceptives.
- If on long-term therapy, increase intake of vitamin D either through sunlight, supplement, or food (e.g., tuna, sardines, salmon, eggs, milk, butter, dry cereals, oatmeal, and sweet potatoes).

BENZODIAZEPINES

Benzodiazepines are the most frequently prescribed sedative-hypnotics and one of the most commonly prescribed drug classes. Benzodiazepines are classified as either anxiolytics or sedative-hypnotics depending on their primary usage. An anxiolytic reduces anxiety, and the benzodiazepine anxiolytics are discussed in Unit 17. This chapter focuses on their use as sedative-hypnotics.

Benzodiazepines have several advantages over barbiturates. They are the only sedative-hypnotics effective and safe for more than 14 nights' consecutive use, they do not produce REM suppression, there is a wider safety margin between therapeutic and toxic doses, they do not induce liver enzymes, they are rarely lethal in overdose (unless used with another CNS depressant), and there is less dependence or abuse potential when used as a sedative-hypnotic. Although they do not suppress REM sleep, they may suppress non-REM sleep, which could cause sleep disturbances such as nightmares. There are five benzodiazepines commonly used as sedative-hypnotics, classified on the basis of the duration of action: long-acting: flurazepam (Dalmane), quazepam (Doral); short-acting: estazolam (ProSom), temazepam (Restoril), triazolam (Halcion).

Action

Benzodiazepines depress activity in the CNS, specifically the hypothalamic, thalamic, and limbic systems of the brain, resulting in a calming effect. Recent research has shown that there are specific benzodiazepine receptors in the brain, which produce their effects by inhibiting stimulation of the brain. This causes inhibition of hyperexcitable nerves in the CNS, which may be responsible for causing seizure activity, control of agitation and anxiety, and reduction of excessive sensory stimulation and sleep induction. Because benzodiazepine receptors are in the same area in the CNS as those that have a role in alcohol addiction, these drugs are used in the treatment and prevention of symptoms of alcohol withdrawal. Benzodiazepines also produce skeletal muscle relaxation.

Uses

Benzodiazepines have a variety of clinical indications. Most frequent uses include preoperative sedation, sleep induction, skeletal muscle relaxation, and relief of anxiety. Additional therapeutic uses include treatment of alcohol withdrawal, agitation, depression, and convulsive disorders.

Side and Adverse Effects

The most common side effects involve the CNS and include drowsiness, morning hangover, dizziness, lethargy, and paradoxical excitation or nervousness. Other less common side effects may include disorientation, palpitations, dry mouth, nausea and vomiting, and nightmares. Prolonged use of triazolam has been associated with memory loss and rage reactions. Although triazolam is still available for use, its safety is being reviewed by the Food and Drug Administration. Benzodiazepine toxicity (overdose) may result in the following symptoms: excessive sedation, confusion, decreased reflexes, and coma. Unless ingested with another CNS depressant (e.g., alcohol), benzodiazepine overdoses rarely result in death. Treatment is symptomatic and supportive, including use of the specific benzodiazepine antagonist, flumazenil (Romazicon).

Interactions and Contraindications

Concurrent administration with other CNS depressants potentiates the effects of benzodiazepines. Monoamine oxidase inhibitors decrease metabolism of benzodiazepines, thus increasing their depressant effects. Cimetidine (Tagamet) decreases benzodiazepine metabolism to prolong its action.

These drugs are contraindicated for persons with severe hepatic or renal dysfunction, sleep apnea, and acute narrow-angle glaucoma. Prolonged administration (more than 3 to 5 weeks consecutive nights) of these sedative-hypnotics is not recommended. Cautious use is indicated for persons with psychiatric disorders, history of suicidal tendencies, history of drug or alcohol abuse or addiction, for geriatric patients, and for those with chronic lung diseases.

Nursing Actions

Assess vital signs and level of consciousness; document as baseline. Obtain patient history regarding renal or hepatic disease, respiratory disorders, psychiatric disorders, alcohol and drug abuse, and drug and food allergies. Determine patient's use of other prescription and over-the-counter drugs, particularly CNS depressants. Monitor serum renal and liver function tests and complete blood count for baseline values. Administer 15 to 30 minutes before bedtime to maximize hypnotic effects. Encourage and utilize nondrug measures to promote relaxation, rest, and sleep (e.g., warm bath, soothing music, back massage, avoiding caffeinated products late in the day). Maintain and document patient safety measures: side rails up, call light within reach, assistance with ambulation. Monitor for symptoms of withdrawal when drug is stopped (mild symptoms of physical dependence occur in approximately 50% of patients taking therapeutic doses for 6 to 12 weeks; severe symptoms are most likely to occur if the drug is taken for more than 4 months, then abruptly discontinued): increased anxiety, psychomotor agitation, irritability, headache, insomnia, tremors, and palpitation. More severe symptoms include confusion, psychosis, and seizures. Gradual discontinuation of the drug will prevent withdrawal.

Patient Teaching
• Take the drugs only when necessary. Do not increase dose or frequency of administration, and do not use for longer than 3 to 5 weeks of consecutive nights.
• Report side effects such as morning hangover; drug selection or dose may need to be changed.
• Do not take with other CNS drugs, especially CNS depressants such as alcohol, tranquilizers, or opioids.
• Do not abruptly discontinue drug (because of possibility of withdrawal symptoms).
• Do not keep drug on bedside table or in a readily accessible place (because of potential for accidental overdose).
• Utilize nondrug measures to promote relaxation, rest, and sleep (e.g., warm baths, soothing music, no caffeinated drinks after dinner).

CHAPTER 10

LOCAL AND GENERAL ANESTHETIC AGENTS

*A*nesthesia is an alteration in the central nervous system (CNS) in which certain drugs produce varying degrees of pain relief, depression of consciousness, skeletal muscle relaxation, and diminished or absent reflexes. An *anesthetic agent* depresses the CNS to produce depression of consciousness, loss of responsiveness to sensory stimulation, or muscle relaxation. *General anesthetic* agents act on the CNS to abolish pain perception and reaction to painful stimuli. The ideal components of anesthesia are (1) amnesia with unconsciousness, (2) analgesia, and (3) muscle relaxation. Because there is no single anesthetic agent capable of safely producing ideal anesthesia, a combination of drugs, known as *balanced anesthesia*, may be used. Balanced anesthesia includes (as needed):

- narcotic analgesics
- induction with an ultrashort-acting barbiturate
- nitrous oxide and/or other inhalation agent with oxygen
- skeletal muscle relaxant (neuromuscular blocking agent)
- other adjunctive drugs: sedative-hypnotics, anticholinergics (e.g., atropine), antiemetics, or antianxiety drugs

Balanced anesthesia minimizes cardiovascular problems, decreases the dose of general anesthetic drug needed, reduces the incidence of postanesthesia nausea and vomiting, minimizes anesthetic effect on organ function (i.e., liver and kidneys), and shortens anesthesia recovery time.

There are four stages of anesthesia: (1) analgesia, (2) excitement and hyperactivity, (3) surgical anesthesia, and (4) medullary paralysis. General anesthesia is administered to maintain stage 3 for as long as necessary and to avoid stage 4, when spontaneous breathing stops and death occurs unless anesthesia is stopped and resuscitative measures begun. With the newer anesthetic agents, it may not be possible to identify each stage separately, but knowing the stages is important for the nurse because patients recovering from anesthesia progress through the same stages in reverse. Therefore, hyperactivity or analgesia may extend into the postanesthesia recovery period.

GENERAL ANESTHETIC AGENTS

There are two subclasses of general anesthetic agents: inhalation and intravenous.

Inhalation agents are volatile (evaporating rapidly) liquids or gases that are vaporized in oxygen and inhaled to induce anesthesia. Intravenous drugs may be used for general anesthesia or for anesthesia induction.

Inhalation Agents

The only inhaled gas currently used as a general anesthetic agent is nitrous oxide. Inhaled volatile liquids are a group of drugs known as halogenated (containing a group of elements with similar properties) anesthetics: halothane (Fluothane), enflurane (Ethrane), isoflurane (Forane), desflurane (Suprane), sevoflurane (Ultane), and methoxyflurane (Penthrane).

Actions and Uses

The mechanism of action of general anesthetic agents is not clearly understood, but they do not appear to act by the receptor mechanism. It is believed that these highly lipid (fat)-soluble agents alter the lipid structure of cell membranes, which impairs physiologic functioning and interrupts CNS intercommunication. Nerve cell membranes have a high lipid content, as does the blood-brain barrier. Anesthetic agents easily cross this blood-brain barrier and concentrate in nerve cell membranes in the brain. This initially produces loss of the senses (sight, touch, taste, smell, hearing, and awareness) and then unconsciousness. Even though the vital cardiac, respiratory, and vasomotor centers are controlled by the medulla, they are usually spared because the medullary center is depressed last. Inhalation agents are absorbed through the alveoli and the majority of the drug is excreted unchanged through the lungs. General anesthetic agents are used to produce unconsciousness and skeletal and smooth muscle relaxation for surgical procedures. Nitrous oxide is the weakest of the general anesthetic agents and is primarily used in conjunction with other more potent anesthetics or for dental procedures. Because methoxyflurane

(Penthrane) can cause significant respiratory depression, its use is limited to short operations, dental procedures, and, in some institutions, as analgesia during childbirth.

Side and Adverse Effects

The side and adverse effects of general anesthetic agents are dose-dependent and vary with the individual drug. The heart, liver, kidneys, respiratory tract, and peripheral circulation are the sites primarily affected. Myocardial depression is a common side effect. All of the halogenated anesthetics are hepatotoxic, although the newer agents (isoflurane, desflurane, and sevoflurane) cause significantly less liver damage, as well as less myocardial depression. Although nausea, vomiting, and confusion may occur, the use of balanced anesthesia has decreased the incidence of these side effects. Hypotension may occur during anesthesia induction, but blood pressure usually returns to normal once surgery has begun. Temporary decrease in renal function may occur, but there are no apparent long-term effects on kidneys.

Malignant hyperthermia is a rare, potentially fatal hypermetabolic reaction that may be precipitated by the use of volatile anesthetic agents and neuromuscular blocking agents. It is characterized by sudden, unexpected onset of hyperthermia (temperature >104°F), severe muscle spasms, carbon dioxide retention (hypercarbia), cyanosis, and metabolic acidosis. Treatment (which must begin immediately) is rapid cooling and intravenous dantrolene (Dantrium), a central-acting skeletal muscle relaxant.

Interactions and Contraindications

If these general anesthetic agents are given with sympathomimetics (e.g., bronchodilators, vasopressors) or tricyclic antidepressants before, during, or shortly after surgery, potentially fatal cardiac arrhythmias may occur. Persons who abuse cocaine are also at risk for cardiac arrhythmias. Their use with cardiac depressants (antiarrhythmics), beta-adrenergic blockers, and calcium-channel blockers may cause increased cardiac depression. Concurrent use of tetracycline may increase potential for renal toxicity.

Enflurane is contraindicated for persons with convulsive disorders because of the potential for seizures. Halothane and methoxyflurane are contraindicated for patients with liver disease because of the increased potential for hepatotoxicity. Cautious use is indicated for patients with individual or family history of malignant hyperthermia, as well as for those with increased intracranial pressure (these drugs dilate cerebral blood vessels and may further increase intracranial pressure).

INTRAVENOUS ANESTHETIC AGENTS

Action and Uses

A number of intravenous anesthetic agents are used for anesthesia induction or as sole anesthesia for short procedures or diagnostic testing. They are highly lipid-soluble and are initially distributed to brain, liver, and kidneys. They are then redistributed to body fat and skeletal muscles, which lowers the circulating concentration, causing a short duration of action.

Barbiturates

The ultrashort-acting barbiturates most commonly used as anesthesia adjuncts are thiopental sodium (Sodium Pentothal), thiamylal sodium (Surital), and methohexital sodium (Brevital). Following intravenous administration, unconsciousness occurs in less than 30 seconds, with a duration of action of 20 to 30 minutes. These drugs have no analgesic properties and can cause excitement in the presence of pain. Blood pressure and cardiac changes are not common unless the drug is administered too rapidly. Adverse effects may include depressed respirations, yawning, coughing, and laryngospasm. Accidental arterial injection can cause clotting and inflammation at the site. Extravasation (leaking of drug into tissues) may cause tissue damage and gangrene.

Benzodiazepines

The short-acting drug in this category most commonly used as anesthesia adjunct is midazolam (Versed), although diazepam (Valium) may also be used. Midazolam is given intramuscularly for preoperative sedation or intravenously for conscious sedation during diagnostic testing, induction of general anesthesia, and maintenance of general anesthesia with nitrous oxide and oxygen for short surgical procedures. Because both midazolam and diazepam are metabolized to active metabolites, they have long half-lives, producing a sedative effect for a number of hours following surgery or procedure. Adverse effects may include respiratory depression, apnea, or even death if administered too rapidly by the intravenous route. Smaller doses must be used if other CNS depressants are given concurrently (e.g., narcotic analgesics, general anesthetics).

Short-Acting Narcotics

Drugs used in this category include fentanyl (Sublimaze), sufentanil (Sufenta), and alfentanil (Alfenta). Concurrent use of these drugs with general anesthetic agents permits lower doses of other induction agents as well as the general anesthetic drug.

These drugs may also be used alone for diagnostic or short procedures. Side and adverse effects are those associated with all narcotic drugs (see Chapter 8).

Ketamine (Ketalar)

Ketamine is an anesthetic agent that abolishes perception of and reaction to pain. It produces *cataleptic anesthesia* (also known as *neuroleptanesthesia* or *dissociative anesthesia*), whereby the patient appears to be awake but neither responds to pain nor remembers the procedure. It produces marked analgesia, sedation, immobility, amnesia, and lack of awareness of surroundings. It is rapidly effective either intravenously or intramuscularly:

> intramuscular = onset of action 3–8 minutes; anesthesia in 10–20 minutes

> intravenous = onset of action 30–60 seconds; anesthesia in 5–10 minutes

Ketamine is usually used for diagnostic or short procedures only, but may be used for induction of anesthesia. Adverse effects include enhanced muscle tone, vomiting, hypersalivation, shivering, and increases in blood pressure, heart rate, and respiratory secetions. Awakening may take several hours. During recovery, vivid unpleasant dreams or hallucinations may occur (more common in adults than in children). Ketamine is contraindicated for patients with coronary artery disease, severe hypertension, cerebral vascular disease, increased intracranial pressure, or psychiatric disorders. Cautious use is indicated for patients with mild hypertension and convulsive disorders, and for those undergoing eye surgery (increased intraocular pressure).

Nursing Actions

Preoperative

Obtain a list of all the over-the-counter and prescription drugs taken by the patient. Encourage the patient to include illicit drugs such as cocaine (because of the potential for serious drug interactions). Have information available for anesthesiology as necessary. Assess for risk factors: obesity, smoking, cardiac or respiratory disease, drug or food allergies, and so on. To alleviate anxiety and promote recovery, teach patient about the procedure and perioperative care involved. Discuss reasons for preoperative medications and NPO (nothing by mouth) status. Discuss pain control measures available postoperatively. Explain the rationale for turning, coughing, and deep breathing. Instruct the patient regarding care and assessments in the postanesthesia recovery room. Be sure the surgical permit is signed by the patient before administration of preoperative sedation, after a thorough explanation by the physician, and with a witness to the signature. Always check respirations prior to administration of preoperative medications (some of the drugs can depress respirations).

Postanesthesia Recovery

Close, frequent observation of the patient and all body systems, particularly ABCs (airway, breathing, circulation) and vital signs. Assess for sudden elevation in temperature. Administer oxygen as necessary. Reduce pain medication by one-half to one-fourth to prevent CNS and respiratory depression. Auscultate breath sounds for possible hypoventilation. Observe for any change in neurologic status. Careful monitoring of intake and output. Check all dressings and drainage tubes for placement and drainage, and intravenous lines for infiltration and correct drip rate. Implement safety measures as appropriate (e.g., side rails, restraints, reorientation to surroundings). Have resuscitative equipment and emergency drugs readily available; know how and when to use them.

LOCAL ANESTHETIC AGENTS

There are a number of local anesthetic agents currently available. Some of the more commonly used topical drugs are benzocaine (Dermoplast, Lanacaine, Solarcaine, Americaine), dibucaine (Nupercaine), butamben (Butesin), prilocaine (Emla), and proparacaine (Alcaine, Ophthetic) (ophthalmic). Drugs that may be used parenterally or topically include bupivacaine (Marcaine), lidocaine (Xylocaine), procaine (Novocain), mepivacaine (Carbocaine), and tetracaine (Pontocaine). Cocaine is one of the oldest local anesthetic agents and is still used in some instances for topical anesthesia of ear, nose, and throat (it is too toxic for systemic use and has high abuse potential).

Action and Uses

Local anesthesia is also called *regional anesthesia* because it causes loss of sensation and motor activity in localized regions of the body. The anesthetic agents work by reversibly inhibiting nerve conduction in specific areas of the body without causing loss of consciousness. Loss of sensation precedes loss of motor function; during recovery, motor function returns before sensation.

Local anesthetic agents are used for surgical, dental, and diagnostic procedures as well as for treatment of certain types of pain. They may also be used to eliminate the gag reflex for insertion of an endotracheal tube.

Routes of Administration

1. Topical (or surface)

   a. eyes

   b. skin—poorly soluble, little systemic absorption; main toxic effect is development of an allergy (usually contact dermatitis)

   c. mucosa—nose, mouth, throat, urethra, rectum, and vagina are highly vascular, causing ready systemic absorption; excessive application may cause systemic toxicity

2. Injection: potency and duration of action increases as lipid solubility of the drug increases. Onset of action is determined by the drug concentration and size of the nerve to be injected. Accidental intravenous administration must be avoided, as the drug concentration is high and potentially fatal. A vasoconstrictor, such as epinephrine, may be combined with the anesthetic agent to help confine the drug to the injected area and prevent systemic absorption. The area affected depends on how and where the drug is injected:

   a. local infiltration—superficial application; used to suture lacerations or minor surgical or dental procedures; the larger the area infiltrated, the greater the potential for systemic toxicity

   b. nerve block—injection of drug along a nerve before it reaches the surgical site; this allows large amounts of anesthetic agent to be delivered to a specific area without affecting the whole body

   c. epidural—the drug is administered outside the dura mater of the spinal column in mid-back; anesthesia is generally from the waist down; this route is preferred to spinal because of fewer side effects such as postanesthesia headache. It is also becoming more popular for the administration of opioids for pain management.

   d. spinal (saddle block) or intrathecal—drug administration is through the dura mater into the subarachnoid space (into spinal fluid) in the mid-back; anesthesia is generally from the waist down

   e. caudal—has limited use today; drug is administered outside the dura mater at base of spine and affects only the pelvic region and legs

The advantages of spinal and epidural anesthesia for major surgery include good muscle relaxation, the patient is awake without depressed respiratory and cardiovascular function (good for patients with diseases of these systems and for the elderly), and few side effects. The most common side effect is hypotension due to vasodilation.

Side and Adverse Effects

Side and adverse effects of local anesthetic agents are usually limited and of little clinical importance. However, if systemic absorption occurs, through excessive topical application of the drug to mucosa, accidental intravenous administration, or injection into a highly vascular area, toxicity can occur. The first set of symptoms to occur are related to CNS stimulation (e.g., anxiety and fear, tingling sensations, tremors, tinnitus, nausea and vomiting), progressing to CNS depression (e.g., hypotension, respiratory depression, bradycardia, arrhythmias, coma, and cardiac arrest). Symptomatic and supportive therapy is usually sufficient to reverse the toxic effects if treatment is not delayed.

Interactions and Contraindications

Bupivacaine may interact with epinephrine or halothane to produce cardiac arrhythmias. All local anesthetic drugs may interact with phenothiazines, tricyclic antidepressants, and monoamine oxidase (MAO) inhibitors to cause hypertension. However, there are few clinically significant drug interactions because the site of action of the anesthetic agents is limited to the site of application or injection.

Local anesthetic agents with epinephrine cannot be used for the following:

- nerve blocks or infiltration in areas supplied by end arteries (fingers, toes, nose, ears, and penis) because of the risk of tissue ischemia leading to gangrene
- obstetric epidural anesthesia (concentration no greater than 1:200,000 may be acceptable) because the vasoconstrictive action in uterine blood vessels may cause decreased placental circulation, decreased intensity of uterine contractions, and prolonged labor
- persons with severe cardiovascular disease or hyperthyroidism (increased risk of arrhythmias, hypertension, and tachycardia)
- intravenous use (potential for cardiac arrhythmias)
- as an adjunctive drug with inhalation anesthesia (increased risk for severe ventricular arrhythmias)

Nursing Actions

Preoperative

Ask the client if he or she has had an allergic reaction to local anesthesia. Assess the patient's understanding of the intended procedure, attitude toward regional anesthesia, and degree of anxiety. Obtain baseline vital signs and laboratory data. Obtain list of all over-the-counter and prescription drugs taken by the patient. Encourage patient to include illicit drugs such as cocaine (because of the potential for serious toxic reaction). Have information available for anesthesiology as necessary. If assisting the anesthesiologist or nurse anesthetist in injecting a local anesthetic agent, show the container to him or her and verbally verify the name of the drug, the concentration (percentage), and whether the solution is plain or contains epinephrine. Have drugs and resuscitation equipment readily available in any location where local anesthetics are administered. Know how to use them.

Postanesthesia Recovery

Remember that motor function returns before sensation. Do not place hot blankets or heating pads directly on the area affected by the local anesthetic. Bedrest may be ordered for 6–12 hours following spinal or epidural anesthesia; do not ambulate until motor and sensory functions have recovered completely. Provide adequate hydration (to prevent spinal headache). Know indications of local anesthesia toxicity and how to determine which stage of toxicity is being exhibited. Report occurrence of symptoms immediately to anesthesiology. Perform close, frequent observation of the patient and all body systems, particularly ABCs (airway, breathing, and circulation) and vital signs. Check all dressings and drainage tubes for placement and drainage, and intravenous lines for infiltration and correct drip rate. If patient has had topical anesthesia to mouth, nose, or throat, withhold food or drink until gag reflex has returned. Implement safety measures as appropriate (e.g., side rails, restraints). Have resuscitative equipment and emergency drugs readily available; know how and when to use them.

CHAPTER 11

SKELETAL MUSCLE RELAXANTS

*S*keletal muscle relaxants used in the perioperative period are divided into two categories: *neuromuscular blocking agents* and *spasmolytics* (antispasm drugs).

Spasmolytic drugs are categorized as centrally acting and peripherally acting. The drug discussed in this chapter is the peripherally acting drug, dantrolene (Dantrium). Neuromuscular blocking agents are classified as nondepolarizing and depolarizing drugs.

Nondepolarizing drugs prevent acetylcholine (see Unit 6) from acting at the neuromuscular junction, so muscles remain in a relaxed state. *Depolarizing* drugs act at the neuromuscular junction to combine with cholinergic receptors (see Unit 6) to cause muscle contraction but not relaxation, thus preventing further neurocommunication (muscle paralysis preceded by muscle spasms). The nondepolarizing drug discussed in this chapter is tubocurarine (Tubocuraine) and the depolarizing agent is succinylcholine (Anectine).

TUBOCURARINE (TUBOCURAINE)

Action

Tubocurarine is a component of curare, a neuromuscular blocking agent extracted from certain plants found in the Amazon rain forest. It is an acetylcholine antagonist that competes for the cholinergic receptor sites at the neuromuscular junction. This antagonism causes a decrease in the response of the muscle to acetylcholine, resulting in relaxed (flaccid) paralysis. Tubocurarine has significant histamine-releasing properties, and no known effect on intellectual functions, consciousness, or pain threshold. The drug does not cross the blood-brain barrier and has no effect in the central nervous system (CNS). For this reason, anesthesia is begun before neuromuscular blockade is started, to prevent the unanesthetized patient from having the frightening experience of paralysis and inability to breathe. The neuromuscular blocking action of tubocurarine may be reversed with anticholinesterases (see Unit 6) such as neostigmine (Prostigmin), pyridostigmine (Mestinon), and edrophonium (Tensilon), which prevent the normal breakdown of acetylcholine at the neuromuscular junction, leading to an accumulation of the neurotransmitter and return of muscle stimulation.

Uses

Tubocurarine is used to produce skeletal muscle relaxation as an adjunct to general anesthesia and to facilitate both endotracheal intubation and mechanical ventilation. In an intensive care setting, tubocurarine is used to minimize patients' movements to conserve energy or to reduce agitation that may increase intracranial pressure (another nondepolarizing drug, pancuronium [Pavulon], may also be used for sedation in the Intensive Care Unit). Tubocurarine is also used to prevent trauma during convulsive therapy, to reduce intensity of muscle contractions in tetanus, and to diagnose myasthenia gravis.

Side and Adverse Effects

The primary adverse effects of tubocurarine result from neuromuscular blockade at all neuromuscular end plates. Prolonged paralysis may lead to decubitus ulcer formation from prolonged immobility. Because of respiratory muscle paralysis with prolonged apnea, assisted ventilation is necessary until the effects of the drug have worn off. Relaxation of arterial muscles results in vasodilation, which may cause flushing, hypotension, bradycardia or tachycardia, or worsening of a pre-existing heart condition. Relaxation of the gastrointestinal tract with decreased muscle tone and motility may lead to vomiting, regurgitation, and aspiration. Histamine release may cause respiratory difficulty, such as wheezing and bronchospasm. Tubocurarine, particularly if used with a general anesthetic agent, may cause malignant hyperthermia (a rare, potentially fatal reaction characterized by sudden, unexpected hyperthermia [temperature >104°F], severe muscle spasms, carbon dioxide retention, cyanosis, and metabolic acidosis).

Interactions and Contraindications

Drugs that increase the action of tubocurarine include skeletal muscle relaxants, aminoglycosides, inhalation anesthetics, ketamine, quinine derivatives, polymyxin B, clindamycin, amphotericin B, diuretics, procainamide, and verapamil. Drugs that may decrease the effectiveness of tubocurarine include carbamazepine, hydantoins (i.e., phenytoin [Dilantin]), and theophylline.

Tubocurarine is contraindicated for persons with conditions that may be made worse by histamine release and vasodilation, such as asthma, bronchospasm, hypotension, and cardiac disease, as well as for those with hyperthermia. Cautious use is indicated in patients with pulmonary disease or lung cancer, dehydration, electrolyte or acid-base imbalance, decreased renal function, and myasthenia gravis. Hypothermia may decrease the action or duration of tubocurarine.

Nursing Actions

Obtain patient history regarding renal, hepatic, cardiovascular, or respiratory diseases. Determine personal or family history of malignant hyperthermia. Perform a predrug administration physical assessment, including vital signs, state of hydration, weight, reflexes and muscle tone, and breath sounds. Assess baseline electrolyte values and renal and hepatic status. Emergency equipment for endotracheal intubation, mechanical ventilation, and oxygen should be immediately available. An anticholinesterase drug such as neostigmine (Prostigmin) is used to reverse the effects of tubocurarine. Know the sequence of muscle paralysis: jaw muscles, eyelid muscles, and other muscles of head and neck, limbs, intercostals and diaphragm, abdomen, and trunk. Facial and diaphragm muscles are the first to recover, followed in order by legs, arms, shoulder girdle, trunk, larynx, hands and feet, and pharynx. Muscle function has usually returned within 90 minutes. Monitor vital signs closely and keep airway clear of secretions following administration of the drug. Perform frequent skin assessments and change patient's position frequently if paralysis is prolonged. Understand that patients may experience sore muscles, constipation, difficulty voiding, and dizziness upon arising. Remember that professional demeanor is very important with patients who have received neuromuscular blocking agents: they are paralyzed but can think and hear.

SUCCINYLCHOLINE (ANECTINE)

Action and Uses

Succinylcholine is a depolarizing neuromuscular blocker that works by causing the muscle cell membrane to become excited (depolarize), leading to rapid muscle contractions followed by flaccid (relaxed) paralysis. Because of these rapid muscle contractions, patients often experience postoperative muscle pain. Succinylcholine is used to produce skeletal muscle relaxation as adjunct to general anesthesia, to facilitate endotracheal intubation and endoscopy, to increase pulmonary compliance in mechanical ventilation, and to reduce intensity of muscle contractions during convulsive therapy. The use of succinylcholine as general anesthesia adjunct or during long-term mechanical ventilation has, for the most part, been replaced by more effective and less toxic neuromuscular blocking agents. Succinylcholine is com-

monly used during delivery by cesarean section. If repeated doses are required prior to delivery, the neonate should be closely monitored for apnea and decreased muscle tone.

Side and Adverse Effects

The primary adverse effects of succinylcholine are similar to tubocurarine and result from neuromuscular blockade at all neuromuscular end plates. Prolonged paralysis may lead to decubitus ulcer formation from prolonged immobility. Because of respiratory muscle paralysis with prolonged apnea, assisted ventilation is necessary until the effects of the drug have worn off. Increased intraocular pressure may cause or aggravate glaucoma. Because of the muscle contractions, patients may complain of severe muscle pain that may last for several days after the drug is given. Slight histamine release may contribute to bronchospasms, wheezing, hypotension, and cardiac arrhythmias in susceptible individuals. Succinylcholine, particularly if used with a general anesthetic agent, may cause malignant hyperthermia.

Interactions and Contraindications

A number of drugs may prolong neuromuscular blockade if given concurrently with succinylcholine. Some of the more common ones include aminoglycosides, iodide, halothane, lidocaine, narcotic analgesics, monoamine oxidase (MAO) inhibitors, phenothiazines, quinine derivatives, procainamide, and propranolol. Digitalis glycosides may increase the risk of cardiac arrhythmias. Anticholinesterases (e.g., neostigmine [Prostigmin], pyridostigmine [Mestinon], and edrophonium [Tensilon]) inhibit the action of plasma pseudocholinesterase (necessary to inactivate succinylcholine), thus prolonging neuromuscular blockade.

The use of succinylcholine is contraindicated for anyone with an individual or family history of malignant hyperthermia. It is also contraindicated for intraocular surgery or for patients with glaucoma. Cautious use is indicated for persons with low serum pseudocholinesterase levels, renal, hepatic, pulmonary, metabolic, or cardiovascular disorders, neuromuscular disease, dehydration, or hyperthermia. Its use may be contraindicated in anyone with hyperkalemia or at risk for hyperkalemia (the intense muscle contractions cause release of potassium into the bloodstream) as well as those with severe burns or trauma.

Nursing Actions

Assess for personal or family history of low pseudocholinesterase levels. Patients at risk for this condition include those with severe burns or trauma, malnutrition or dehydration, severe liver disease, cancer, severe anemia, or myxedema (hypothyroidism). Determine individual or family history of malignant hyperthermia. Perform a predrug administration physical assessment including vital signs, state of hydration, weight, reflexes and muscle tone, and breath sounds. Assess baseline electrolyte values and renal and hepatic status. Emergency equipment for endotracheal intubation, mechanical ventilation, and oxygen should be immediately available. Know the sequence of muscle paralysis: eyelid muscles, jaw, limbs, abdomen, glottis, intercostals, and diaphragm. Recovery generally occurs in reverse order. Monitor vital signs closely and keep airway clear of secretions following administration of the drug. Inform patients that they may experience muscle stiffness and pain for as long as 24 to 30 hours after receiving the drug. They may also experience hoarseness and sore throat. Remember that professional demeanor is very important with patients who have received neuromuscular blocking agents: they are paralyzed but can think and hear.

DANTROLENE (DANTRIUM)

Action

Dantrolene is a peripherally acting muscle relaxant that exerts its effect by direct action within the skeletal muscle fiber. It does not interfere with neuromuscular communication and has no CNS effects. Dantrolene reduces the amount of calcium released from the muscle fibers, thereby causing the muscle contraction (or spasm) to relax. This interference with calcium release from the muscle fibers may prevent an increase in intracellular calcium, which activates the acute muscle spasms of malignant hyperthermia. Dantrolene has no effect on contraction of cardiac or intestinal smooth muscle.

Uses

Intravenous dantrolene is the drug of choice, with supportive measures such as rapid cooling, for the immediate treatment of malignant hyperthermia. Oral dantrolene may be used 2 to 3 days preoperatively as prophylaxis for patients with an individual or family history of malignant hyperthermia. Dantrolene may be given postoperatively for 1 to 3 days following an occurrence of malignant hyperthermia to prevent recurrence of symptoms. Other uses include symptomatic treatment of skeletal muscle spasms secondary to spinal cord injury, stroke, cerebral palsy, and multiple sclerosis.

Side and Adverse Effects

The most common side effect is muscle weakness sufficient to affect overall functional capacity of the patient. This may be manifested by symptoms of drooling, drowsiness, slurred speech, dizziness, malaise, and fatigue. More serious adverse effects include potentially fatal hepatic necrosis (especially in women over 35 years old and taking estrogens),

seizures, erratic blood pressure, and pleural effusion with pericarditis. Gastrointestinal side effects include diarrhea, gastrointestinal bleeding, anorexia, abdominal cramps, and difficulty swallowing. Diarrhea is usually transient, but if it is severe, the drug may have to be withheld. Intravenous dantrolene may cause edema and thrombophlebitis.

Interactions and Contraindications

Concurrent use of dantrolene with alcohol or other CNS depressants may cause CNS depression. Verapamil and other calcium-channel blockers increase risk of ventricular fibrillation and cardiovascular collapse (from hyperkalemia). Women over the age of 35 who are taking estrogens and dantrolene concurrently are at greater risk for hepatotoxicity (mechanism of action unknown). These interactions do not usually occur during acute treatment of malignant hyperthermia.

There are no contraindications to the use of dantrolene as acute treatment or prevention of malignant hyperthermia. For preoperative prevention of malignant hyperthermia, cautious use is indicated in patients with pre-existing neuromuscular disease with respiratory depression, as there is an increased risk of perioperative complications.

Nursing Actions

Assess patient for personal or family history of malignant hyperthermia. Avoid intravenous extravasation (infiltration into the tissue) to prevent tissue necrosis. Monitor intravenous site frequently. During intravenous infusion, monitor vital signs, electrocardiogram, and serum electrolytes.

REVIEW QUESTIONS: UNIT 3

1. Lack of adequate REM sleep can cause serious psychological problems, including psychosis.

    A. True

    B. False

2. Barbiturates are known as liver enzyme inducers. This means that:

    A. an additional enzyme must be administered concurrently to prevent toxicity.

    B. barbiturates will be metabolized very slowly.

    C. barbiturates increase the liver's ability to metabolize themselves, producing drug tolerance.

3. Some patients may be on long-term barbiturate therapy. Which of the following dietary nutrients may need to be increased in the diet?

   A. Vitamin K

   B. Vitamin D

   C. Potassium

   D. Calcium

4. Benzodiazepines are more commonly prescribed as hypnotics over the barbiturates because benzodiazepines :

   A. induce liver enzymes.

   B. provide pain relief also.

   C. do not suppress REM sleep.

   D. have no potential for physical dependence.

5. Patient teaching regarding benzodiazepine use as hypnotics includes:

   A. do not use for longer that 3 to 5 weeks of consecutive nights.

   B. take the drug with the evening meal to prevent bedtime wakefulness.

   C. keep the drug at bedside to monitor number of pills taken.

   D. these drugs will not cause sleep disturbances, such as nightmares.

6. The antidote/antagonist specific for benzodiazepine overdose is:

   A. nalozone (Narcan).

   B. flumazenil (Romazicon).

   C. neostigmine (Prostigmin).

   D. naltrexone (ReVia, Trexan).

7. General anesthetic agents are primarily excreted through the:

   A. kidneys.

   B. liver.

   C. gastrointestinal tract.

   D. lungs.

8. Which of the following nursing actions is most appropriate to aid in excretion of a general anesthetic agent from a postsurgical patient?

   A. Assist to turn, cough, and deep breathe

   B. Increase intravenous fluid rate

   C. Offer oral fluids as soon as possible

   D. Use passive range of motion exercises

9. Care for a patient who has received local anesthesia includes knowledge that:

   A. sensation returns before motor function.

   B. motor function returns before sensation.

   C. sensation and motor function return simultaneously.

   D. close, frequent assessment of vital signs is not as important as for a patient receiving general anesthesia.

10. A patient has had topical local anesthesia applied to her mouth and throat for a diagnostic procedure. What is the most important information you need to know before offering her something to drink?

    A. Presence of adequate urine output

    B. Ability to hold the glass by herself

    C. Return of her gag reflex

    D. Number of hours since the procedure

11. Which of the following drugs should be readily available to reverse the muscle paralysis of turbocurarine?

    A. Naloxone (Narcan)

    B. Flumazenil (Romazicon)

    C. Neostigmine (Prostigmin)

    D. Naltrexone (ReVia, Trexan)

12. Which of the following is the drug of choice to prevent or treat malignant hyperthermia?

    A. Diazepam (Valium)

    B. Acetaminophen (Tylenol)

    C. Edrophonium (Tensilon)

    D. Dantrolene (Dantrium)

13. A postsurgical patient who received succinylcholine as part of his anesthesia asks why his muscles and throat are so sore. The nurse's best response is:

   A. "This is a normal response to the muscle relaxant you received during surgery and should go away in 24 to 48 hours."

   B. "I'm very worried about this. I will call your doctor right away."

   C. "You must have been fighting the anesthesia and had to be restrained."

   D. "I'll get you some pain medication."

LONG-TERM AND HOME HEALTH CARE

OBJECTIVES

1. Explain why long-term care patients are at greater risk for adverse drug effects.

2. Identify drugs that contribute to falls, immobility, confusion, and incontinence.

3. Explain the actions, side and adverse effects, interactions, and contraindications of drugs used to treat confusion and urinary incontinence.

4. Identify nursing interventions relevant to each major classification of drugs used to treat confusion and urinary incontinence.

5. Discuss the drugs used in the palliative care of terminally ill patients and related nursing implications.

CHAPTER 12

FALLS, IMMOBILITY, CONFUSION

*O*lder Americans constitute only 12% of the population but are thought to consume nearly one-third of all prescription drugs. Most older people take at least one prescription drug daily and studies have repeatedly documented large numbers of people who routinely take multiple drugs. *Polypharmacy* is the term used when people take multiple drugs at the same time. Adverse drug reactions occur seven times more often in older people than in their younger counterparts. Reasons for this disproportionate rate of adverse drug reactions are that, compared to younger adults, older people:

- More often have multiple diagnoses that are treated with multiple drugs.
- Tend to metabolize and excrete drugs more slowly owing to less efficient renal and hepatic function.
- May be more or less sensitive to specific drugs.
- Are more likely to take drugs that have a narrow margin of safety.
- Are more likely to take the same drug over a very long period of time.

It is essential for nurses, especially those in long-term care settings, to understand the risks and benefits of drug therapy in this patient population.

Falls, immobility, confusion, and incontinence are common problems in the long-term care setting that may be partially attributed to drug therapy. This chapter will discuss drugs implicated in falls, immobility, confusion, and incontinence as well as specific drugs employed to treat these same problems.

FALLS AND IMMOBILITY

As people get older, the risk of falls and the severity of fall-related injuries steadily increases. Drugs that have been associated with an increased risk of falls include psychotropics (neuroleptics, antidepressants, sedatives), antihypertensives, and diuretics. A common adverse effect of all of these agents is orthostatic hypotension. When the patient shifts from a lying or sitting position to a standing position, blood pools in the lower extremities, blood pressure falls, blood flow to the brain is inadequate, and the patient becomes dizzy or loses consciousness. Other situations that may bring on this drop in blood pressure include prolonged standing and taking a hot shower or bath.

In addition to orthostatic hypotension, psychotropics may decrease alertness so that the patient is less attentive to obstacles in the environment. The sedated patient tends to decrease physical activity, eventually becoming weaker and more prone to falls. Table 12–1 summarizes some drug actions that may contribute to falling and decreased mobility.

Nursing Actions

People who are fearful of falling may restrict their activity, creating a vicious cycle in which they become weaker and progressively more prone to falls. When patients are taking drugs that pose a risk for falls, it is important to assess the person's mobility. Observe him or her changing positions and note unsteadiness. Assess pulse and blood pressure in the lying, sitting, then standing positions. A pulse increase of 20 or more, or a drop of 20 mm Hg in blood pressure reflects orthostatic hypotension.

If a patient is receiving psychotropics and seems excessively sedated, notify the physician. Assist with mobility if the patient is unsteady.

Patient Teaching
• When getting up, rise slowly, exercise your legs before standing, and be sure you are steady before beginning to walk.
• Your medications may cause your body to adapt more slowly to position changes and you must allow for this.
• Grab bars in the bathroom are recommended to reduce the risk of falls.
• Use a shower chair rather than standing in the shower.
• Avoid very warm showers or baths; warm water dilates your blood vessels and could make you feel faint.
• Regular physical activity will help you maintain muscle strength and balance.
• If you become dizzy, either lie down or sit down and put your head between your knees to improve blood flow to the brain.

TABLE 12–1

Drugs Associated with Falls and Decreased Mobility

Classification	Action	Adverse Effect
Psychotropics	CNS* depression: decreases alertness and activity; extrapyramidal effects; lowers blood pressure	Muscle weakness, impaired coordination, poor judgment, delayed response time Orthostatic hypotension
Diuretics	Diuresis reduces blood volume, lowering blood pressure	Orthostatic hypotension
Antihypertensives	Dilation of blood vessels lowers blood pressure; some have sedative effects; decreased energy and physical activity	Orthostatic hypotension
Antianginals	Dilation of blood vessels lowers blood pressure	Orthostatic hypotension

*CNS, central nervous system

CONFUSION

Confusion is a state of disturbed thinking that can be acute or chronic. Acute confusion is sometimes called *delirium*. *Dementia* is the term used for chronic, irreversible confusion. The most common types of dementia are Alzheimer's disease and vascular dementia.

Delirium

Among the many risk factors for delirium are infections, circulatory disorders, metabolic disorders, neoplasms, trauma, and medications. Drug classifications and specific agents that are known to contribute to delirium include:

- analgesics
- anticholinergics
- antidepressants
- antihistamines
- antiparkinsonian drugs
- cimetidine
- digitalis glycosides
- diuretics
- neuroleptics
- sedatives/hypnotics

Nursing Actions

Sometimes confusion is resolved by simply changing a drug, reducing the dosage, or discontinuing a drug. Unfortunately, when older people develop confusion, thorough assessments of contributing factors are not always done. When a patient becomes confused, you should always suspect medications as possible culprits. Review the drug profile and look up drug adverse effects and interactions. If a drug or combination of drugs is known to contribute to confusion, bring this to the attention of the physician.

When patients are confused, safety is a priority. Keep the bed in low position. Follow agency policies in relation to side rails. Use restraints only as a last resort. Encourage a family member to stay with the patient. Frequently reorient the patient to time, place, and person. Reduce environmental stimuli and use simple, direct communication. Use a calm, slow, and gentle approach when providing care.

Dementia

Although dementia is generally considered irreversible, various pharmacologic agents have been employed in an effort to improve cognitive function or to slow the progress of the cognitive decline.

Alzheimer's Disease

To date, the most effective drugs for the treatment of Alzheimer's disease are the cholinesterase inhibitors tacrine and donepezil. These drugs do not reverse the effects of the disease but seem to slow its progression in many patients in the early stages. By preventing the breakdown of acetylcholine by cholinesterase, they increase the amount of acetylcholine, which is an important neurotransmitter. Tacrine (Cognex) was the first cholinesterase inhibitor marketed for treatment of Alzheimer's disease. Donepezil (Aricept) has become the drug of choice because tacrine may cause liver damage. Frequent adverse effects of both of these drugs are nausea, diarrhea, vomiting, and dizziness (Table 12–2).

Because there is no cure for Alzheimer's disease, a wide variety of agents are being studied for their actions in the prevention and treatment of the disease. Some of these agents are included in Table 12–3. As of this writing, it is not known whether any will prove to be useful.

TABLE 12–2
Cholinesterase Inhibitors

Prototype	Specific Considerations
tacrine (Cognex)	Frequent adverse effects: nausea, vomiting, diarrhea, and dizziness. Contraindicated with severe, active liver disease; active gastrointestinal ulcers; urinary or gastrointestinal obstruction. **Pregnancy Category X.** Interactions: may enhance theophylline and increase adverse effects of NSAIDs*; may interfere with anticholinergics; effects are enhanced by cimetidine.
donepezil (Aricept)	In addition to nausea, diarrhea, vomiting, and dizziness, donepezil also may cause insomnia, muscle cramps, fatigue, and anorexia. Patients with cardiac disease may develop bradycardia. Unlike tacrine, does not harm the liver.

*NSAIDs, nonsteroidal anti-inflammatory drugs

TABLE 12–3
Experimental Drugs Under Study for the Treatment of Alzheimer's Disease (AD)

Drug Classification and Examples	Possible Benefits with Alzheimer's Disease	Comments
Neurotrophic factors NGF (nerve growth factor)	Helps neurons regenerate after injury and stimulates growth of axons and dendrites	Improves memory in lab animals. Human testing has been hindered by problems crossing the blood-brain barrier.
Estrogen	May interact with NGF to protect cholinergic neurons. May prevent formation of beta amyloid. May act as antioxidant to protect neurons.	Studies have found that women who take estrogen seem to have reduced risk of AD. Estrogen use in early stage AD is now being studied to see if it will affect the course of the disease.
Calcium channel blockers	There is evidence of excess calcium in the neurons of AD patients. If this excess contributes to AD, decreasing the intracellular calcium may bring about improvement. Calcium channel blockers block the movement of calcium into neurons, which may prevent or slow the progression of AD.	Clinical testing of calcium channel blockers is underway.
Antioxidants vitamin E deprenyl acetyl-L-carnitine selegiline (Eldepryl)	Oxygen free radicals are by-products of metabolism that are harmful to cells. This could be a factor in the neuron damage seen with AD. Substances that disarm oxygen free radicals are called antioxidants.	There is limited evidence that selegiline or vitamin E slows the progression of AD. Researchers caution that selegiline has many side effects and that the dosage of vitamin E used in research is far greater than the usual recommended dosage.
Anti-inflammatory agents NSAIDs other than aspirin, prednisone	There is some evidence that people who have taken NSAIDs other than aspirin for as little as 2 years have less risk for AD.	Much more study is needed before this NSAIDs can be recommended for prevention of cognitive decline. The effects of prednisone in early stage AD is under study.

(Continued on p. 76)

Drug Classification and Examples	Possible Benefits with Alzheimer's Disease	Comments
Other: kampo medicine	Kampo medicine is a traditional Japanese medicine made of roots and herbs. One study showed improved memory.	Further study of these less traditional treatments is needed. However, kampo and ginkgo do not require prescriptions and you may encounter patients who are taking these without medical advice. Be sure to note this on your drug history.
ginkgo biloba	One controlled study suggested ginkgo delayed the progression of AD in relation to cognitive performance and social function.	
dronabinol	Limited evidence that dronabinol improves appetite in AD patients and decreases disturbed behavior.	

NSAIDs, nonsteroidal anti-inflammatory drugs

Vascular Dementia

There is no specific agent that improves cognitive function with vascular dementia. Some physicians recommend one enteric-coated aspirin each day to decrease the risk of recurrent stroke. Aspirin inhibits platelet clumping, thereby decreasing the risk of formation of blood clots that could cause strokes. Gastrointestinal distress is the most common adverse effect of aspirin. If taken in high doses over time, aspirin may cause more serious adverse effects from toxicity. Aspirin interacts with many other drugs, so you must be aware of all drugs the patient is taking.

INCONTINENCE

Urinary incontinence is a problem affecting many people, but the incidence increases with age and disabilities. Because older people are more likely to take medications, they are more likely to be exposed to agents that can cause incontinence.

Some drugs affect the mechanics of urination, whereas others create functional problems that affect the patient's ability to control the passage of urine. Among the many agents that can contribute to incontinence are xanthines, alpha-adrenergic agonists and blockers, anticholinergics, antihistamines, antiparkinsonian, antipsychotics, high ceiling diuretics, opiate agonists, sedative/hypnotics, and sympathomimetics (Table 12–4).

TABLE 12–4

Drugs that Affect Urinary Continence

Drug Classification	Action	Effect
Alpha-adrenergic blockers	Decrease urethral closing pressure in women	Leakage of urine under stress
Anticholinergics	Decrease bladder contractility; can cause confusion and contribute to immobility	Bladder becomes distended; overflow incontinence results
Diuretics	Increase urine volume; bladder fills more quickly	Patient unable to access toilet in time to prevent incontinence
Sedatives/hypnotics	Altered sensorium: confusion, sedation; decreased mobility	Patient fails to recognize or respond to need to void. Patient unable to get to toilet in time.

Data from Duthrie, E. H., & Katz, P. R. (1998). *Practice of Geriatrics*, 3rd ed. Philadelphia: W. B. Saunders, p. 191.

When a patient develops urinary incontinence, your assessment should always include a list of the drugs the patient is taking. If a drug may be contributing to the problem, consult the physician about alternatives.

Pharmacologic Treatment of Urinary Incontinence

Some drugs contribute to urinary incontinence; others may be helpful in relieving the problem. Drug therapy is usually reserved for incontinence that does not respond to conservative treatment. Table 12–5 identifies some drugs that may be used for each type of urinary incontinence.

TABLE 12–5

Drugs Used to Treat Incontinence

Drug Classification	Appropriate Use
Estrogen cream	Stress incontinence due to atrophic vaginitis
Alpha-adrenergic agonists phenylpropanolamine (sustained release), pseudoephedrine	Stress incontinence
Alpha-adrenergic blockers prazosin (Minipress), terazosin (Hytrin), doxazosin (Cardura), finasteride (Propecia)	Urge incontinence due to urethral obstruction. Overflow incontinence due to underactive detrusor or urethral obstruction (only if some voiding is possible).
Antidepressants imipramine (Tofranil), doxepin (Sinequan)	Stress incontinence Urge incontinence with detrusor overactivity and normal bladder contractility
Anticholinergics	Urge incontinence with detrusor overactivity and normal bladder contractility
Smooth muscle relaxants oxybutynin (Ditropan), dicyclomine (Antispas), calcium channel blockers	Urge incontinence with detrusor overactivity and normal bladder contractility
Cholinergic bethanechol (Urecholine)	Overflow incontinence with underactive detrusor

Data from Duthie, E., & Katz, P. (1998) *Practice of Geriatrics*, 3rd ed. Philadelphia: W.B. Saunders.

As you can see, a wide range of drugs may be prescribed for the patient with urinary incontinence, depending on the underlying cause. All of the classifications identified in this chapter are covered in detail elsewhere in this book. Many of them have significant systemic actions that require ongoing assessment and patient teaching for safe use.

Nursing Actions

A few general guidelines when patients are taking drugs for urinary incontinence are as follows:

* Document incontinent episodes (or have the patient do so) to assess for improved control of voiding.
* Assess for bladder distention.
* Drug therapy may be combined with other measures such as Kegel exercises.
* Be sensitive to the patient's concerns about incontinent episodes.
* As long as incontinence is a problem, provide assistance as needed with personal hygiene.

Patient Teaching

For patients taking drugs with side effects such as orthostatic hypotension:

* You may feel dizzy when changing positions.
* To avoid falls, rise slowly and exercise your legs before standing.
* If you feel dizzy, lie down or sit down and lower your head to improve blood flow.

DRUG THERAPY DURING TERMINAL ILLNESS

*M*aintaining the best possible quality of life is a challenge for health care providers when patients near the end of life. A critical component of quality of life is comfort. Promoting comfort involves physical, psychological, and spiritual interventions. For the terminally ill person, comfort is closely related to relief of symptoms. Drug therapy is just one tool we have to relieve symptoms and promote comfort.

Symptoms and mood states encountered among patients who were dying have been described by Pickett and Yancey (1996). Among the physical symptoms were pain, nausea and vomiting, anorexia, dyspnea, delirium, fatigue, constipation or diarrhea, and urinary incontinence. Mood states included anxiety, depression, and anger. This chapter reviews some of these symptoms commonly encountered at the end of life and describes drugs that may be helpful.

PAIN

Pain is one of the most common symptoms of many disease processes. Although it is a protective mechanism, unrelieved pain affects quality of life and has limited purpose. Patients nearing the end of life may have both acute and chronic pain that requires attention.

Management of pain is thoroughly covered in Chapter 14 of the textbook, and analgesics are addressed in Chapter 8 of this supplement. There are, however, some important considerations when dealing with patients in the terminal stage of illness.

- The goal of pain management is to identify a safe and effective dose.
- When a patient has pain for 12 or more out of 24 hours, analgesics should be given around-the-clock rather than PRN.
- Notify the physician if the prescribed analgesics are not effective.
- Opioids are often needed for effective management of moderate to severe pain.
- Combinations of opioids and nonopioids may be especially effective.

- Once severe pain is under control, noninvasive routes (oral, transdermal, rectal, sublingual) for analgesics are recommended for the terminally ill patient.
- The risk of respiratory depression decreases as opioids are used over time.
- Be alert for respiratory depression if the patient is becoming increasingly sedated. However, remember that respiratory and mental status will decline as the patient nears death.
- Side effects of opioids can be managed with metoclopramide (Reglan) for nausea and vomiting, diphenhydramine (Benadryl) for itching, and laxatives for constipation.
- Fears about addiction to opioids have been greatly exaggerated.
- Concern about addiction should be secondary to concern about pain relief for the terminally ill patient.
- Use of placebos is deceitful and must be discouraged.
- With terminal illness, nonpharmacologic measures such as relaxation and imagery are best used WITH analgesics, not in place of them.

DYSPNEA

Dyspnea (shortness of breath) is a problem with a variety of cardiac and pulmonary conditions. Patients with dyspnea feel like they are suffocating and are understandably anxious. Drugs that may be effective in relieving dyspnea are as follows:

- opioids (morphine sulfate, oxycodone, nebulized morphine, hydromorphone)
- bronchodilators
- diuretics
- anxiolytics

COUGH

Cough in the terminally ill person may be due multiple factors, including lung cancer, chronic pulmonary disease, respiratory infections, and heart failure. Persistent coughing taxes the muscles of the thorax and abdomen and can be exhausting. Drugs that may be effective in relieving cough are as follows:

- cough suppressants: codeine, dextromethorphan
- mucolytics: to thin secretions so they can be cleared more easily
- bronchodilators
- anxiolytics

NAUSEA AND VOMITING

Nausea and vomiting have numerous causes, including drug adverse effects, specific cancers, anxiety, pain, infection, bowel obstruction, radiation, renal failure, and some electrolyte imbalances. Whenever possible, the underlying cause should be treated while managing the nausea and vomiting. Many antiemetics (drugs that relieve nausea and vomiting) are available, such as the following:

- metoclopramide (Reglan)
- dexamethasone (Decadron)
- prochlorperazine (Compazine)
- diazepam (Valium)

DELIRIUM

Delirium is an acute disturbance in mental function. Specific manifestations vary, but the patient may be confused, agitated, or combative and may have delusions or hallucinations. Delirium can be attributed to drug adverse effects, fluid and electrolyte imbalances, pain, infections, circulatory impairment, and endocrine disorders. If cerebral edema is a contributing factor, corticosteroids may be helpful. Agents that may be used to manage delirium include the following:

- antipsychotics
- benzodiazepines

ANXIETY

Anxiety is a vague feeling of uneasiness or apprehension. Unlike fear, in which a specific threat is known, the cause of anxiety is often not readily identified. In patients who are terminally ill, anxiety may be related to uncontrolled pain, dyspnea, thoughts about impending death, and even some drug effects. Anxiolytics (drugs used to treat anxiety) are

covered in Chapter 50. Specific anxiolytic drugs recommended for the terminally ill patient include the following:

- alprazolam (Xanax), a short-acting benzodiazepine
- amitriptyline (Elavil)
- lorazepam (Ativan)

DEPRESSION

Depression is a feeling of sadness or despair. Like anxiety, it may be related to uncontrolled pain, thoughts about impending death, and some drugs. For the terminally ill, tricyclic antidepressants such as amitriptyline (Elavil) or desipramine (Norpramin) are most often used.

FATIGUE

Fatigue is an almost universal symptom experienced by people with advanced diseases. Patients describe a lack of energy that is not alleviated by rest. Fatigue may be attributed to the disease process itself, effects of treatments, poor nutrition, and depression. Drug therapy for fatigue is limited. If fatigue is a side effect of opioid therapy, corticosteroids may be helpful. In some situations, amphetamines have been used.

CONSTIPATION

Constipation is the passage of dry, hard stools. Bowel movements are generally less frequent than the patient's usual pattern. Constipation is an adverse effect of many drugs, especially opioids, which are commonly used in end of life pain management. Other contributing factors are immobility, dehydration, and intestinal obstruction. Bulk laxatives are not recommended because of the risk of intestinal obstruction. The following are recommended:

- laxatives: magnesium sulfate (Milk of Magnesia), senna (Senokot), bisacodyl (Dulcolax)
- stool softener: docusate (Colace)

If laxatives and stool softeners alone are not effective, suppositories may be needed also.

SUMMARY

As patients near the end of life, there is much that nurses can do to improve the quality of the remaining time. Good management of troubling symptoms is an important part of the nurse's role. Although this chapter has emphasized drug therapy, many other supportive actions are appropriate as well.

The importance of employing drugs to promote comfort is only one aspect of drug therapy at the end of life. In the face of circulatory, renal, or hepatic failure, patients may respond to drugs differently. When a patient does not metabolize or excrete drugs efficiently, serum levels of drugs may rise to toxic levels quickly. Patients, families, and health care providers may question whether it is necessary to continue drugs that have no short-term benefit and cause unpleasant side effects (some antihypertensives, for example).

REFERENCES

Ferrell, B. R., Grant, M., Virani, R., & Marugg, C. (1999). Guidelines: Critical areas of end of life care. Report of project entitled *Strengthening Nursing Education to Improve Pain Management and End of Life Care*. Supported by a grant from the Robert Wood Johnson Foundation.

Pickett, M., & Yancey, D. (1998). Symptoms of the dying. *In* McCorkle, R., Grant, M., Frank-Stromborg, M., & Baird, S. (Eds.). *Cancer Nursing: A Comprehensive Textbook*, 2nd ed. (pp. 1157–1182). Philadelphia: W.B. Saunders.

REVIEW QUESTIONS: UNIT 4

Case Study

Mrs. Seigel is an 80-year-old female with stress incontinence. (See the Care Plan in Chapter 21 of the textbook). After doing Kegel exercises for 2 months, she notes improvement but still has episodes of incontinence. Her physician prescribes phenylpropanolamine 25 mg PO BID and estrogen cream to be used intravaginally at HS.

The following questions relate to this situation.

1. How could estrogen cream improve stress incontinence?

2. True or False: Estrogen cream is not absorbed into the system.

3. Phenylpropanolamine is classified as a/an

    _____.

4. The goal of pain management during terminal illness is:

    A. identify a safe and effective dose of analgesics.

    B. prevent excessive sedation.

    C. avoid development of drug addiction.

    D. control pain without opioids.

5. A type of drug that can help relieve cough is:

    A. ACE inhibitor.

    B. antidepressant.

    C. mucolytic.

    D. bronchoconstrictor.

6. What action is common to metoclopramide (Reglan), dexamethasone (Decadron), prochlorperazine (Compazine), and diazepam (Valium)?

    A. Tranquilizer

    B. Anti-inflammatory

    C. Muscle relaxant

    D. Antiemetic

7. Corticosteroids may be used to treat delirium caused by:

    A. cerebral edema.

    B. kidney failure.

    C. carbon monoxide.

    D. electrolyte imbalances.

8. Alprazolam (Xanax) and lorazepam (Ativan) may be used during terminal illness to treat:

    A. insomnia.

    B. dyspnea.

    C. constipation.

    D. anxiety.

9. Bulk laxatives are not recommended in terminal illness because of the risk of:

    A. diarrhea.

    B. ruptured appendix.

    C. excess gas formation.

    D. intestinal obstruction.

10. Older Americans consume nearly _____ of all prescription drugs.

    A. Three-fourths.

    B. One-half.

    C. One-third.

    D. One-fourth.

11. Because of age-related changes in renal and hepatic function, the older person:

    A. metabolizes drugs more slowly.

    B. requires higher drug dosages.

    C. is less likely to have drug toxicities.

    D. can take multiple drugs without interactions.

12. Mr. Garcia is taking an anti-inflammatory, a diuretic, antacids, and a bronchodilator. He complains of dizziness when he first stands up. Which drug is most likely causing the problem?

    A. Anti-inflammatory

    B. Diuretic

    C. Antacid

    D. Bronchodilator

13. Mr. Garcia's blood pressure is 130/72 and his pulse is 80 when he is supine. On standing, the blood pressure is 100/54 and his pulse is 60. This is characteristic of:

    A. fluid retention.

    B. allergic drug reaction.

    C. orthostatic hypotension.

    D. normal effects of position change.

14. Adverse drug effects can cause:

    A. delirium.

    B. dementia.

15. Cholinesterase inhibitors may improve symptoms of Alzheimer's disease by:

    A. destroying pathogens.

    B. repairing damaged neurons.

    C. stimulating cerebral circulation.

    D. increasing acetylcholine in the brain.

16. Aspirin may be given to patients with vascular dementia in an effort to prevent:

    A. stroke.

    B. varicose veins.

    C. congestive heart failure.

    D. peptic ulcer disease.

Match the type of bladder control problem on the right with the drug on the left that may cause it.

17. _____ Diuretics

18. _____ Anticholinergics

19. _____ Sedatives/hypnotics

20. _____ Alphaadrenergic blockers

A. Unable to reach toilet quickly enough

B. Bladder becomes distended; overflows

C. Urine leaks under stress

D. Patient unaware of need to void

21. Stress incontinence due to atrophic vaginitis may be relieved by:

    A. imipramine (Tofranil).

    B. estrogen cream.

    C. oxybutynin (Ditropan).

    D. bethanechol (Urecholine).

DRUGS USED TO TREAT CANCER

OBJECTIVES

1. List the types of antineoplastic agents.

2. Explain the barriers to effective chemotherapy for cancer.

3. Identify the major side and adverse effects associated with cancer chemotherapy.

4. Discuss nursing implications for the patient receiving cancer chemotherapy.

CHAPTER 14

ANTINEOPLASTICS

*C*ancer is the second leading cause of deaths in the United States. It is not a single disease, but rather is a term used to describe a large group of diseases characterized by uncontrolled growth and spread of abnormal cells. Drugs can cure some types of cancer. In other cases, drugs may be able to suppress growth of cancer cells enough to reduce symptoms, improve quality of life, and prolong life.

Some barriers to effective cancer treatment include the following:

- Antineoplastic drugs are not selective. Drugs that are toxic to cancer cells are also toxic to normal cells, as evidenced by the many side and adverse effects encountered with these drugs.
- It is impossible to know when all cancer cells have been destroyed.
- Not all cancers are equally responsive to drug therapy. Large, solid tumors are least responsive.
- Cancer cells are capable of developing resistance to antineoplastics.
- Drugs do not easily reach some tumors, such as those in the brain, because the blood-brain barrier inhibits the passage of most antineoplastic drugs.

Drugs used in the treatment of cancer are referred to as antineoplastic agents. The general term *chemotherapy* is commonly used as well to refer to cancer treatment with drugs. The types of drugs employed in the treatment of cancer include antitumor antibiotics, alkylating agents, antimetabolites, plant alkaloids, hormonal agents, and others. Biologic response modifiers (BRMs) are also used to treat certain types of cancer. BRMs are addressed in Chapter 27.

Some antineoplastics are *cell cycle phase specific*, meaning they are effective against cancer cells only during a specific phase of reproduction. Others are *cell cycle phase nonspecific*, meaning they can affect cancer cells regardless of the phase of cell division. All hormonal agents and BRMs are cell cycle phase nonspecific. Other antineoplastics are evenly divided between specific and nonspecific agents.

COMMON SIDE AND ADVERSE EFFECTS OF ANTINEOPLASTICS

Antineoplastic agents share a number of common side and adverse effects that not only can make life difficult but may also be fatal (See Table 14–1).

TABLE 14–1

Common Side and Adverse Effects of Antineoplastics

Side/Adverse Effect	Nursing Considerations
Suppressed bone marrow production of red blood cells, white blood cells, and platelets	
Anemia: deficiency of red blood cells.	Assess for fatigue, pallor, tachycardia. Encourage adequate rest.
Leukopenia: deficiency of white blood cells.	Assess for frequent and/or persistent infections. Protect from people with infections, monitor for fever, avoid rectal route for temperatures.
Thrombocytopenia: deficiency of platelets.	Assess for easy bruising and bleeding. Protect from trauma, apply pressure to injection sites, use soft toothbrush and electric razor.
Nausea and vomiting	Give antiemetics as ordered. Create a pleasant environment. Do not serve fluids with meals. Assess for dehydration (thready, rapid pulse; low BP; concentrated urine).
Anorexia	Provide small, frequent meals. Assist with oral hygiene as needed. Respect food preferences. Monitor weight to evaluate adequacy of food intake. Offer nutritional supplements as ordered.
Xerostomia	Encourage additional fluids. Advise sugarless gum or hard candy, ice chips, artifical saliva. Avoid very dry foods.
Stomatitis	Encourage or assist with frequent oral hygiene. Assess oral cavity for lesions. Encourage dental care.

(Continued on p. 84)

Side/Adverse Effect	Nursing Considerations
Diarrhea	Administer antidiarrheal drugs as ordered. Assess for side effects, especially constipation. Assist with perineal care if needed.
Constipation	Document stool frequency and characteristics. Encourage fluids and high-fiber foods. Encourage exercise as tolerated. Administer laxatives, stool softeners, enemas as ordered.
Cardiomyopathy, heart failure	Monitor for heart failure: dyspnea, edema, increasing pulse pressure. Elevate head of bed. Avoid overtiring. Protect edematous extremities from trauma. Administer oxygen, diuretics, inotropics as ordered.
Pulmonary inflammation and fibrosis	Assess activity tolerance, respiratory rate and effort. Protect from respiratory infections. Use humidifiers as ordered. Assist with turning, coughing, deep breathing to prevent pneumonia. Elevate head of bed if dyspneic.
Numbness, tingling, loss of deep tendon reflexes in extremities	Assess for abnormal sensations, absence of sensation, and loss of reflexes. Protect affected areas and inspect frequently for injury.
Alopecia (hair loss)	Assess patient feelings. If desired, conceal hair loss with hairpiece, scarf, cap, turban. Refer to American Cancer Society for free hairpieces and strategies for managing hair loss.
Phlebitis	Though central lines are most often used, if a peripheral line is employed, assess infusion sites for redness and tenderness. Report any signs of extravasation immediately.
Photosensitivity	Avoid sun exposure. Use sunscreen and wide-brimmed hat when outdoors.
Teratogenesis	Be aware of potential harm to fetus. Reinforce physician's instructions regarding avoidance of pregnancy during and after therapy.
Sterility/erectile dysfunction	Be aware of potential for sterility and/or erectile dysfunction. Be sensitive to patient's concerns about these effects. Identify resources for information and assistance re: banking sperm, treatment of erectile dysfunction.

ANTITUMOR ANTIBIOTICS

Antitumor antibiotics are used only to treat cancer, not for infections. All are given parenterally. They act by altering DNA so that RNA and protein synthesis are inhibited. Most of the side and adverse effects of these drugs are like the general effects already described: nausea, vomiting, stomatitis, anorexia, alopecia, and bone marrow depression. Cardiotoxicity and pulmonary toxicity are especially dangerous adverse effects of some antitumor antibiotics. Cardiotoxicity may be manifested by acute symptoms (dysrhythmias during and after drug administration), or by delayed effects (congestive heart failure, cardiomyopathy).

Specific antitumor antibiotics, their uses, and adverse effects are presented in Table 14–2.

TABLE 14-2

Antitumor Antibiotics

Drug	Uses	Adverse Effects
dactinomycin (Actinomycin D)	Wilms' tumor, rhabdomyosarcoma, choriocarcinoma, Ewings' sarcoma, Kaposi's sarcoma, testicular cancer.	**Bone marrow depression**, nausea, vomiting, diarrhea, alopecia, folliculitis, inflammation of gastrointestinal mucosa. Dermatitis (skin inflammation) in areas that have been treated with radiation.
doxorubicin (Adriamycin, Rubex)	Hodgkin's disease; non-Hodgkin's lymphoma; some leukemias; soft tissue and bone sarcomas; lung, stomach, breast, ovary, testes, and thyroid carcinomas.	**Cardiotoxic effects**: cardiac dysrhythmias shortly after administration; may persist up to 2 weeks. Congestive heart failure and cardiomyopathy may occur later. With breast cancer, dexarazoxane (Zinecard) can be given to reduce cardiotoxicity. Other adverse effects: bone marrow suppression, anorexia, nausea and vomiting, local tissue necrosis with extravasation, alopecia, stomatitis, conjunctivitis, pigmentation of extremities, reddish color to urine and sweat.
liposomal daunorubicin (DaunoXome)	HIV-related Kaposi's sarcoma	Same as doxorubicin.
idarubicin (Idamycin)	Acute myelogenous leukemia	**Bone marrow depression,** cardiotoxicity, nausea, vomiting, stomatitis, alopecia, local tissue trauma with extravasation.
mitoxantrone (Novantrone)	Some leukemias, some lymphomas, breast cancer	**Bone marrow depression**, nausea, vomiting, inflammation of mucous membranes, cardiotoxicity (less than doxorubicin), blue-green color to urine, skin, and sclera.
bleomycin (Blenoxane)	Testicular carcinomas, some lymphomas, some squamous cell carcinomas	**Pulmonary inflammation and fibrosis,** nausea and vomiting, stomatitis, alopecia, skin reactions. 1% of lymphoma patients have a hypersensitivity reaction with fever, chills, confusion, hypotension, and wheezing.
mitomycin (Mutamycin)	Adenocarcinoma of stomach and pancreas	**Bone marrow depression**, nausea, vomiting, stomatitis, alopecia, nephrotoxicity, pulmonary toxicity.
plicamycin	Testicular carcinoma	**Bleeding** related to decrease in platelets and some clotting factors, nausea, vomiting, stomatitis, renal injury, serum calcium imbalance.

HIV, human immunodeficiency virus.

ALKYLATING AGENTS

Alkylating agents are nitrogen mustard, nitrosureas, and other compounds including cisplatin, carboplatin, and busulfan. These agents interact with DNA, inhibiting its replication and resulting in cell death. The most important adverse effect is bone marrow suppression. Other adverse effects of alkylating agents are alopecia, nausea and vomiting, and inflammation of the gastrointestinal mucosa (See Table 14-3).

Nitrogen Mustards

Nitrogen mustards used in the treatment of cancer are cyclophosphamide (Cytoxan), mechlorethamine (Mustargen), chlorambucil (Leukeran), melphalan (Alkeran), and ifosfamide (Ifex). Cyclophosphamide, chlorambucil, and melphalan can be given orally; others are only administered parenterally.

Side and Adverse Effects

General adverse effects common to these drugs are bone marrow suppression, severe nausea, vomiting, alopecia, acute hemorrhagic cystitis, renal damage, sterility, immune suppression, and hypersensitivity.

Nitrosureas

Examples of nitrosureas are carmustine (BCNU), lomustine (CCNU), streptozocin (Zanosar). The nitrosureas are among a limited number of antineoplastic agents that cross the blood-brain barrier. This makes them useful in the treatment of brain tumors, in addition to a variety of other cancers. In addition to the intravenous route, carmustine can be administered via implantation into the cavity left by excision of a brain tumor.

Side and Adverse Effects

All but streptozocin can cause serious bone marrow depression. The nitrosureas also may cause severe nausea and vomiting and damage to the kidneys, liver, and lungs.

Other Alkylating Agents

Other alkylating agents are cisplatin (Platinol), carboplatin (Paraplatin), and busulfan (Myleran).

Nursing Actions

The risk of nephrotoxicity is greatest with cisplatin. It can be reduced by maintaining good hydration before and 24 hours after cisplatin is given and concurrent administration of diuretics and amifostine (Ethyol). There is a risk of hemorrhagic cystitis with cyclophosphamide and ifosfamide. It can be prevented by extensive hydration. Monitor pulmonary status in patients taking busulfan because of the risk of pulmonary infiltrates and fibrosis. If the patient experiences nausea and vomiting, administer antiemetics. Assess for fluid volume deficit. Administer intravenous fluids as ordered. Because of the risk of neurotoxicity, assess hearing and mental status. Instruct the patient to report tinnitus. Monitor blood studies for bone marrow depression. Assess for signs of anemia, leukocytopenia, and thrombocytopenia.

TABLE 14-3

Alkylating Agents

Drug	Uses	Side and Adverse Effects
Nitrogen Mustards cyclophosphamide (Cytoxan)	Hodgkin's disease, non-Hodgkin's lymphoma, multiple myeloma, solid tumors of the head, neck, ovary, and breast	**Bone marrow depression**, severe nausea, vomiting, alopecia, acute hemorrhagic cystitis, sterility, immunosuppression, pulmonary fibrosis, cardiotoxicity, hypersensitivity reactions
mechlorethamine (Mustargen)	Hodgkin's disease, non-Hodgkin's lymphoma	**Bone marrow depression**, severe tissue damage with extravasation, nausea, vomiting, diarrhea, alopecia, stomatitis, amenorrhea, sterility
chlorambucil (Leukeran)	Chronic lymphocytic leukemia, Hodgkin's disease, non-Hodgkin's lymphoma, ovarian cancer	**Bone marrow depression,** hepatotoxicity, sterility, pulmonary infiltrates and fibrosis, mild nausea and vomiting
melphalan (Alkeran)	Multiple myeloma, ovarian and breast carcinoma	**Bone marrow depression**; rarely, severe nausea and vomiting
ifosfamide (Ifex)	Germ-cell cancer of testes	**Bone marrow depression**, nausea, vomiting, metabolic acidosis, CNS toxicity, **hemorrhagic cystitis** (risk of cystitis reduced by good hydration and concurrent administration of mesna [Mesnex])
Nitrosureas carmustine (BCNU)	Brain tumors, Hodgkin's disease, non-Hodgkin's lymphoma, multiple myeloma, malignant melanoma, hepatoma, adenocarcinoma of the stomach, colon, and rectum	**Bone marrow depression**, severe nausea and vomiting, hepatotoxicity, nephrotoxicity, pulmonary toxicity, phlebitis
lomustine (CCNU)	Lymphomas; melanomas; carcinoma of breast, lung, colon; brain tumors; Hodgkin's disease	**Bone marrow depression**, nephrotoxicity, hepatotoxicity, neurotoxicity, nausea and vomiting, pulmonary fibrosis
streptozocin (Zanosar)	Metastatic islet-cell tumors	**Nephrotoxicity**, nausea and vomiting, hypo- or hyperglycemia, diarrhea, chills, fever; mild to moderate bone marrow depression
Other cisplatin (Platinol)	Testicular cancer, carcinoma of ovary, bladder, head, and neck	**Nephrotoxicity**, severe nausea and vomiting, neurotoxicity, bone marrow depression, ototoxicity; risk of nephrotoxicity reduced with good hydration, diuretics, and concurrent administration of amifostine (Ethyol)
carboplatin (Paraplatin)	Approved only for ovarian cancer; also being used for small cell lung cancer, endometrial cancer, and squamous cell cancer of head and neck	**Bone marrow depression**, nausea and vomiting, nephrotoxicity, neurotoxicity, ototoxicity, anaphylaxis
busulfan (Myleran)	Chronic myelogenous leukemia	**Bone marrow depression, pulmonary infiltrates and fibrosis**, nausea, vomiting, alopecia, gynecomastia, sterility, skin hyperpigmentation, cataracts, hepatitis

Data from Lehne, R. A. (1998). *Pharmacology for Nursing Care*, 3rd ed. Philadelphia: W. B. Saunders.

ANTIMETABOLITES

Antimetabolites exert their antineoplastic effects by interfering with essential metabolic processes, resulting in cell death or impaired replication. Antimetabolites include antifolates, antipurines, and antipyrimidines.

Antifolates: Methotrexate (Folex)

Actions and Uses

Antifolates prevent folic acid from being converted to an active form. Methotrexate (Folex) is the only antifolate used as an antineoplastic agent. This drug is used to treat choriocarcinoma, non-Hodgkin's lymphoma, acute lymphocytic leukemia of childhood, sarcomas of the head and neck, and osteogenic sarcoma.

Side and Adverse Effects

The most serious adverse effects are bone marrow depression, pulmonary fibrosis, and oral and gastrointestinal ulcers. It can also cause nausea and vomiting and is nephrotoxic in high doses. Liver and hematologic toxicity have occurred. Methotrexate has been associated with fetal death and malformations.

Nursing Actions

The risk of nephrotoxicity is reduced by keeping the patient well hydrated and the urine alkaline. Advise patients not to become pregnant during or for 6 months after treatment with this drug because it is teratogenic.

Antipurines

Actions and Uses

Antipurines disrupt many metabolic processes including synthesis of nucleic acids. The prototype antipurine is mercaptopurine (Purinethol), which is used most often to treat acute lymphocytic leukemia, and sometimes to treat acute and chronic myelogenous leukemia. Other antipurines are thioguanine, pentostatin (Nipent), fludarabine (Fludara), and cladribine (Leustatin). All are used for various types of leukemia.

Side and Adverse Effects

Bone marrow depression is the most serious adverse effect. Mercaptopurine also can cause liver dysfunction, nausea, vomiting, and ulcerations in the mouth and gastrointestinal tract. Because the drug may harm a fetus, women should avoid pregnancy while taking it.

Antipyrimidines

Actions and Uses

Antipyrimidines interfere with the synthesis of DNA and RNA. Cytarabine (Cytosar-U) is the prototype. It is used for acute myelogenous leukemia. Other antipyrimidines that are similar in actions and adverse effects are fluorouracil (Adrucil), floxuridine (FUDR), gemcitabine (Gemzar).

Side and Adverse Effects

The most serious adverse effect is bone marrow depression. Other adverse effects are nausea, vomiting, fever, stomatitis, hepatotoxicity, and conjunctivitis. Neurotoxicity and pulmonary edema may occur with high doses.

PLANT ALKALOIDS (MITOTIC INHIBITORS)

Vincristine (Oncovin) and vinblastine (Velban) are derived from the periwinkle plant. Vinorelbine (Navelbine) has similar structure and actions to vincristine and vinblastine but is a semisynthetic. The specific actions and adverse effects are noted in Table 14–4.

TABLE 14–4

Plant Alkaloids

Drug	Use	Side and Adverse Effects
vincristine (Oncovin)	Hodgkin's disease, non-Hodgkin's lymphoma, acute lymphocytic leukemia, Wilms' tumor, rhabdomyosarcoma, Kaposi's sarcoma, breast cancer, and bladder cancer	**Peripheral neuropathy** with alterations in sensation, weakness, decreased reflexes, constipation, and urinary hesitancy. Severe tissue injury with infiltration. Alopecia may occur, but nausea and vomiting are rare.
vinblastine (Velban)	Hodgkin's disease, non-Hodgkin's lymphoma, and carcinoma of the breast and testes	**Bone marrow suppression** most important adverse effect; can also cause nausea, vomiting, alopecia, stomatitis, tissue necrosis with extravasation, and neurotoxicity (less than vincristine).
vinorelbine (Navelbine)	Only approved for treatment of non-small-cell lung cancer	Incidence of **bone marrow depression** is about 50%. Can cause alopecia, constipation, nausea, vomiting, necrosis with extravasation, and peripheral neuropathy (less than vincristine).

HORMONAL AGENTS

Some hormones and hormone antagonists are used in the treatment of cancer. They include androgens, gonadotropin-releasing hormone analogues, androgen receptor blockers, estrogens, estrogen mustard, antiestrogens, progestins, and glucocorticoids.

Actions and Uses

Glucocorticoids are employed for lymphomas and some leukemias. The other hormonal agents are indicated for treatment of breast, endometrial, and prostate cancers. These agents are primarily used in combination with other drugs or treatments, or when other approaches have failed. When used for advanced cancers, the goal is more palliative than curative. That is, the drug may slow the growth of the cancer, relieve symptoms, or extend survival time.

Most of these drugs are covered elsewhere in this book. For details, see the following chapters:

- Estrogens and progestins: Chapter 45
- Androgens: Chapter 46
- Glucocorticoids: Chapter 43

Table 14–5 summarizes examples and the antineoplastic uses of these drugs.

TABLE 14–5

Hormones and Hormone Antagonists Used as Antineoplastics

Hormone/ Hormone Antagonist	Uses and Adverse Effects	Specific Considerations
Glucocorticoids prednisone (Deltasone, et al.)	Uses: in combination with other drugs to treat acute and chronic lymphocytic leukemias, Hodgkin's disease, non-Hodgkin's lymphoma. Relieves some symptoms of cancer and cancer therapy, e.g., suppresses chemotherapy-induced nausea and vomiting.	Long-term therapy has many serious adverse effects, including increased susceptibility to infection, osteoporosis, fluid and electrolyte imbalances, adrenal insufficiency, peptic ulcer disease, and muscle weakness. See Chapter 43 for a detailed discussion of nursing implications of glucocorticoid therapy.
Antiestrogens tamoxifen (Nolvadex) anastrozole (Arimidex)	Treatment of breast cancer.	Nausea, vomiting, menstrual irregularities, hot flushes. May increase the risk of endometrial cancer. In addition, anastrozole can cause headache, diarrhea or constipation, peripheral edema, dyspnea, hypertension, and pain
Gonadotropin-releasing hormone agonists leuprolide (Lupron)	Both used to treat prostate cancer. Leuprolide is also used to treat endometriosis.	

goserelin (Zoladex)	Goserelin is dispensed by a pellet that is injected into the abdominal wall. Leuprolide can be given SC or IM.	Causes hot flushes. May cause erectile dysfunction and loss of libido. Initially, patient may have bone pain and worsening urinary obstruction.
Androgen receptor blockers flutamide (Eulexin) bicalutamide (Casodex) Nilutamide (Nilandron)	In combination with gonadotropin-releasing hormone agonist or orchiectomy to treat prostate cancer	May cause breast pain and enlargement, nausea, vomiting, and diarrhea. Risk of hepatotoxicity with flutamide and nilutamide.
Estrogens diethylstilbestrol diphosphate (Stilphostrol) ethinyl estradiol (Estinyl)	Prostate cancer	Fluid retention, nausea, depression, thromboembolic disorders, gynecomastia, hypercalcemia. See Chapter 45 for additional information.
Estrogen Mustard estramustine (Emcyt)	Advanced prostate cancer	Risk of myocardial infarction and thrombotic stroke. Causes gynecomastia, nausea, vomiting, diarrhea, fluid retention, and hypercalcemia.
Progestins medroxyprogesterone acetate (Depo-Provera) megestrol acetate (Megace)	Both used for advanced endometrial cancer. Megestrol also used for advanced breast cancer.	Fluid retention, weight gain, hypercalcemia (with bone metastasis). See Chapter 45 for additional information. Megestrol improves appetite in cachexic patients.

OTHER ANTINEOPLASTIC AGENTS

A variety of other drugs now are used in the treatment of cancers, and new agents are constantly being evaluated. Some of these drugs are included in Table 14–6.

TABLE 14–6

Miscellaneous Antineoplastic Agents

Drug	Use	Side and Adverse Effects
asparaginase (Elspar) pegaspargase (Oncaspar)	Acute lymphocytic leukemia	Injury to pancreas, liver, and kidneys; coagulation disorders; CNS depression; nausea and vomiting; anaphylaxis (less common with pegaspargase than with asparaginase)
paclitaxel (Taxol)	Metastatic ovarian and breast cancers	Bone marrow depression, anaphylaxis, peripheral neuropathy, bradycardia, myocardial infarction, muscle and joint pain, alopecia, mild gastrointestinal distress.
docetaxel (Taxotere)	Breast cancer	Bone marrow depression (neutropenia, anemia), hypersensitivity including anaphylaxis, severe fluid retention, nausea, diarrhea, stomatitis, fever, neurotoxicity (pain, numbness, tingling).
hydroxyurea (Hydrea)	Chronic myelocytic leukemia, ovarian cancer	Bone marrow depression, nausea and vomiting, and dysuria. Rarely, stomatitis and neurotoxicity.
mitotane (Lysodren)	Inoperable adrenocortical carcinoma	CNS depression or toxicity, nausea, vomiting, adrenal insufficiency, dermatitis, visual disturbances, orthostatic hypotension, nephrotoxicity.
procarbazine (Matulane)	Advanced Hodgkin's disease, non-Hodgkin's lymphoma, brain tumors	Bone marrow depression, nausea and vomiting, peripheral neuropathy, CNS depression, secondary leukemias, sterility. Hypertensive crisis if combined with other sympathomimetics; disulfiram-like reaction with alcohol.
dacarbazine (DTIC-Dome)	Metastatic malignant melanoma	Bone marrow depression, nausea and vomiting, flu-like syndrome, hepatic necrosis, photosensitivity, burning pain at injection site.
altretamine (Hexalen)	Persistent or recurring ovarian cancer	Bone marrow depression, nausea and vomiting, neurotoxicity (peripheral and CNS).

CNS, central nervous system.

REVIEW QUESTIONS: UNIT 5

1. Antineoplastics are drugs used to treat:

    A. parasitic infestations.

    B. elevated blood glucose.

    C. cancer.

    D. nausea.

2. A deficiency of white blood cells is called:

    A. leukopenia.

    B. leukocytosis.

    C. leukemia.

    D. leukoplakia.

3. It is important to protect patients from trauma when they have:

    A. anemia.

    B. stomatitis.

    C. xerostomia.

    D. thrombocytopenia.

4. The hair loss that occurs with some antineoplastics is called:

    A. pattern baldness.

    B. teratogenesis.

    C. alopecia.

    D. alkalosis.

5. The most dangerous adverse effect of many antineoplastics is:

    A. bone marrow depression.

    B. nausea and vomiting.

    C. alopecia.

    D. diarrhea.

6. Because nitrosureas cross the blood-brain barrier, they can be used to treat:

    A. leukemias.

    B. brain tumors.

    C. lung cancer.

    D. myocardial tumors.

7. Good hydration is important when giving cisplatin (Platinol) to prevent:

    A. dehydration.

    B. pneumonia.

    C. nephrotoxicity.

    D. hearing loss.

8. Peripheral neuropathy is characterized by:

    A. altered sensation.

    B. diarrhea.

    C. muscle spasms.

    D. hyperactive reflexes.

DRUGS THAT AFFECT THE AUTONOMIC AND CENTRAL NERVOUS SYSTEMS

OBJECTIVES

1. Name and list the physiologic effects of sympathetic neurotransmitters.
2. Name and list the physiologic effects of parasympathetic neurotransmitters.
3. Identify the effects of the stimulation of alpha- and beta-adrenergic receptors.
4. Differentiate between direct-acting and indirect-acting cholinergic drugs.
5. Identify actions, uses, side and adverse effects, interactions, and contraindications of selected adrenergic, antiadrenergic, cholinergic, and anticholinergic drugs.
6. Discuss nursing actions and patient teaching associated with the use of adrenergic, antiadrenergic, cholinergic, and anticholinergic drugs.
7. Define the types of seizures.
8. Identify classifications of, rationales for, and examples of anticonvulsant drugs.
9. Identify actions, uses, side and adverse effects, contraindications, and interactions for selected anticonvulsant drugs.
10. Discuss nursing actions and patient teaching associated with the use of anticonvulsant drugs.
11. Identify actions, uses, side and adverse effects, interactions, and contraindications of selected drugs used to treat Parkinson's disease.
12. Discuss nursing actions and patient teaching associated with drugs used to treat Parkinson's disease.
13. Explain the effects of stimulants on the central nervous system.
14. Define narcolepsy and attention deficit–hyperactivity disorder.
15. Identify actions, uses, side and adverse effects, contraindications, and interactions for selected central nervous system stimulants.
16. Discuss nursing actions and patient teaching associated with use of central nervous system stimulants.

As discussed in Unit 3, the nervous system is composed of all nerve tissues: brain, spinal cord, nerves, and ganglia (groups of nerve cells located outside the central nervous system) and is divided into the central nervous system and the peripheral nervous system. Drugs affecting the central nervous system (CNS) are classified as either depressants or stimulants. The CNS depressant drugs not covered in this unit are discussed in Units 2 and 3.

The autonomic nervous system is the division of the peripheral nervous system that includes sensory and motor nerves, which primarily control internal organs that usually function automatically, without conscious thought or effort. The autonomic nervous system is divided into two branches: the sympathetic nervous system (SNS) and the parasympathetic nervous system (PNS). The sympathetic nervous system and the parasympathetic nervous system act on the same organs but produce opposite responses in order to maintain homeostasis (balance).

The sympathetic nervous system (SNS) is also known as the adrenergic system because one of its primary neurotransmitters (substances released by a neuron that produce activity in target cells), epinephrine, is also called adrenaline. Drugs that mimic the effects of epinephrine and the other primary neurotransmitter, norepinephrine, are called adrenergic drugs, or sympathomimetics. They are also known as adrenergic agonists because they *initiate* a response at the adrenergic receptor sites. Drugs that block the effect of the neurotransmitters are called *adrenergic blockers* or *sympatholytics*. These are adrenergic antagonists because they *prevent* a response at the receptor sites.

The SNS is stimulated by physical or emotional stress, such as strenuous exercise, pain, trauma, or intense emotions (e.g., fear). Because the specific body responses increase the capacity for strong muscle activity in response to a real or imaginary threat, the SNS reaction is often called the "fight, flight, or fright" response. These body responses, which are protective mechanisms designed to help the person get away from the stress or to cope with it, include the following:

- increased blood pressure and cardiac output
- increased circulation to brain, heart, and skeletal muscles
- increased oxygen consumption
- bronchodilation
- increased rate and depth of respiration
- increased breakdown of muscle glucose for energy
- increased blood glucose level
- increased blood coagulation
- increased muscle strength
- increased mental activity and ability to think clearly
- pupil dilation to aid vision
- decreased blood flow to viscera, skin, and other organs not needed for "fight, flight, or fright"

The parasympathetic nervous system (PNS) is called the cholinergic system because it primary neurotransmitter is acetylcholine. Drugs that mimic acetylcholine are called cholinergic drugs, or parasympathomimetics. They are cholinergic agonists since they *initiate* a cholinergic response. Anticholinergic drugs, or parasympatholytics, block the effect of acetylcholine. They are also called cholinergic antagonists because they *inhibit* the effect of acetylcholine at the receptor sites.

Functions stimulated by the PNS are described as resting, reparative, or vegetative: "digest and rest." These functions include digestion, excretion, cardiac deceleration, and near vision. Specific body responses include the following:

- peripheral blood vessel dilation (no effect on systemic blood vessels)
- decreased heart rate (possibly bradycardia)
- increased gastrointestinal enzymes and gastrointestinal motility
- bronchoconstriction
- increased secretions from lungs, sweat glands, stomach, and intestines
- pupil constriction
- contraction of smooth muscle in urinary bladder
- contraction of skeletal muscle
- no apparent effect on blood coagulation, blood glucose, mental activity, or muscle strength

Drugs that affect the SNS and PNS act not only on target receptors, but also on nearly all SNS or PNS receptors. For this reason, most of the side and adverse effects are either normal responses to autonomic stimulation or exaggerations of normal responses. If you are thoroughly familiar with the body's response to SNS and PNS stimulation, you will be able to predict certain side effects and adverse reactions. This will enable you to determine correct nursing actions and provide appropriate patient teaching.

CHAPTER 15

ADRENERGICS

*D*rugs that stimulate the sympathetic nervous system are called *adrenergics, adrenergic agonists,* or *sympathomimetics* because they mimic the effects of the sympathetic neurotransmitters, epinephrine and norepinephrine. These substances, which are also known as *catecholamines*, are either endogenous (occurring naturally within the body) or exogenous (administered as medications). They act on adrenergic receptors located on smooth muscle cells in the heart, bronchioles, gastrointestinal tract, urinary bladder, and eyes. The four main adrenergic receptors are $alpha_1$, $alpha_2$, $beta_1$, and $beta_2$. Alpha-adrenergic receptors are located in blood vessels. When $alpha_1$ receptors are stimulated, release of norepinephrine causes arterioles and venules to constrict, causing blood pressure to rise. When $alpha_2$ receptors are stimulated, release of norepinephrine is inhibited, causing vasodilation, which results in a decrease in blood pressure.

$Beta_1$ receptors are located primarily in the heart. Stimulation of these receptors increases heart rate and the force of heart muscle contraction. $Beta_2$ receptors are located mainly in smooth muscle of lungs, the arterioles of skeletal muscles, and uterine muscle. Stimulation of $beta_2$ receptors causes relaxation of lung smooth muscle (bronchodilation), increased blood flow to skeletal muscles, and relaxation of uterine muscle (decreased uterine contractions).

Another neurotransmitter, dopamine, acts on special receptors located in arteries in the kidneys, mesentery, brain, and heart. When these receptors are stimulated, vasodilation occurs and blood flow increases. Only dopamine can activate these special receptors.

Sympathomimetic drugs are classified into three categories according to their effects on organ cells:

1. Direct-acting: directly stimulate the receptor (e.g., epinephrine and norepinephrine)

2. Indirect-acting: stimulate the release of norepinephrine from nerve endings, which then binds to the receptors and causes a physiologic response (e.g., amphetamines)

3. Mixed-acting: stimulate receptor sites and cause release of norepinephrine from nerve endings (e.g., ephedrine)

USES

The clinical indications for adrenergic drugs arise mainly from effects on the heart, blood vessels, and bronchi. These uses include the following:

- **emergency drugs** to treat acute cardiovascular, respiratory, and allergic disorders
- **cardiac stimulants** in cardiac arrest and heart block
- to **raise blood pressure** in hypotension and shock if fluid volume replacement is not sufficient
- **bronchodilators** for bronchospasms and bronchoconstriction (e.g., asthma, bronchitis)
- **vasoconstriction** to relieve edema in respiratory tract, skin, and other tissues
- **decongestion** in allergic disorders
- **topically** for vasoconstriction, hemostasis, pupil dilation, and decongestion
- to **stop preterm labor**
- to **decrease appetite (anorexiants)**

Table 15–1 lists some of the more common adrenergic drugs and their primary clinical uses.

TABLE 15–1

Adrenergic Drugs

Generic/Trade Name	Major Clinical Use
Alpha and Beta Activity	
epinephrine (Adrenalin)	Allergic reactions, cardiac arrest, hypotension and shock, local vasoconstriction, bronchodilation, cardiac stimulation, ophthalmic conditions
ephedrine (Efedrin)	Bronchodilation, cardiac stimulation, nasal decongestion
dopamine (Intropin)	Hypotension and shock
Alpha Activity	
norepinephrine betartrate (Levophed)	Hypotension and shock
metaraminol (Aramine)	Hypotension and shock
oxymetazoline (Afrin)	Nasal decongestion
phenylephrine (Neo-Synephrine)	Hypotension and shock, nasal decongestion, ophthalmic conditions
phenylpropanolamine (Dexatrim, Propagest)	Nasal decongestion, appetite suppression
tetrahydrozoline (Visine)	Nasal decongestion, ophthalmic vasoconstriction
xylometazoline (Otrivin)	Nasal decongestion
Beta Activity	
albuterol (Proventil)	Bronchodilation
dobutamine (Dobutrex)	Cardiac stimulation
isoproterenol (Isuprel)	Bronchodilation, cardiac stimulation
isoetharine (Bronkosol)	Bronchodilation
metaproterenol (Alupent)	Bronchodilation
pirbuterol (Maxair)	Bronchodilation
terbutaline (Brethine)	Bronchodilation, inhibit preterm labor (unlabeled use)

SIDE AND ADVERSE EFFECTS

Side and adverse effects are related to SNS stimulation. They may include the following:

Alpha-Adrenergic Drugs

- Central nervous system: restlessness, headache, insomnia, excitement, and euphoria
- Cardiovascular system: palpitations or arrhythmias, tachycardia, and hypertension
- Other: anorexia, dry mouth, nausea, and vomiting

Beta-Adrenergic Drugs

- Central nervous system: headache, nervousness, dizziness, and tremors
- Cardiovascular system: tachycardia, palpitations, arrhythmias, and unpredictable blood pressure changes
- Other: nausea, vomiting, muscle cramps, and sweating

Two of the most life-threatening toxic effects (usually from overdose) involve the central nervous system (convulsions) and the cardiovascular system (cardiac arrhythmias and severe hypertension). Intracranial bleeds and other body hemorrhages may occur from hypertension. Seizures are usually managed with diazepam (Valium) and hypertension treated with a rapid-acting adrenergic blocker (alpha: phentolamine [Regitine]; beta: labetalol [Trandate, Normodyne]).

INTERACTIONS AND CONTRAINDICATIONS

Alpha-adrenergic and beta-adrenergic agents given together antagonize each other, thereby reducing therapeutic effects. Urinary alkalizers (e.g., sodium bicarbonate, which makes urine less acid) and general anesthetic agents (e.g., halothane) reduce excretion of adrenergic drugs, increasing their effects and increasing the risk of cardiac arrhythmias. Many other-the-counter preparations contain adrenergic drugs (e.g., ephedrine), so concurrent use with prescription agents may produce overdoses with potentially life-threatening central nervous system and cardiovascular effects. Digitalis increases the potential for arrhythmias; tricyclic antidepressants may precipitate acute hypertensive crisis and possible respiratory depression and arrhythmias. Monoamine oxidase inhibitors, antihistamines, and thyroid preparations reduce metabolism of adrenergic drugs, thereby increasing their effects. Antihypertensive agents, beta-blockers, and antipsychotic drugs are antagonistic to adrenergics, reducing their therapeutic effects.

Alpha-adrenergic drugs can falsely elevate serum corticosteroid levels and falsely decrease serum glucose levels.

Contraindications to the use of adrenergic drugs include severe hypertension, ventricular tachycardia, narrow-angle glaucoma, cardiac arrhythmias, and angina pectoris. Local anesthetic agents containing epinephrine should not be used in fingers, toes, nose, ears, or penis because of potential tissue damage from vasoconstriction. Cautious use is indicated for the elderly and for persons with diabetes mellitus, hyperthyroidism, pregnancy and lactation, heart disease, arteriosclerosis, uncorrected hypovolemia, and asthma. Concurrent use of these drugs with halothane anesthetic agents may precipitate cardiac arrhythmias. Careful use is also indicated for persons with insomnia, anxiety, or psychosis because of their stimulant effects on the central nervous system.

NURSING ACTIONS

Prior to administration of the drug, check for drug and food allergies. Obtain medical and drug history, especially regarding respiratory, cardiovascular, endocrine, or psychiatric disorders and the use of over-the-counter or prescription medications, which may contain other adrenergic agents. When the drug is given for hypotension and shock or anaphylaxis, observe for increased blood pressure, urine output, and level of consciousness, improved tissue perfusion and skin color, easier breathing, and stronger pulse. When the drug is given as a bronchodilator or for anaphylaxis, observe for reduced or absent wheezing, less labored breathing, and decreased respiratory rate. When the drug is given for its nasal decongestant effects, observe for decreased nasal congestion and greater ability to breathe through the nose. To give epinephrine subcutaneously, use a tuberculin syringe (for accurate measurement of small doses), aspirate (to prevent accidental administration into a blood vessel), and massage the injection site (to accelerate drug absorption and provide faster relief of symptoms). Do not give epinephrine and isoproterenol together or within 4 hours of each other; both are potent cardiac stimulants and, if given too close together, could precipitate cardiac arrhythmias. Observe for excessive central nervous system stimulation (nervousness, anxiety, tremors) and cardiac arrhythmias and hypertension.

Patient Teaching

- Take drug *exactly* as prescribed to prevent occurrence of side effects.
- Use caution when driving or using heavy machinery, as these drugs may cause blurred vision.
- Excessive use of nasal decongestants may cause rebound nasal congestion, inflammation, or ulceration of nasal mucosa.
- Inhaled solutions of isoproterenol may turn saliva and sputum a harmless pink color.
- Report adverse reactions, such as fast pulse, palpitations, chest pain, insomnia, tremors, and anxiety.
- Notify the health care provider if a previously effective dose becomes ineffective.

C H A P T E R   1 6

ANTIADRENERGICS

ACTION

Antiadrenergic drugs decrease or block the effects of sympathetic nerve stimulation, endogenous epinephrine and norepinephrine, and adrenergic drugs. These drugs are also known as *adrenergic blockers* or *blocking agents*, and *sympatholytics*.

They act by preventing these substances from occupying their appropriate receptor sites in tissue and organs. Because a base level of sympathomimetic activity is necessary to maintain normal body functioning (e.g., regulation of blood pressure, blood glucose, and stress response), the goal of antiadrenergic therapy is to suppress pathologic stimulation, not the normal physiologic response to stress, activity, and other stimuli.

Alpha$_2$ adrenergic agonists inhibit the release of norepinephrine in the brain and decrease the effects of the stimulation of the sympathetic nervous system throughout the body. The major clinical effect is to lower blood pressure. Activation of pancreatic alpha$_2$ receptors suppresses insulin secretion.

Alpha-adrenergic blockers occupy alpha$_1$ receptor sites in skin, mucosa, intestines, and kidneys to prevent alpha-adrenergic vasoconstriction. These drugs dilate arterioles and veins to increase peripheral blood flow, decrease blood pressure, constrict pupils, and increase gastrointestinal motility. They also prevent alpha-adrenergic contraction of smooth muscle in nonvascular tissue (e.g., muscles in prostate and urinary bladder).

Nonselective alpha-adrenergic blockers occupy peripheral alpha$_1$ receptors to cause vasodilation (hypotension) and alpha$_2$ receptors to cause cardiac stimulation; the hypotension may be accompanied by tachycardia and possibly cardiac arrhythmias.

Beta-blockers occupy beta-adrenergic receptor sites and prevent receptors from responding to sympathetic nerve impulses, effects of epinephrine and norepinephrine, and beta-adrenergic drugs. Some of the specific beta-blocking effects include decreased heart rate, decreased cardiac output, decreased supine and standing blood pressure, bronchoconstriction, less effective glucose metabolism, and decreased intraocular pressure (decreased formation of aqueous humor).

USES

Alpha$_2$ adrenergic agonists are used to treat hypertension. Alpha$_1$ blockers (antagonists) are used to treat hypertension, benign prostatic hypertrophy (BPH), and vasospastic disorders such as frostbite and Reynaud's disease. Nonselective alpha-adrenergic antagonists are used to treat pheochromocytoma (a rare adrenal tumor that secretes epinephrine and norepinephrine) and severe hypertension (due to excessive catecholamines or adrenergic drugs), and to prevent tissue necrosis from extravasation (leaking of an intravenously administered drug into the surrounding tissue) of potent vasoconstricting drugs (e.g., epinephrine) into subcutaneous tissue. Beta-adrenergic blockers are used to treat hypertension, hypertensive crises or emergencies, angina, cardiac arrhythmias, prevention of myocardial infarction (MI) or reinfarction, glaucoma, and overdose of adrenergic drugs. *Nonselective beta-blockers* block both beta$_1$ (cardiac) and beta$_2$ (primarily bronchial and vascular smooth muscle) receptors. *Cardioselective beta-blockers* produce more effects on beta$_1$ than on beta$_2$ receptors.

Table 16–1 lists some of the more common antiadrenergic drugs and their clinical uses.

TABLE 16-1

Antiadrenergic Drugs

Generic (Trade) Name	Major Clinical Use
Alpha agonists	
clonidine (Catapres)	Hypertension
methyldopa (Aldomet)	Hypertension
Alpha blockers	
doxazosin (Cardura)	Hypertension, benign prostatic hypertrophy
prazosin (Minipress)	Hypertension, benign prostatic hypertrophy
terazosin (Hytrin)	Hypertension, benign prostatic hypertrophy
Nonselective alpha-blockers	
phenoxybenzamine (Dibenzyline)	Frostbite, Reynaud's disease, hypertension caused by pheochromocytoma
phentolamine (Regitine)	Hypertension caused by pheochromocytoma, prevention of tissue necrosis from extravasation of vasoconstrictive drugs
Beta-blockers (nonselective)	
carteolol (Cartrol, Ocupress)	Hypertension, glaucoma
metipranolol (OptiPranolol)	Glaucoma
penbutolol (Levatol)	Hypertension
propranolol (Inderal)	Hypertension, angina pectoris, cardiac arrhythmias, myocardial infarction, hypertrophic obstructive cardiomyopathy, migraine prophylaxis, thyrotoxicosis, pheochromocytoma
nadolol (Corgard)	Hypertension, angina pectoris
sotalol (Betapace)	Cardiac arrhythmias
timolol (Blocadren, Timoptic)	Hypertension, myocardial infarction, glaucoma
Beta blockers (cardioselective)	
acebutolol (Sectral)	Hypertension, ventricular arrhythmias
atenolol (Tenormin)	Hypertension, angina pectoris, myocardial infarction
betaxolol (Betoptic)	Hypertension, glaucoma
esmolol (Brevibloc)	Supraventricular tachyarrhythmias
metoprolol (Lopressor)	Hypertension, myocardial infarction
Alpha-beta blockers	
carvedilol (Coreg)	Hypertension
labetalol (Trandate, Normodyne)	Hypertension, including hypertensive crises

SIDE AND ADVERSE EFFECTS

- Alpha-adrenergic agonists and blocking agents: hypotension, tachycardia, sedation, drowsiness, and edema
- Beta-adrenergic blocking agents: bradycardia and heart block, congestive heart failure, (edema, dyspnea, fatigue), bronchospasm (wheezing, dyspnea), fatigue, dizziness, central nervous system effects (mental depression, insomnia, vivid dreams, hallucinations), and hypotension

INTERACTIONS AND CONTRAINDICATIONS

Alpha-adrenergic agonists and blocking agents have increased effects when given in conjunction with other antihypertensives, central nervous system depressants (additive effect), and epinephrine (stimulates alpha and beta receptors, which increases vasodilation, further decreasing blood pressure). Because of their sodium- and water-retaining properties, concurrent use of estrogens or nonsteroidal anti-inflammatory drugs (NSAIDs) may cause an increase in edema and congestive heart failure as well as decreasing the antihypertensive effect of the alpha-blocking drugs.

Beta-blocking agents have increased effects when given with other antihypertensives, phenoxybenzamine (Dibenzyline) and phentolamine (Regitine), chlorpromazine (Thorazine), cimetidine (Tagamet), and furosemide (Lasix). Concurrent use of digoxin may increase the potential for bradycardia and heart block. Antacids decrease the absorption of oral beta-blockers. Isoproterenol stimulates beta-adrenergic receptors to antagonize the effects of beta-blockers and atropine increases heart rate; these two drugs may be used to treat excessive bradycardia due to beta-blocker overdose.

The use of alpha blockers is contraindicated for patients with angina, myocardial infarction, and stroke. Methyldopa (Aldomet) is contraindicated for persons with active liver disease. Beta-blockers are contraindicated in the presence of bradycardia, heart block, congestive heart failure, and asthma and other allergic or pulmonary conditions characterized by bronchoconstriction.

NURSING ACTIONS

Prior to starting the drug, assess the client's status in relation to condition for which the drug is going to be given (i.e., baseline blood pressures for hypertension or urinary patterns for benign prostatic hypertrophy). Check blood pressure in both lying and standing positions to evaluate for postural (orthostatic) hypotension. Assess for conditions that contraindicate the use of antiadrenergic drugs (e.g., active liver disease, congestive heart failure, heart block) and for the use of other prescription and over-the-counter drugs. When the drug is to be discontinued, taper the dose down gradually over 1 to 2 weeks (long-term blockade of beta-adrenergic receptors increases receptor sensitivity to epinephrine and norepinephrine, leading to increased risk of severe hypertension, angina, arrhythmias, and myocardial infarction). Antidotes for bradycardia are atropine or isoproterenol; for CHF, digitalis and diuretics; for hypotension, vasopressors (e.g., dopamine, epinephrine); for bronchoconstriction, bronchodilators (e.g., isoproterenol, ephedrine). Give the first dose of doxazosin, prazosin, or terazosin at bedtime to prevent fainting from severe orthostatic hypotension. When increasing the dose of a beta-blocker, check blood pressure and pulse frequently to monitor for therapeutic and adverse effects. Some patients with a pulse rate of 50 to 60 bpm may be continued on the drug if they are not hypotensive and have no arrhythmias. Observe for the following therapeutic effects:

- hypertension: decreased blood pressure
- benign prostatic hypertrophy: improved urination
- pheochromocytoma: decreased pulse rate, blood pressure, sweating, palpitations, and blood glucose level
- Reynaud's disease or frostbite: improved skin color, skin temperature, and quality of peripheral pulses

Patient Teaching

- The side effects of palpitations and dizziness usually disappear with continued use of the drug but may occur under conditions that promote vasodilation (e.g., alcohol ingestion, high environmental temperature, exercise, large meal, or increasing drug dose).
- Do not abruptly stop taking the drug (because of the risk for rebound hypertension, possibly severe, or angina).
- Change positions slowly, especially from lying down to standing up (to prevent a rapid drop in blood pressure and fainting).
- Take the drug at same time every day (especially beta-blockers) to maintain therapeutic blood level.
- Count pulse once a day; if it is less than 50 bpm for several days in a row, report this to the health care provider (but do not stop the drug!).
- Avoid concurrent use of over-the-counter asthma and cold remedies, decongestants, and appetite suppressants (these drugs increase blood pressure). Over-the-counter analgesics such as ibuprofen (Motrin, Advil), ketoprofen (Orudis), and naproxen (Naprosyn) may increase blood pressure by causing edema (sodium and water retention).
- Report weight gain of more than 2 lbs per week, ankle edema, difficulty breathing, or excessive fatigue (may be drug-induced congestive heart failure) to the health care provider.

CHAPTER 17

CHOLINERGICS

*A*cetylcholine is a neurotransmitter that acts on body cells that respond to stimulation of the parasympathetic nervous system. The parts of the cell that respond to neurotransmitters are receptors. There are two types of cholinergic receptors: *nicotinic* and *muscarinic*. Nicotinic activation causes skeletal muscle contraction and, in the brain, promotes the release of acetylcholine in the cerebral cortex. Activation of muscarinic receptors can stimulate or suppress cells in the heart and blood vessels, gastrointestinal tract, respiratory tract, urinary tract, and the eye.

Cholinergic drugs mimic the effects of acetylcholine, or increase the concentration of acetylcholine by stimulating its production or preventing its breakdown. Because their effects are like those of parasympathetic stimulation, cholinergic drugs are also called *parasympathomimetics*. Table 17–1 lists the cholinergic drugs, their uses, and specific considerations.

TABLE 17–1

Cholinergic Drugs

Drug	Uses	Specific Considerations
bethanechol (Urecholine)	Treats urinary retention and postoperative decrease in gastrointestinal activity.	Routes: PO or SC only (*NOT* IM or IV). Administer before meals to reduce gastrointestinal distress. Can cause central nervous system stimulation and circulatory collapse. Expect urination within 1 hour. Anticipate need for catheterization if not effective.
neostigmine (Prostigmin)	Long-term treatment of myasthenia gravis, to reverse neuromuscular blocking agents, and to relieve urinary retention.	Give with milk or food. If patient has trouble swallowing, give 30–45 minutes before meals. IV form must be given very slowly. Check pulse before parenteral dose. If pulse is < 60, anticipate order for atropine to increase heart rate before giving neostigmine.
edrophonium (Tensilon)	Used to diagnose myasthenia gravis, to differentiate myasthenic crisis from cholinergic crisis, and to reverse effects of neuromuscular blockers.	Routes: IM, IV. Have atropine available as an antidote. Monitor for extreme muscle weakness related to cholinergic crisis.
pyridostigmine (Mestinon)	Preferred drug for long-term treatment of myasthenia gravis.	Routes: PO, IM, IV. Give PO drug with food or milk. If patient has difficulty swallowing, give 30–45 minutes before meals. Atropine may be ordered with pyridostigmine to reduce side effects. Schedule largest dosage to coincide with times of greatest fatigue.
tacrine (Cognex)	Used to delay progression of symptoms in early Alzheimer's disease.	Risk of liver toxicity. Monitor liver function results. Evaluate mental status. Effects reduced by smoking; enhanced by cimetidine. Take at regular intervals; can be taken with meals.
donepezil (Aricept)	Used to delay progression of symptoms in early Alzheimer's disease.	Advantage over tacrine is lack of liver toxicity. May aggravate chronic pulmonary disease.

ACTIONS AND USES

Cholinergic drugs are classified as direct-acting or indirect-acting. *Direct-acting cholinergic drugs* are synthetic substances that have longer durations of action than acetylcholine. Their target organs and actions as summarized earlier include the following:

- Heart: decreased rate
- Blood vessels: dilation
- Gastrointestinal tract: increased tone and contractility, increased salivary and gastrointestinal secretions, sphincter relaxation
- Bladder: increased tone and contractility, sphincter relaxation
- Bronchi: increased tone and contractility
- Lungs: increased secretions
- Eye: miosis (pupil constriction), contraction of ciliary muscle

Examples of direct-acting cholinergics are bethanechol (Urecholine), and pilocarpine. Bethanechol is used to treat urinary retention by causing contraction of the bladder muscle and relaxing the urinary sphincters. Topical or implanted pilocarpine (Isopto Carpine, Ocusert) is used in the treatment of glaucoma (see Chapter 48).

Indirect-acting cholinergics are also called *anticholinesterase* agents because they work by preventing the breakdown of acetylcholine by cholinesterase (an enzyme). Normally, excessive accumulation of acetylcholine is prevented by cholinesterase. Effects of indirect-acting drugs are as follows:

- Skeletal muscle: improved force of contraction
- Brain: enhanced transmission of impulses

Indirect-acting cholinergics are used to reverse the neuromuscular blocking effects of some drugs used in surgery, and in the treatment of myasthenia gravis and Alzheimer's disease.

SIDE AND ADVERSE EFFECTS

Side and adverse effects of cholinergic drugs are related to parasympathetic stimulation. They may include the following:

- Cardiovascular: bradycardia, dysrhythmias, hypotension
- Central nervous system: headache, drowsiness, seizures, loss of consciousness
- Respiratory: bronchospasm, increased secretions, failure
- Gastrointestinal: increased salivation, nausea, vomiting, diarrhea, abdominal cramping
- Bladder: increased frequency and urgency of urination
- Other: increased sweating, pupil constriction, rash

Cholinergic crisis is related to overdose and is manifested by severe weakness that affects the muscles of chewing, swallowing, and breathing. Paralysis of leg muscles occurs as well. Overdose is treated with atropine sulfate.

INTERACTIONS AND CONTRAINDICATIONS

Drugs that decrease the effects of cholinergic agents are anticholinergics and antihistamines. Quinidine and procainamide can also antagonize the drug effects.

Cholinergics are contraindicated with mechanical obstruction of the gastrointestinal or urinary tract.

NURSING ACTIONS

Monitor vital signs, respiratory status, mental status, muscle strength, and elimination. Have atropine available as an antidote for cholinergic overdose.

Patient Teaching
<ul><li>Report any palpitations, dizziness, difficulty breathing, or gastrointestinal distress.</li><li>You may notice increased salivation and sweating.</li></ul>

ANTICHOLINERGICS

*A*s the name implies, *anticholinergic drugs* block the effects of acetylcholine, which normally delivers messages that result in parasympathetic effects. Therefore, anticholinergics are also called *cholinergic blockers* or *parasympatholytic* agents. Table 18–1 lists the anticholinergic drugs, their uses, and specific considerations.

TABLE 18–1

Anticholinergics

Drug	Uses	Specific Considerations
atropine Ophthalmic preparations: homatropine hydrobromide (Homapin) and Mydrapred Ophthalmic (a combination of atropine and prednisolone)	Bradycardia, peptic ulcer disease and diarrhea. Given preoperatively to reduce respiratory and gastrointestinal secretions and to reduce the risk of cardiac dysrhythmias. Decreases renal and biliary spasms when given with opioids to treat colic. Ophthalmic preparation dilates the pupil for eye examination and treatment of iris inflammation; prevents accommodation of lens so refraction can be evaluated.	Oral drugs are best absorbed 30 minutes before meals. Therapeutic dosages of oral or parenteral atropine produces mild central nervous system excitement. Ophthalmic preparations have minimal systemic effects unless permitted to drain into the tear duct. Occluding the tear duct reduces absorption. May be given with open-angle glaucoma *IF* a miotic drug is also given.
scopolamine	Motion sickness, cycloplegia and mydriasis of eye, preanesthetic sedation, obstetric amnesia.	Therapeutic doses (except ophthalmic preparations) cause sedation. Otherwise, considerations are like atropine (above).
trihexyphenidyl (Artane) biperiden (Akineton) procyclidine (Kemadrin) benztropine (Cogentin)	Reduces muscle spasms in Parkinson's syndrome and in patients who have extrapyramidal drug effects. With Parkinson's, usually started with small doses and gradually increased.	Similar to atropine, except no ophthalmic preparations or uses. Children may have paradoxical stimulation with restlessness, tremors, and euphoria.
flavoxate (Urispas)	For cystitis and prostatitis, to relieve pain, spasm, and urinary frequency and urgency.	Side effects usually minor. Not recommended before age 12.

ACTIONS AND USES

Anticholinergic drugs bind to receptor sites that normally receive acetylcholine. This prevents acetylcholine from activating parasympathetic responses. The greatest effects occur in organs with muscarinic receptors (heart, blood vessels, gastrointestinal tract, respiratory tract, urinary tract, eye), but large doses can block nicotinic receptors in skeletal muscle as well.

To review, organs affected by anticholinergics and the effects are

- Heart: increased rate
- Respiratory tract: bronchodilation, decreased secretions
- Gastrointestinal tract: decreased muscle tone and motility, which can lead to constipation

- Eye: mydriasis (pupil dilation); diminished response to light; increased intraocular pressure in people with glaucoma
- Central nervous system: stimulation initially, then depression
- Smooth muscle: relaxation
- Other: decreased salivation and sweat production, relaxation of bladder and ureters, relaxation of smooth muscle in gallbladder and bile ducts.

Because they have such a wide range of effects, anticholinergics have many uses, such as the following:

- Gastrointestinal conditions: spastic conditions and some acute inflammatory disorders
- Genitourinary disorders: relief of painful smooth muscle spasms and urinary frequency associated with cystitis, urethritis, and prostatitis
- Eye: topical ophthalmic preparations dilate the pupil and prevent contraction of the ciliary muscle during examinations and surgical procedures
- Respiratory tract: relaxation of bronchoconstriction associated with asthma or chronic bronchitis
- Heart: bradycardia and heart block
- Other: decrease salivation in Parkinson's syndrome, reduce risk of bradycardia and hypotension during surgery, reduce respiratory secretions during surgery

SIDE AND ADVERSE EFFECTS

In general, the side and adverse effects of anticholinergics are directly related to their pharmacologic actions. For example, atropine may be used to treat bradycardia. Since it increases the heart rate, a possible adverse effect is tachycardia. Other effects that can be problematic are as follows:

- Central nervous system: initially stimulation (restlessness, confusion, tremor, hallucinations), then depression (drowsiness, sedation, slow respiratory rate)
- Gastrointestinal tract: dry mouth, constipation, paralytic ileus
- Urinary tract: urine retention
- Eye: mydriasis (pupil dilation), blurred vision, sensitivity to light
- Skin: warm, dry

Elderly patients are especially susceptible to adverse effects of anticholinergics because they metabolize them more slowly, often have multiple medical problems and take multiple drugs that are affected by anticholinergics.

Children are generally more sensitive to anticholinergics. Some ophthalmic preparations have caused behavioral disturbances and psychotic reactions in children.

INTERACTIONS AND CONTRAINDICATIONS

Cholinergic drugs interfere with the effects of anticholinergics because their actions are directly opposite. Drugs that enhance the effects of anticholinergics include antihistamines, phenothiazines, thioxanthenes, tricyclic antidepressants, and disopyramide.

Anticholinergics are contraindicated with tachycardia, myocardial infarction, narrow-angle (angle closure) glaucoma, hiatal hernia, and urinary or gastrointestinal tract obstruction. Note that patients with open-angle glaucoma can safely be given anticholinergics (as in preoperative situations) if they are also given miotics to constrict the pupils.

NURSING ACTIONS

After administering eye drops, gently press the inner canthus for 1 to 2 minutes to reduce systemic absorption. After administering ophthalmic ointment, tell the patient to close the eye and roll the eyeball to distribute the drug.

Monitor the heart rate for tachycardia (above 100 beats per minute). Assess bowel sounds and palpate the abdomen for distention. Record bowel movements and urine elimination. Inquire about urinary hesitancy and palpate the bladder for distention. Monitor body temperature for fever related to decreased sweating.

The antidote for anticholinergic poisoning is physostigmine salicylate (Antilirium), usually given slowly by the intravenous route.

Patient Teaching
• If this drug makes you drowsy, avoid activities, such as driving, that require alertness.
• In addition to taking extra fluids, sugarless gum and hard candy help to relieve dry mouth.
• To prevent constipation, take in at least eight 8-ounce glasses of fluid daily (unless contraindicated), increase fiber intake, and exercise daily.
• You may need to wear dark glasses outdoors because your eyes will be more sensitive to light.
• Your eyes will adjust more slowly to changes in light.
• Becoming overheated could cause heat stroke because your body cannot cool itself by sweating as efficiently as usual.
• Notify your health care provider if you have palpitations, problems with urination, excessive sleepiness, or confusion.

ANTICONVULSANTS

*A*nticonvulsant drugs, also called *antiepileptic drugs* (AEDs), are used to treat seizure disorders. A seizure disorder is a disorder of the brain that appears to involve excessive electrical discharges from nerves located in the area of the brain known as the cerebral cortex. The terms *seizure, convulsion,* and *epilepsy* are frequently used interchangeably, but they do not have the same meaning. A *seizure* is a brief episode of abnormal electrical activity in nerve cells in the brain that may or may not be accompanied by outward changes in appearance or behavior. A *convulsion* is characterized by spasmodic contractions of involuntary muscles. *Epilepsy* is a chronic, recurrent pattern of seizures. In about 50% of all cases of epilepsy, the cause is unknown (idiopathic, or primary, epilepsy), and about 50% of cases are secondary to trauma, infection, brain anoxia, cerebral vascular accident, or other illnesses.

Seizures are classified into two main types: partial (focal) seizures and generalized seizures:

- **Partial seizures** (or **psychomotor seizures**) begin in a specific area of the brain and produce symptoms that range from simple motor and sensory manifestations to complex abnormal movements and bizarre behavior (e.g., chewing or lip smacking).
- **Generalized seizures**, which are subdivided into **nonconvulsive** and **convulsive**, are bilateral and symmetric and have no obvious point of origin in the brain.
  — **Nonconvulsive seizures** are known as **absence** (or **petit mal**), **myoclonic,** and **atonic** seizures.
    - **Absence seizures** are characterized by abrupt changes in consciousness that last only a few seconds. The person may have a blank, staring expression with or without blinking of the eyelids, twitching of head or arms, or other motor movements.
    - **Myoclonic seizures** are short and involve contractions of a muscle or group of muscles.
    - **Atonic seizures** are a sudden loss of muscle or postural tone, also known as "drop attacks."

The most common type of convulsive seizure is the *tonic-clonic* or *major motor seizure*, also known as a *grand mal seizure*. The *tonic phase* involves loss of consciousness, sustained contraction of skeletal muscles, abnormal postures, and absence of respirations with cyanosis. The *clonic phase* is characterized by rapid rhythmic and symmetric jerking movements of the body. These seizures may be preceded by an *aura*, or brief warning, such as a flash of light or specific sound. *Status epilepticus* is a life-threatening emergency characterized by generalized tonic-clonic convulsions occurring at very close intervals. There is a high risk for permanent brain damage and death from status epilepticus because of hypotension, hypoxia, and cardiac arrhythmias.

A variety of AEDs are used to control epilepsy. The major classifications include hydantoins, barbiturates, benzodiazepines, succinimides, oxazolidinediones, iminostilbenes, and certain miscellaneous drugs. These drugs, despite their pharmacologic differences, their therapeutic uses, and their potential for adverse effects, all possess the ability to depress abnormal electrical discharges within the central nervous system (CNS) to inhibit seizure activity. The exact mechanism and site of action of these drugs is not known. It is believed that they act in two ways to control seizure activity. First, they may act directly on abnormal neurons to decrease nerve excitability and responsiveness to stimuli so that the seizure threshold is raised, and seizure activity is decreased. Second, they prevent the spread of impulses from abnormal neurons to normal neurons in the surrounding tissue. This helps prevent or minimize seizures by limiting excessive electrical activity to a small portion of the brain.

NURSING ACTIONS

The following nursing actions and patient teaching relate to anticonvulsants in general. Drug-specific nursing actions and patient teaching are included with the different classifications.

Obtain a thorough health history, including medical disorders, use of other medications, and drug and food allergies. Review the history of type and frequency of seizures. Monitor baseline and periodic liver and renal function tests and complete blood cell count (CBC). Obtain baseline and periodic urinalyses to assess for albuminuria (a symptom of nephrosis). Monitor serum drug concentrations. Warn patients not to substitute generic brands without the approval of health care provider, as the effect of generic drugs can be 10% above or below the effect of the trade name drug. Assist the patient to identify, and how to avoid, seizure triggers, such as alcohol ingestion, fever, emotional or physical stress, and sensory stimuli (e.g., flashing lights, loud noises). Protect the patient from harm during seizure: place a pillow or piece of clothing under the head; loosen tight clothing, especially around neck and chest; when the seizure stops, turn the patient to his or her side to facilitate drainage of secretions from the mouth and throat. **Never try to place a tongue blade or other object between the patient's teeth.**

Patient Teaching

- Take the drug exactly as prescribed. It must be taken regularly to achieve and maintain adequate blood levels. Do not take additional doses (because of increased risk of adverse reactions) and do not stop the drug abruptly (because of increased risk of seizures).
- Report continuing seizure activity, excessive drowsiness, or signs of adverse effects to the health care provider. Drug dose and timing may need adjustment.
- Avoid driving a vehicle or performing activities requiring physical and mental alertness if drowsiness occurs.
- Do not take other drugs (prescription or over-the-counter) without approval of health care provider. Inform the dentist or other health care providers of anticonvulsant use.
- You may take the drug with food to decrease gastrointestinal side effects if not specifically indicated otherwise.
- Carry a Medic-Alert device at all times with information regarding the use of anticonvulsant drugs.

HYDANTOINS

Uses

The hydantoin AEDs are used primarily for control of tonic-clonic and partial complex seizures. Drugs in this category include phenytoin (Dilantin), ethotoin (Peganone), mephenytoin (Mesantoin), and fosphenytoin (Cerebyx). Phenytoin is the drug of choice and one of the most effective anticonvulsants for treating all types of seizures, with the exception of absence seizures (phenytoin may worsen absence seizures). Phenytoin is also used for prevention and treatment of seizures during or following neurosurgery or head trauma. Occasionally, phenytoin is used for status epilepticus, although it is not considered a first-line drug for this purpose. Unlabeled uses include control of cardiac arrhythmias, control of seizures associated with eclampsia of pregnancy, and treatment of trigeminal neuralgia.

Side and Adverse Effects

A number of side and adverse effects are associated with hydantoins.

- **Central nervous system** (common during the first week or two of therapy): drowsiness, sedation, ataxia, nystagmus, diplopia, fatigue, irritability, nervousness, dizziness, slurred speech, tremors, and headache
- **Gastrointestinal**: nausea, vomiting, and anorexia
- **Skin disorders** (which may occur with almost all anticonvulsant drugs and may be of sufficient severity to warrant discontinuation of the drug): rash, exfoliative dermatitis, and Stevens-Johnson syndrome (a severe reaction characterized by oral and anogenital mucosal lesions, malaise, headache, fever, joint pain, and conjunctivitis)
- **Gingival hyperplasia** (overgrowth of gum tissue) often occurs, especially in children
- **Blood dyscrasias**: aplastic or hemolytic anemia, leukopenia, agranulocytosis, and thrombocytopenia
- **Other**: hepatotoxicity, hypocalcemia, and lymphadenopathy resembling malignant lymphoma

Interactions and Contraindications

Phenytoin interacts with many other drugs. Drugs that increase the effects of phenytoin are CNS depressants and other anticonvulsants. Tricyclic antidepressants and antipsychotic drugs lower the seizure threshold and precipitate seizures so that phenytoin drug dosages may need to be increased. Other drugs that increase the potential for phenytoin toxicity by inhibiting its liver metabolism or by displacing it from plasma protein-binding sites include alcohol, benzodiazepines, chloramphenicol, cimetidine, ibuprofen, isoniazid, miconazole, phenothiazine antipsychotic drugs, and salicylates.

Drugs that decrease the effects of phenytoin by decreasing its absorption or by increasing its metabolism include alcohol (chronic ingestion), antacids, antineoplastics, folic acid, nitrofurantoin, rifampin, sucralfate, and theophylline.

Phenobarbital and phenytoin have variable interactions with unpredictable effects. These two drugs are often used together for seizure control. Although phenobarbital induces drug metabolism in the liver (see Chapters 2 and 9) and may increase metabolism of other anticonvulsant drugs, its interaction with phenytoin is different. The two drugs given together usually have a synergistic effect, although the interaction varies with dose, route, time of administration, degree of liver enzyme induction already present, and other factors; thus, the occurrence of significant interactions is unpredictable.

Phenytoin decreases the effects of oral anticoagulants, corticosteroids, and oral contraceptives as well as decreasing absorption of folic acid, calcium, and vitamin D.

Phenytoin is contraindicated or must be used cautiously in persons with CNS depression, hepatic or renal damage, and bone marrow depression.

 Pregnancy Category D.

Nursing Actions

If possible, avoid the intramuscular route of administration because of potential for tissue irritation and sloughing. During intravenous administration, closely monitor the rate of administration, as a rate faster than 50 mg/minute may cause hypotension or cardiac arrhythmias. Check the intravenous site frequently for redness or irritation. Report pulse <60 bpm, BP <120/80, and respirations <12/minute. Do not mix intravenous phenytoin with other drugs or intravenous solutions except normal saline (possibility of drug precipitation). Give medication exactly as ordered. Do not substitute prompt-release form for extended-release form. Because of the hyperglycemic effect of these drugs, diabetic patients should monitor blood glucose levels frequently.

Patient Teaching

- Phenytoin may harmlessly color urine pink, red, or brown.
- Use appropriate contraception during therapy. If pregnancy is suspected, notify the health care provider immediately (potential for severe birth defects).
- Do not take the drug within 2 to 3 hours of taking an antacid (decreased phenytoin absorption).
- You may take the drug with food (but not milk) to minimize gastrointestinal distress.
- Maintain very good oral hygiene to reduce the possibility of gingival hyperplasia.
- Increase intake of vitamin D either through sunlight, supplement, or food (e.g., tuna, sardines, salmon, eggs, milk, butter, dry cereals, oatmeal, sweet potatoes).
- Maintain adequate folic acid (folate) intake through supplements or diet (e.g., green, leafy vegetables, fresh fruits, whole grains, liver).

BARBITURATES

The two barbiturates most commonly used as antiepileptic drugs are phenobarbital (Solfoton, Luminal) and primidone (Mysoline), which is metabolized in the liver to phenobarbital. A major advantage is that phenobarbital has the longest half-life of all usual AEDs, which allows for once-a-day dosing. This is useful for patients who have trouble remembering to take their medication or for those with unpredictable schedules.

Uses

Phenobarbital is used to treat tonic-clonic and partial seizures. It is a first-line drug for the management of status epilepticus and is an effective prophylactic drug for control of febrile seizures. Phenobarbital may also be used in the management of pre-eclampsia and eclampsia of pregnancy, meningitis, and toxic reactions.

Side and Adverse Effects

- **Central nervous system**: the primary adverse effect of barbiturates is dose-dependent respiratory depression. Overdose may result in death from respiratory failure. Other CNS effects are drowsiness, lethargy, headache, confusion, dizziness, morning hangover, and paradoxical excitation or restlessness.
- **Blood dyscrasias** (with long-term use): megaloblastic anemia, thrombocytopenia, leukopenia, agranulocytosis, and folic acid and vitamin D deficiency.
- **Other**: laryngospasm, bronchospasm, liver damage, exfoliative dermatitis, ataxia. There may be adverse effects related to liver enzyme induction, tolerance and cross-tolerance, and dependence and abuse potential.
- **Allergy/hypersensitivity**: not common, but can be severe due to the edema of mucous membranes of mouth, lips, tongue, face, and viscera.
- **Stevens-Johnson syndrome**: a potentially fatal adverse effect characterized by fever, cough, muscle aches and pains, headache, and the appearance of wheals or blisters on the skin, mucous membranes, and other organs.

Interactions and Contraindications

Alcohol, antihistamines, benzodiazepines, opioids, and tranquilizers enhance the depressant and adverse effects of barbiturates. Monoamine oxidase (MAO) inhibitors inhibit the metabolism of barbiturates, prolonging their effects. Liver enzyme induction decreases the effect of oral anticoagulants, oral contraceptives, theophylline, corticosteroids, anticonvulsants, and digitoxin. Concurrent use with fluoxetine (Prozac) may produce hypertension, diaphoresis, ataxia, flushing, nausea, dizziness, and anxiety.

Contraindications include severe respiratory disorders, severe liver or kidney disease, and a history of alcohol or other drug abuse. Barbiturates should not be given to laboring women because of the potential for neonatal respiratory depression. Cautious use is advised in patients with a history of depression, psychosis, or suicidal tendencies. **Pregnancy category D.**

Nursing Actions

Do not administer intramuscularly unless absolutely necessary (because of pain and possible necrosis at the injection site). If an intramuscular route is selected, use a large muscle mass, rotate injection sites, and monitor sites for irritation. Administer intravenous phenobarbital slowly; too rapid administration may cause laryngospasms, apnea, and hypotension. Check the intravenous site frequently for infiltration; extravasation (leaking of the drug into tissues) may cause tissue necrosis. Assess for the effectiveness of other drugs given concurrently with barbiturates (e.g., oral anticoagulants, oral contraceptives, other AEDs). Monitor for and report chronic toxicity symptoms: ataxia, slurred speech, irritability, poor judgment, confusion, insomnia, malaise.

Patient Teaching

- Take medication exactly as prescribed. The drowsiness experienced during first few weeks of therapy usually decreases with continued use.
- Do not take other prescription or over-the-counter drugs without the approval of a health care provider.
- Do not abruptly stop taking the drug (because of the possibility of seizures or withdrawal syndrome).
- Report fever, sore throat or mouth, malaise, easy bruising or bleeding, petechiae, jaundice, or rash.
- Use alternative methods of contraception in addition to or instead of oral contraceptives. Report possible pregnancy to the health care provider immediately.
- Increase intake of vitamin D either through sunlight, supplement, or food (e.g., tuna, sardines, salmon, eggs, milk, butter, dry cereals, oatmeal, sweet potatoes).
- Maintain adequate folic acid (folate) intake through supplements or diet (e.g., green, leafy vegetables, fresh fruits, whole grains, liver).

BENZODIAZEPINES

Uses

Benzodiazepines are used as first-line drugs for the treatment of status epilepticus and as second-line drugs for the treatment of epilepsy. The benzodiazepine most often used to treat status epilepticus is diazepam (Valium), although lorazepam (Ativan) may also be used for this purpose. The two benzodiazepines used primarily as second-line AEDs are clonazepam (Klonopin) and clorazepate (Tranxene). The major value of clonazepam is in the treatment of absence, myoclonic, and tonic-clonic seizures. Clorazepate is a long-acting benzodiazepine used primarily as an additional drug for patients whose seizures continue despite treatment with a single medication.

Unlabeled uses for clonazepam include treatment of restless leg syndrome, abnormal movements associated with Parkinson's disease, acute manic episodes of bipolar disorder, and adjunct therapy for schizophrenia.

A new form of diazepam, diazepam rectal gel (Diastat), is now available for the management of selected patients with epilepsy on stable regimens of AEDs who require intermittent use of diazepam to control episodes of increased seizure activity.

Side and Adverse Effects

- **Central nervous system**: drowsiness, morning hangover, dizziness, lethargy, and paradoxical excitation or nervousness. Long-term anticonvulsant use may result in behavioral and personality changes, including hyperactivity, irritability, moodiness, and aggressive behavior.
- **Other:** disorientation, palpitations, dry mouth, nausea and vomiting, and nightmares.
- **Toxicity (overdose)**: excessive sedation, confusion, decreased reflexes, and coma. Unless ingested with another CNS depressant (e.g., alcohol), benzodiazepine overdoses rarely result in death. Treatment is symptomatic and supportive, including use of the specific benzodiazepine antagonist, flumazenil (Romazicon).

Tolerance to clonazepam develops in approximate 30% of patients who initially respond favorably to the drug, and their seizures recur, usually within 1 to 6 months after starting therapy. Some patients respond to an increased dose, but others do not.

Interactions and Contraindications

Concurrent administration with other CNS depressants potentiates the effects of benzodiazepines. MAO inhibitors decrease metabolism of benzodiazepines, thus increasing their depressant effects. Cimetidine decreases benzodiazepine metabolism to prolong its action.

These drugs are contraindicated for persons with severe hepatic or renal dysfunction, sleep apnea, and acute narrow-angle glaucoma. Cautious use is indicated for persons with psychiatric disorders, history of suicidal tendencies, history of drug or alcohol abuse or addiction, geriatric patients, and those with chronic lung diseases.

Nursing Actions

Physical and psychological dependence may occur in patients with history of drug and alcohol abuse. Monitor for symptoms of withdrawal if the drug is stopped abruptly: increased anxiety, psychomotor agitation, irritability, headache, insomnia, tremors, palpitations, confusion, psychosis, and recurrence of seizures. Intravenous diazepam should not be infused, mixed, or diluted with other solutions (possibility of drug precipitation). Diazepam interacts with plastic; use of plastic containers or intravenous administration sets decreases the availability of the drug. Monitor for symptoms of overdose: confusion, excessive drowsiness, irritability, sweating, muscle and abdominal cramps, decreased reflexes, and coma.

Patient Teaching

- Report return of seizure activity immediately; the drug dose will be adjusted or the drug changed to another AED.
- Take the drug exactly as prescribed; do not abruptly stop taking the drug (because of return of seizure activity or occurrence of withdrawal symptoms).
- Do not take other prescription or over-the-counter drugs without the approval of a health care provider.
- Report suspected pregnancy immediately (because of the possibility of fetal malformations).

SUCCINIMIDES

Uses

Succinimide anticonvulsants are used primarily to manage absence seizures. The major drugs in this category are ethosuximide (Zarontin) and methsuximide (Celontin). There is new evidence that ethosuximide may be useful for controlling myoclonic seizures or partial complex seizures.

Side and Adverse Effects

- **Central nervous system** (most common adverse effects): drowsiness, lethargy, dizzi-

ness, headache, euphoria, and hiccups, although some tolerance does build up to these effects.
- **Gastrointestinal**: nausea, vomiting, anorexia, abdominal cramps, diarrhea, epigastric pain.
- **Genitourinary**: urinary frequency, vaginal bleeding; renal and liver function impairment.
- **Skin**: rashes, hair loss.
- **Other**: blood dyscrasias (e.g., thrombocytopenia, leukopenia, aplastic anemia, bone marrow depression), muscle weakness, gingival hyperplasia, Stevens-Johnson syndrome.

Interactions and Contraindications

Succinimides increase the effect of hydantoins and decrease the effects of primidone and phenobarbital. Valproic acid may either increase or decrease succinimide levels.

Patients with signs of infection (fever, sore throat) should use succinimides cautiously because of the possibility of fatal blood dyscrasias. Cautious use is also indicated in persons with renal and liver disease.

Patient Teaching

- Do not abruptly discontinue the drug; absence seizures will recur. Tonic-clonic seizures may also occur.
- Report gastrointestinal symptoms, drowsiness, dizziness, or other neurologic symptoms; drug dose may need adjustment.
- Promptly report signs and symptoms of infection; blood tests may need to be done to check for blood dyscrasias.
- Drug may harmlessly color urine pink, red, or brown.

OXAZOLIDINEDIONES

Oxazolidinediones may be used to treat absence seizures, but due to frequent and severe adverse effects (hepatic or renal damage, blood dyscrasias, myasthenia gravis–like syndrome) have largely been replaced by newer drugs that have pharmacologically similar effects (e.g., ethosuximide [Zarontin]). The drugs in the oxazolidinedione category include trimethadione (Tridione) and paramethadione (Paradione).

IMINOSTILBENES

Carbamazepine (Tegretol), an iminostilbene derivative, is chemically related to the tricyclic antidepressants and unrelated to other anticonvulsants. Its anticonvulsant mechanism of action is unknown. It is the second most frequently prescribed AED in the United States, after phenytoin.

Uses

Carbamazepine is a first-line drug for treatment of simple and complex partial seizures, and generalized tonic-clonic seizures. It is also the specific analgesic for the treatment of trigeminal neuralgia.

Side and Adverse Effects

Adverse effects include dizziness, drowsiness, ataxia, gastrointestinal upset, immune system dysfunction, bone marrow depression, thrombophlebitis, congestive heart failure, coronary artery disease, dyspnea, kidney and liver impairment, muscle and joint pain, increased intraocular pressure and impotence. Psychotic symptoms, confusion, or agitation may occur.

Interactions and Contraindications

Drugs that increase the effects (and potential toxicity) of carbamazepine include cimetidine, danazol, isoniazid, verapamil, antihistamines, serotonin selective reuptake inhibitors (SSRIs), felbamate, and tricyclic antidepressants.

Drugs that decrease the effects of carbamazepine include barbiturates, primidone, hydantoins, charcoal, theophylline, acetaminophen, and anticoagulants. Carbamazepine decreases the effects of valproic acid, oral contraceptives, doxycycline, haloperidol, and succinimides. Concurrent use with lithium increases CNS toxicity. Reversal of neuromuscular blocking effect of nondepolarizing neuromuscular blockers may occur. Antidiuretic effects of vasopressin, lypressin, or desmopressin may be potentiated.

Carbamazepine is contraindicated in persons who are hypersensitive to tricyclic antidepressants or have a history of bone marrow depression. MAO inhibitors should be discontinued at least 14 days before administration of carbamazepine. Cautious use is indicated for persons with glaucoma or adverse blood reactions to other drugs. This drug may cause confusion and agitation in the elderly.

Patient Teaching
• Take drug exactly as prescribed.
• Do not abruptly stop taking the drug (possibility of status epilepticus).
• Exposure to sunlight may cause photosensitivity reaction; use sunscreen and protective clothing.
• Utilize alternative methods of contraception in addition to or instead of oral contraceptives.
• Report skin lesions or changes in skin pigmentation to health care provider. Drug may need to be discontinued.

MISCELLANEOUS ANTICONVULSANTS

Gabapentin (Neurontin)

Gabapentin is indicated as adjunct therapy for the treatment of partial seizures in adults. It is also being used experimentally to manage symptoms of amyotrophic lateral sclerosis (Lou Gehrig's disease). Gabapentin is an amino acid whose mechanism of action as an anticonvulsant is unknown. Common adverse effects include fatigue, dizziness, and drowsiness; these usually subside with continued use. There are no known interactions and no significant changes in serum levels of other AEDs taken concurrently. To promote the maximum effect of the drug, time between doses should not exceed 12 hours. The first dose of gabapentin should be taken at bedtime to minimize the dizziness, fatigue, and ataxia that occur initially.

Lamotrigine (Lamictal)

Lamotrigine is chemically unrelated to other AEDs. Its exact mechanism of action is unknown. Lamotrigine is used as adjunct therapy to treat partial seizures in adults. Common adverse effects include dizziness, headache, ataxia, rash, nausea and vomiting, double or blurred vision, and photosensitivity. Dosage may need to be adjusted in the elderly and those with hepatic impairment.

Vigabatrin (Sabril) and Tiagabine (Gabitril)

Vigabatrin and tiagabine are adjunctive AEDs used for the treatment of complex partial seizures in adults and resistant partial seizures in children. Adverse effects in adults are fatigue, drowsiness, dizziness, irritability, headache, depression, confusion, poor concentration, abdominal pain, and anorexia. Adverse effects in children may include agitation and insomnia. Drug interactions are not common.

Valproic Acid (Depakene, Depakote)

Valproic acid is used alone or with other AEDs for simple and complex absence seizures and with other AEDs for absence, myoclonic, and generalized tonic-clonic seizures. Other approved uses include bipolar disorder and migraine headache prophylaxis. The exact mechanism of action is unknown. Adverse gastrointestinal effects are most common and include nausea and vomiting, anorexia, abdominal cramps, indigestion, and diarrhea or constipation. Central nervous system effects include drowsiness, fatigue, ataxia, anxiety, headache, nystagmus, and behavior disturbances. Mild blood dyscrasias may occur and bleeding, bruising, or coagulation disorder may require discontinuation of the drug. Adverse endocrine effects include hyperglycemia, gynecomastia (breast enlargement in males), acute pancreatitis, or menstrual irregularities. Drug interactions include competition for protein-binding sites with carbamazepine, clonazepam, phenobarbital, phenytoin, and aspirin.

Topiramate (Topamax)

Topiramate appears to block the spread of seizures rather than raise the seizure threshold. It is used as adjunct therapy in treating adults with partial seizures and has orphan drug status for Lennox-Gastaut syndrome. Age, gender, race, baseline seizure frequency, and concurrent AED therapy do not appear to affect the effectiveness of the drug. Adverse effects are generally dose related and include fatigue, drowsiness, dizziness, uncoordinated movements, difficulty concentrating, speech and language difficulties, and nystagmus. Cautious use is indicated for persons with liver and kidney disorders and with a history of kidney stones. Concurrent use of topiramate with other AEDs may require dosage adjustment of any or all of the drugs.

ANTIPARKINSONIAN

PARKINSON'S SYNDROME

Parkinson's syndrome is a chronic, progressive, degenerative condition that affects the central nervous system. The basic defect is a deficiency of dopamine (a neurotransmitter) in relation to the amount of acetylcholine in the basal ganglia. Dopamine is needed for normal neuromuscular activity. The classic signs of Parkinson's are as follows:

- tremor: trembling or shaking, mostly in the upper extremities, during voluntary movements or at rest
- rigidity: stiffness
- bradykinesia: extremely slow movements

Patients with advanced disease often have jerky movements and gait disturbances. Other signs and symptoms are loss of dexterity and power in affected limbs, changes in handwriting, lack of facial expression, rubbing the thumb against the fingertips (called "pill rolling"), and drooling.

Drug therapy for Parkinson's syndrome is intended to increase dopamine or decrease acetylcholine in the brain. The two primary classifications of drugs used are dopaminergics and anticholinergics. Anticholinergics are covered in Chapter 18.

DOPAMINERGICS

Dopaminergic drugs used to treat Parkinson's include levodopa (L-dopa), carbidopa (Lodosyn), amantadine (Symmetrel), bromocriptine (Parlodel), pergolide (Permax), and selegiline (Eldepryl).

Action and Uses

Dopaminergics treat Parkinson's syndrome by increasing the amount of dopamine in the brain by various mechanisms. Carbidopa by itself is ineffective, but it is given with levodopa because it reduces the metabolism of levodopa. Sinemet is a commercially prepared combination of levodopa and carbidopa. After the patient has taken levodopa for a few years, it is common for symptoms to return. Therefore, it is usually reserved until symptoms are significant.

Amantadine, bromocriptine, pergolide, and selegiline are more often used with levodopa rather than alone. Most of these drugs have other uses in addition to the treatment of Parkinson's.

Side and Adverse Effects

Dopaminergic agents all have the potential for some effects on the central nervous system (CNS), usually stimulation. CNS effects could include dyskinesia (abnormal, involuntary movements), agitation, ataxia, bradykinesia (slow movement), confusion, hallucinations, insomnia, and dizziness. Other effects that may be seen with specific dopaminergic agents are as follows:

- levodopa: anorexia, nausea and vomiting, orthostatic hypotension, cardiac dysrhythmias, and abrupt changes in motor function
- amantadine: bluish skin color on legs
- bromocriptine and pergolide: nausea, hypotension
- selegiline: abdominal discomfort

Interactions and Contraindications

The effects of dopaminergic agents may be enhanced by tricyclic antidepressants and monoamine oxidase-A (MAO-A) inhibitors. These combinations can result in serious cardiac dysrhythmias and hypertension. Interestingly, even though anticholinergics may be used to treat Parkinson's syndrome, they decrease the amount of levodopa absorbed. The effects of levodopa are also reduced if given with oral iron preparations, vitamin B_6, alcohol, or antianxiety agents. Antipsychotic drugs and metoclopramide (Reglan) decrease the effectiveness of all dopaminergic agents.

Levodopa is contraindicated with narrow-angle glaucoma, hemolytic anemia, severe angina, transient ischemic attacks, and in patients who have had melanoma.

Nursing Actions

Assess the patient's motor function: gait, balance, and handwriting. Assist with rising if dizziness occurs.

Patient Teaching

For levodopa

- Change positions slowly when taking levodopa to prevent sudden decreases in blood pressure.
- Levodopa can cause gastrointestinal distress, but this usually resolves after taking the drug for a while.
- Levodopa is best taken with or after meals to reduce gastrointestinal side effects.
- It often takes several weeks before the drug effects are apparent; maximum effects may take up to 6 months.

For selegiline

- Take selegiline in the morning and at noon to reduce insomnia at night.

For bromocriptine

- Take with or after meals to reduce gastrointestinal distress.

For amantadine

- You may have some dizziness and feel excitable, but these effects will go away as you get accustomed to the drug.
- Some people develop a bluish discoloration on their legs; this will go away when your health care provider discontinues the drug.

ANTICHOLINERGICS

Anticholinergics increase the proportion of dopamine in relation to acetylcholine by decreasing acetylcholine. Anticholinergics are discussed in detail in Chapter 18. Specific agents used for Parkinson's syndrome are:

- benztropine (Cogentin)
- biperiden (Akineton)
- procyclidine (Kemadrin)
- trihexyphenidyl (Artane)
- diphenhydramine (Benadryl)
- ethopropazine (Parsidol)

CHAPTER 21

CNS STIMULANTS

*C*entral nervous system (CNS) stimulants are drugs that affect a specific area of the brain or spinal cord. Stimulation of the CNS may either increase nerve cell activity or block nerve cell activity. Since many of the actions of CNS stimulants are the same as those of the sympathetic nervous system neurotransmitters epinephrine and norepinephrine, these drugs are sometimes referred to as *sympathomimetic* agents (see Chapter 15).

Central nervous system stimulants decrease appetite, improve mood, increase energy and alertness, and decrease fatigue. Numerous drugs can stimulate the CNS (e.g., cocaine), but only a few are used therapeutically, and their indications for use are limited to treatment of narcolepsy, attention deficit hyperactivity disorder (ADHD), obesity, and reversal of respiratory depression. These drugs are classified as amphetamines, anorexiants, analeptics, and xanthines.

AMPHETAMINES

Action and Uses

Amphetamines increase the amounts of epinephrine, norepinephrine, dopamine, and serotonin in the brain to produce euphoria or mood elevation, increase mental alertness and productivity, decrease fatigue and drowsiness, and prolong wakefulness. They produce tolerance and psychological dependence and have high abuse potential.

Amphetamines are used to treat narcolepsy (a disorder characterized by sudden, periodic "sleep attacks" in which the person goes to sleep at any time, in any place); ADHD, which occurs primarily in children and is characterized by short attention span, hyperactivity, difficulty completing assigned tasks, restlessness, and impulsive behavior; and obesity. Drugs in this category include amphetamine, dextroamphetamine (Dexedrine), methamphetamine (Desoxyn), methylphenidate (Ritalin), and pemoline (Cylert).

ANOREXIANTS

Action and Uses

Anorexiants work primarily by broadly stimulating the CNS and are believed to suppress appetite control centers in the brain, but this has yet to be proven. There is also evidence that they may increase fat metabolism, decrease absorption of dietary fat, and increase glucose uptake in the cells. Anorexiants are used in the treatment of obesity to suppress appetite. Obesity increases the risk of hypertension, coronary artery disease, gallbladder disease, type II diabetes mellitus, sleep apnea, gout, and certain types of cancer. The use of anorexiant drugs is controversial, particularly in the wake of the removal of dexfenfluramine (Redux) and the fenfluramine (Pondimin) half of the "fen-phen" combination from the market. Tolerance develops rapidly to these drugs, and prolonged use is contraindicated. They are generally prescribed for no longer than 8 to 12 weeks as an adjunct to a comprehensive weight loss plan that includes diet and exercise. Drugs in this category include dextroamphetamine (Dexedrine), benzphetamine (Didrex), diethylpropion (Tenuate), phendimetrazine (Adipost), phentermine (Adipex, et al.), mazindol (Mazanor), and phenylpropanolamine (Dexatrim). All but phenylpropanolamine require a prescription. Two new anorexiants are sibutramine, which inhibits the reuptake of norepinephrine, serotonin, and dopamine, and orlistat, which alters fat metabolism.

The following side and adverse effects, interactions, contraindications, nursing actions, and patient teaching relate to amphetamines and anorexiants.

Side and Adverse Effects

Side and adverse effects are related to excessive stimulation of most body systems and primarily occur at doses higher than the therapeutic range or in overdoses of the drug.

- **Central nervous system**: nervousness, restlessness, hyperactivity, anxiety, headache, tremors, difficulty concentrating, confusion
- **Cardiovascular**: hypertension, tachycardia, palpitations, angina, arrhythmias
- **Gastrointestinal:** abdominal pain, nausea, vomiting, diarrhea, dry mouth
- **Genitourinary**: diuresis, increased urinary frequency

Overdoses may produce convulsions and psychotic behavior.

112

Interactions and Contraindications

Amphetamines and anorexiants with tricyclic antidepressants, other CNS stimulants, digoxin, and fluoxetine (Prozac) have an additive potential for toxic effects such as cardiac arrhythmias, tachycardia, hypertension, insomnia, and convulsions.

MAO inhibitors increase release of catecholamines (epinephrine and norepinephrine), causing arrhythmias and severe hypertension.

Beta-blockers increase alpha-adrenergic effects to produce hypertension, bradycardia, arrhythmias, and heart block.

Amphetamines and anorexiants are contraindicated for persons with cardiovascular disorders (hypertension, angina, arrhythmias), anxiety, agitation, glaucoma, hyperthyroidism, or with a history of substance abuse. These drugs are contraindicated during and within 14 days of administration of MAO inhibitors. **Pregnancy category X** (phenylpropanolamine has not shown evidence of causing harm to the fetus during pregnancy, but its absolute safety has not been established).

Nursing Actions

Obtain patient history regarding drug and food allergies, cardiovascular disease, renal or hepatic dysfunction, hyperthyroidism, glaucoma, psychiatric disorders, or substance abuse. Check the use of other prescription and nonprescription drugs, particularly those which may interact with amphetamines and anorexiants. Administer the drug at least 6 hours before bedtime to prevent insomnia. Monitor for drug tolerance (develops within a few weeks); the drug should be discontinued when this occurs. Assist obese patient to set reasonable weight reduction goals; weigh weekly and chart progress. Be alert for signs of overdose: panic, hallucinations, fever, combativeness, circulatory collapse, convulsions, and coma. Initiate a periodic pill count if you have doubts about patient's use (or misuse) of the drug.

For amphetamines used in children, take height and weight measurements as baseline and monitor for appropriate growth at specified intervals. Assess the child's behavior and record to provide a baseline for comparison. Instruct parents of children being treated for ADHD to provide for periodic "drug-free" holidays to allow for normal growth and development. This may be on weekends or during school vacations (as recommended by health care provider).

For anorexiants, if the drug is being given for the treatment of obesity, it should be administered 30 to 45 minutes before meals.

Patient Teaching

- Take the medication exactly as prescribed. Do not increase the dose or frequency of administration.
- Avoid other CNS stimulants such as caffeine (coffee, tea, chocolate, cola).
- Do not take over-the-counter medications without the approval of the health care provider (because many contain CNS-stimulating properties).
- Avoid alcohol use while on the medication.
- Do not abruptly stop taking the drug (because you may have adverse reactions from physical dependency) without checking with the health care provider.
- Take the medication at least 6 hours before bedtime to prevent insomnia.
- For treatment of obesity, take the anorexiant drug 30 to 45 minutes before meals.
- Use of hard candy, chewing gum, or sips of water may help minimize dry mouth.
- If pregnancy is suspected, notify the health care provider immediately.
- Notify the health care provider if restlessness, insomnia, dizziness, diarrhea, or nervousness occur; the dosage of drug may need to be adjusted.

ANALEPTICS

Analeptic drugs are used primarily to stimulate respiration when the natural reflex is lost due to overdoses of opioids, alcohol, barbiturates, and general anesthetic agents. However, their use has decreased with the advent of more appropriate reversal agents (e.g., naloxone [Narcan], an opioid antagonist) and more reliable and effective means of mechanical ventilatory support. The primary drug in this category is doxapram (Dopram).

Action and Uses

Doxapram is a respiratory stimulant that relaxes bronchial smooth muscle, dilates pulmonary arteries, increases tidal volume, and slightly increases respiratory rate to reduce excess carbon dioxide (hypercapnia), which may arise in patients at risk for postoperative pulmonary complications (e.g., chronic obstructive lung disease) or respiratory depression in the postoperative recovery period not caused by skeletal muscle relaxants. It may also be used in conjunction with supportive measures and reversal medications to treat respiratory depression from overdose of CNS depressants. It may be used to treat neonatal apnea that does not respond to xanthine therapy.

Side and Adverse Effects

Side and adverse effects include fever or feeling of bodily warmth, disorientation, dizziness, anxiety, itching, numbness, headache, nausea and vomiting, diarrhea, dyspnea or tachypnea, tachycardia or bradycardia, phlebitis, seizures, spontaneous urination, or urinary retention. Hemoglobin, hematocrit, and red blood cell count may be elevated, while white blood cells may be decreased. There may also be elevated blood urea nitrogen and albuminuria. Additional side and adverse effects are all of those associated with all CNS stimulants.

Interactions and Contraindications

The effects of drug interactions with analeptics are the same as those of the amphetamines.

⚠ Doxapram is usually contraindicated in neonates because of the benzyl alcohol in the injectable form of the drug (although it may be used cautiously to treat neonatal apnea that does not respond to xanthines). Other contraindications include convulsive disorders, head injury, cardiovascular disease, hypertension, and cerebral vascular accident.

Nursing Actions

Perform a thorough respiratory assessment prior to medication administration. Check the patient's history for cardiovascular disease, convulsive disorders, or mechanical respiratory disorders (e.g., chronic obstructive pulmonary disease). Repeat respiratory assessments as often as indicated. Monitor lab values for changes. Assess for side and adverse effects. Do not "piggy-back" intravenous doxapram with solutions containing thiopental, bicarbonate, or aminophylline (a precipitate or gas will form).

XANTHINES

The xanthine drugs are caffeine, aminophylline, and theophylline. This category of drugs may also categorized as analeptics, so actions, uses, side and adverse effects, interactions, and contraindications are the same. Theophylline and aminophylline are discussed in Chapter 24.

Caffeine is the only xanthine/analeptic drug available without a prescription. Over-the-counter doses are lower than those used in the health care setting. Nonprescription caffeine-containing drugs include Anacin, Excedrin, Dristan AF, No-Doz, and Vivarin. Prescription drugs, used for treatment of migraine headaches, include Cafergot, Esgic, and Fioricet. A combination of caffeine and sodium benzoate may be used as a respiratory stimulant to treat neonatal apnea not responsive to other therapies. Caffeine is also contained in chocolate, coffee, tea, soft drinks, and cocoa. The CNS effects most frequently noted are increased motor activity and mental alertness, decreased fatigue, emotional or mood elevation, and mild euphoria.

Caffeine should be used with caution in patients who have a history of peptic ulcers (caffeine stimulates gastric acid production and release), cardiac arrhythmias, or recent myocardial infarction.

Patient Teaching

- Do not overuse caffeine-containing products.
- Avoid concurrent use of prescription caffeine drugs and other caffeine-containing products.
- Take medication exactly as directed or prescribed.
- Caffeine produces tolerance to its stimulating effects, requiring higher doses to produce the desired effects.
- Psychological and physiologic dependence may occur; the drug may have to be withdrawn gradually.

REVIEW QUESTIONS: UNIT 6

1. Beta receptors are located primarily in the_____. Stimulation of these receptors produces_____ and _____.

2. Activation of beta receptors produces what effect on the lungs?
   A. Bronchoconstriction
   B. Bronchodilation
   C. No effect

3. A patient who is using an isoproterenol inhaler for treatment of asthma tells you that her saliva and sputum are "pink." Based on his knowledge of this drug, the nurse responds:
   A. "I will call your health care provider right away."
   B. "The drug may be causing a small amount of bleeding in your airway."
   C. "This is a type of allergic reaction to the drug."
   D. "This is a normal, harmless effect of the drug."

4. Patient teaching regarding the use of alpha-adrenergic drugs to relieve nasal congestion includes information that:

    A. excessive use may cause rebound nasal congestion when the drug is discontinued.

    B. it is permissible for the patient to increase the dose if a previous dose is ineffective.

    C. concurrent use of any over-the-counter cold or allergy medication is safe.

    D. these drugs do not produce any effects that could affect driving a car.

5. Instruct patients who are taking antiadrenergic drugs for the treatment of hypertension not to abruptly stop taking the medication because of the risk for:

    A. edema.

    B. postural hypotension.

    C. urinary retention.

    D. rebound hypertension.

6. A patient is started on prazosin to treat his hypertension. Which of the following patient teaching instructions should be stressed?

    A. Rise slowly from a lying or sitting position.

    B. Take the drug on an empty stomach.

    C. Force fluids to 2,000 mL per day.

    D. Medication must always be taken in the morning.

7. Which side effect should a patient be aware of when taking clonidine?

    A. Anxiety

    B. Diarrhea

    C. Drowsiness

    D. Irritability

8. A patient who is taking doxazosin for the treatment of hypertension asks whether it is all right to take Advil for arthritis pain. Based on knowledge of the drug, the nurse's best response is:

    A. "You may continue to take the Advil without any problems."

    B. "You should not take Advil because it may cause fluid retention and increase your blood pressure."

    C. "I don't know. I'll have to ask your health care provider."

    D. "You shouldn't take Advil, but you could take Motrin without problems."

9. Which of the following statements made by a patient taking phenytoin indicates understanding of the nurse's teaching?

    A. "I will increase the dose if my seizures don't stop."

    B. "I don't need to contact my health care provider before taking an over-the-counter cold remedy."

    C. "I will take good care of my teeth and see my dentist regularly."

    D. "I cannot take this drug with food."

10. Teaching for patients taking carbamazepine includes which one of the following points?

    A. Use sunscreen and protective clothing when out of doors.

    B. This drug has no significant side effects.

    C. Changes in skin pigmentation are normal and of no concern.

    D. Your urine may turn a harmless blue color.

11. Nutrition teaching regarding foods high in vitamin D and folic acid is necessary for patients taking which of the following anticonvulsant drugs?

    A. Clonazepam and clorazepate

    B. Diazepam and lorazepam

    C. Carbamazepine and valproic acid

    D. Phenytoin and phenobarbital

12. Parent teaching for children taking methylphenidate for ADHD should include which of the following?

    A. Give your child the drug at bedtime.

    B. Drowsiness may be a side effect.

    C. If necessary, the child may take over-the-counter cold products without problems.

    D. Provide for periodic "drug-free" holidays.

13. Patient teaching for prescription drugs containing caffeine should include the information that physical and psychological dependence may occur.

    A. True

    B. False

14. An appropriate clinical indication for the use of amphetamines is:

    A. long-term treatment for obesity.

    B. narcolepsy.

    C. respiratory depression.

    D. hypothyroidism.

DRUGS THAT AFFECT THE RESPIRATORY SYSTEM

OBJECTIVES

1. List the drug classifications used to treat disorders of the respiratory system.

2. Explain the actions, side and adverse effects, interactions, and contraindications of drugs used to treat respiratory disorders.

3. Describe nursing assessment data to be collected when patients are on specific drugs that affect the respiratory tract.

4. Identify nursing actions, including patient teaching, relevant to each major classification of drugs used to treat respiratory disorders.

Anatomy and Physiology of the Respiratory System

The primary function of the respiratory system is to supply oxygen for the metabolic needs of the cells and to remove carbon dioxide, which is a waste product of cell metabolism. The respiratory system also plays a role in regulating the pH of the blood. The process of respiration requires the movement of air into and out of the lungs (ventilation), the exchange of gases between the lungs and the blood (external respiration), transport of gases to and from body tissues, the exchange of gases between blood and tissue cells (internal respiration), and the utilization of oxygen by the cells (cellular respiration).

The major structures of the respiratory system are the nose, pharynx, larynx, trachea, bronchi, and the lungs. Alveoli are tiny air sacs at the ends of bronchioles where external respiration takes place. Movement of the diaphragm and chest muscles alters the diameter of the chest cavity, causing air to flow into and out of the lungs. The thoracic cage formed by the spine, the ribs, and the sternum support and protect the lungs. Breathing is controlled by the respiratory center, which is located in the medulla, part of the brain stem.

Normal function of the respiratory system depends on an adequate oxygen supply, patent airway, sufficient alveolar surface area for gas exchange, adequate blood supply, and hemoglobin to carry oxygen, an intact and flexible rib cage, and stimulation from the breathing center.

Respiratory disorders can interfere with any component of respiration, placing the patient at risk for inadequate oxygenation with resulting impairment in cellular metabolism. For example, bronchial constriction impairs the flow of air into and out of the lungs. In patients with pneumonia, the alveoli fill with infected fluid so that gases cannot be exchanged. Patients with brain stem injuries may lack the stimulus for respirations.

Drugs Used to Treat Respiratory Disorders

Drugs used to treat respiratory disorders work by affecting one of more of the factors needed for normal function. To illustrate, drugs can decrease secretions in the respiratory tract, thin mucoid secretions for easier expectoration, relax constricted bronchi, and block the response to allergens. Classifications included in this chapter are cold remedies, expectorants and mucolytics, antihistamines, bronchodilators, and antiasthmatics.

CHAPTER 22

COLD REMEDIES

*T*he common cold is an upper respiratory infection caused by one of many viruses. Patients typically complain of rhinorrhea (runny nose), sneezing, cough, sore throat, headache, malaise, and myalgia. Fever is more common in children than in adults.

Pharmacologic treatment is symptomatic since there is no specific cure for the common cold. Cold remedies usually consist of some combination of a nasal decongestant, antitussive, analgesic, and an antihistamine. Some remedies contain caffeine to counteract the drowsiness caused by the antihistamine. If these drugs are ineffective, intranasal glucocorticoids may be used to control symptoms of rhinitis. See Chapter 8 for information about analgesics. Other agents employed as cold remedies are discussed here.

NASAL DECONGESTANTS

Nasal decongestants are used to relieve the stuffiness and runny nose associated with colds and rhinitis (inflammation of the nasal mucosa). Nasal decongestants are readily available over the counter, that is, without a prescription. See Table 22–1 for prototype decongestants.

Action and Uses

Nasal decongestants constrict blood vessels in the nasal passages, thereby reducing stuffiness associated with dilated vessels and allowing drainage. Topical preparations act more rapidly and pose less risk of adverse effects than oral preparations. Nasal decongestants are used to treat symptoms associated with colds and allergic rhinitis.

Side and Adverse Effects

Adverse effects of nasal decongestants include rebound congestion, central nervous system stimulation, and systemic vasoconstriction. When topical decongestants are used regu-

larly over a period of time, congestion becomes more and more severe as the effect of each dose wears off. This phenomenon is called *rebound congestion*. With oral decongestants, the patient may experience restlessness, irritability, and insomnia due to central nervous system stimulation. Vasoconstriction can affect blood vessels throughout the body, not just nasal tissues. This effect can raise blood pressure and increase the workload of the heart, causing problems in the patient with hypertension or coronary artery disease.

Nursing Actions

Monitor respiratory status, heart rate, and blood pressure. Assess nasal air flow by occluding one nare at a time and asking the patient to sniff inward through the other nare.

Patient Teaching
• If you have hypertension or a cardiac condition, consult with a physician or pharmacist before using these preparations.
• Cleanse the applicator after each use to avoid introduction of pathogens into the drug container.
• To avoid rebound congestion, limit the use of topical decongestants to 5 days.
• Topical decongestants are packaged for use as drops or sprays. Drops are more effective than sprays.
• Drops are most effective when administered while you are lying down with your head tilted back.
• Oral decongestants have a stimulating effect that may cause you to feel restless and to have difficulty sleeping.

TABLE 22–1

Decongestants

Decongestant	Route	Specific Considerations
phenylephrine (Neo-Synephrine)	Topical, oral (in combination agents)	May cause tachycardia and palpitations. Risk of dysrhythmias with digoxin. Contraindicated with MAO inhibitors. Present in many combination agents.
phenylpropanolamine (Propagest)	Oral	Hemorrhagic stroke may be associated with excessive dosage.
ephedrine	Topical	Significant CNS stimulation.
pseudoephedrine (Afrin, Drixoral)	Oral	Less CNS stimulation than ephedrine.
naphazoline (Privine)	Topical	Can cause severe rebound congestion.

CNS, central nervous system; MAO, monoamine oxidase.

ANTITUSSIVES

Action and Uses

The productive cough is an important mechanism that helps remove secretions and foreign matter from the respiratory tract. However, cough that is nonproductive is tiring and uncomfortable. Antitussives are agents used to reduce coughing. They can act on the cough center located in the medulla of the brain or on the peripheral nervous system. The two main types of antitussives are opioids and nonopioids. See Table 22-2 for prototype antitussives.

Side and Adverse Effects

Opioids, when given alone, are classified under Schedule II of the Controlled Substances Act because of the potential for abuse. Mixed drugs that contain opioids are classified as Schedule V because they have less abuse potential. Opioids can cause severe respiratory depression because of the effects on the central nervous system (CNS). They also may

cause drowsiness, constipation, nausea, and vomiting. Nonopioid antitussives typically have few side effects, which may include sedation, dizziness, and constipation.

Nursing Actions

Assess whether the cough is productive. Document the characteristics of the mucus: amount, color, presence of blood, and consistency. Encourage fluids unless contraindicated to thin secretions for easier expectoration.

Patient Teaching
• A productive cough is protective and should not be suppressed.   • Take safety precautions, since drugs may cause dizziness and drowsiness.   • Mobility, high-fiber foods, and extra fluids (unless contraindicated) reduce the risk of constipation.

TABLE 22–2

Prototype Antitussives

Type	Prototype	Specific Considerations
Opioid	Codeine	Follow policies for storing and administering controlled substance. Dosage for cough is only one-tenth that required for analgesia. Watch for respiratory depression. Excessive respiratory depression is treated with naloxone.
Nonopioid	Dextromethorphan	No potential for abuse. In most cases, just as effective as opioids.

ANTIHISTAMINES

Histamine is a substance released from mast cells and basophils as part of the allergic response or other physiologic mechanism. The two types of receptors that can receive histamine are called H_1 and H_2 receptors. H_2 stimulation is evident in the secretion of gastric acid, and so will be addressed in Chapter 34. H_1 stimulation results in dilation of small blood vessels, increased capillary permeability, bronchoconstriction, itching and pain, mucus secretion, and sedation. See Table 22–3 for antihistamine prototypes.

Action and Uses

The release of histamine and the subsequent physiologic responses explain many signs and symptoms of respiratory disorders. Therefore, antihistamines are commonly indicated for patients with such conditions. They are useful in the treatment of motion sickness, insomnia, and other allergies in addition to those affecting the respiratory tract. Antihistamines that block H_1 receptors are called *H_1 receptor antagonists*. These are the agents we commonly think of as "antihistamines." H_2 receptor antagonists block H_2 receptors and are discussed in Chapter 34.

Side and Adverse Effects

Antihistamines are classified as first- or second-generation with the important difference being that sedation is common with first-generation agents, but not with second-generation agents. As you might suspect, this is because first-generation antihistamines cross the blood-brain barrier, whereas second-generation antihistamines do not. Other CNS effects which are more common in the elderly are dizziness, confusion, and fatigue.

Antihistamines exert mild anticholinergic effects characterized by dry mouth, constipation, and a risk for urinary retention and palpitations. Other gastrointestinal effects can include nausea, vomiting, anorexia, and diarrhea.

Two second-generation antihistamines, astemizole and terfenadine, caused fatal dysrhythmias in some people and are no longer used. This occurred when patients consumed excessive amounts of the drug or were unable to metabolize the drug normally. Metabolism could have been impaired by liver disease and by interaction with some other drugs, specifically erythromycin, clarithromycin, ketoconazole, and itraconazole.

Nursing Actions

Since most antihistamines are available over the counter, patient teaching is important.

Patient Teaching

- Avoid potentially hazardous activities if drowsiness occurs.
- If mixed with alcohol or other drugs that depress the CNS, antihistamines may cause excessive sedation.
- Check with the physician or pharmacist before taking antihistamines with antibiotics.
- Sipping liquids or sucking hard sugar-free candy may relieve mouth dryness.
- If you have prostate enlargement, antihistamines may cause you to have more difficulty urinating.
- Increased fluids, physical activity, and fiber may minimize constipation.
- If you have nausea, vomiting, diarrhea, or constipation, try taking the drug with meals.
- These drugs are contraindicated in the third trimester of pregnancy and in breastfeeding mothers.

TABLE 22–3

Antihistamines

Type	Prototype(s)	Specific Considerations
First Generation		
Alkylamines	brompheniramine (Dimetane), chlorpheniramine (Chlor-Trimeton)	Least sedating of the first-generation antihistamines
Ethanolamines	clemastine (Tavist), diphenhydramine (Benadryl)	One of the most sedating
Ethylenediamines	pyrilamine (Nisaval)	
Phenothiazines	promethazine (Phenergan)	One of the most sedating
Piperidines	cyproheptadine (Periactin)	
Second Generation	cetirizine (Zyrtec) fexofenadine (Allegra) loratadine (Claritin)	None cause sedation. Can be taken with meals.

Lehne, R. A. (1998). *Pharmacology for Nursing Care*, 3rd ed. Philadelphia: W. B. Saunders, p. 692.

INTRANASAL GLUCOCORTICOIDS

When symptoms of allergic rhinitis do not respond to other drugs, intranasal glucocorticoids may be ordered. Systemic glucocorticoid therapy is discussed in Chapter 43 and carries a number of risks with long-term therapy. At recommended doses, the intranasal preparation poses little risk. The anti-inflammatory action eliminates rhinorrhea, sneezing, and nasal itching. If excessive drying of the nasal mucosa occurs, the patient may have a burning sensation. Examples of glucocorticoids for intranasal use are beclomethasone (Beconase), budesonide (Rhinocort), dexamethasone (Decadron Phosphate, Turbinaire), flunisolide (Nasalide), fluticasone (Flonase), and triamcinolone (Nasacort). Beclomethasone and flonase are the least irritating.

Intranasal glucorticoids are administered via a metered inhaler one to four times a day until symptoms are controlled. Tell the patient that it takes 1 to 3 weeks for maximal effect. The dosage will then be reduced as low as possible while still achieving the effects.

CHAPTER 23

MUCOLYTICS AND EXPECTORANTS

EXPECTORANTS

As the name suggests, expectorants facilitate the removal of mucus from the respiratory tract. Examples of drugs used for this purpose are guaifenesin (Anti-Tuss, Robitussin), terpin hydrate, and potassium iodide. Only guaifenesin is addressed here.

Action and Uses

Expectorants cause respiratory secretions to be thinner and more readily cleared from the respiratory tract.

Side and Adverse Effects

Adverse effects of guaifenesin are dizziness, headache, and rash. Toxic effects include nausea and vomiting.

Nursing Actions

Assess the patient's ability to expectorate secretions. Auscultate breath sounds.

Since patients can obtain this medication over the counter, patient teaching is the most important nursing activity.

Patient Teaching
• Seek medical care if the symptoms persist for more than 1 week.
• Guaifenesin is not intended to treat cough caused by smoking or chronic respiratory disorders.
• If you feel dizzy, avoid driving and other possibly hazardous activities.

MUCOLYTICS

Actions and Uses

Mucolytics are used to thin mucus so that it can be more readily removed from the respiratory tract. One preparation employed for this purpose is acetylcysteine (Mucomyst), which is given by inhalation. Acetylcysteine breaks down mucus, which reduces its viscosity so that it is more readily removed by coughing, postural drainage, or suctioning.

Side and Adverse Effects

The only serious adverse effect of acetylcysteine is bronchospasm, which is constriction of the bronchi that interferes with movement of gases into and out of the lungs.

Nursing Actions

If the patient experiences wheezing during a treatment, the treatment should be stopped and a bronchodilator administered. Have suction equipment on hand during treatments in case the patient is unable to expectorate the secretions.

CHAPTER 24

BRONCHODILATORS

*B*ronchospasm is constriction of the bronchi, a symptom that occurs in asthma, chronic obstructive pulmonary disease, and acute allergic responses. It interferes with ventilation and, if severe, is life-threatening. Drug classifications employed to treat bronchospasm include methylxanthines, sympathomimetics, and inhaled muscarinics. See Table 24–1 for prototype bronchodilators.

ACTIONS AND USES

Bronchodilators relieve bronchospasm by various mechanisms that permit relaxation of the bronchial smooth muscle. In addition to bronchodilation, sympathomimetics decrease mucus secretion, increase mucus clearance by cilia, and stabilize mast cells. Mast cells are the source of histamine and other chemicals that trigger the inflammatory response. "Stabilizing" them decreases the output of these chemicals.

SIDE AND ADVERSE EFFECTS

Side effects are most prominent with methylxanthines and sympathomimetics because they have important systemic actions.

Methylxanthines

Methylxanthines stimulate the central nervous system (CNS) and thus they may cause irritability, headache, insomnia, and tremors. Cardiovascular effects include tachycardia, palpitations, and hypotension. At toxic levels, seizures and fatal cardiac dysrhythmias may occur. The effects on the gastrointestinal system may include nausea, vomiting, diarrhea, and epigastric pain.

Sympathomimetics

You may recall that sympathomimetics act on adrenergic receptors. Adrenergic receptors in the bronchi are primarily β_2 receptors, whereas receptors in the heart are primarily β_1 receptors. When treating bronchospasm, sympathomimetics that exert effects primarily on the bronchi with minimal cardiac effects are preferred. Such drugs are said to be selective β_2 agonists. Even selective β_2 agonists often produce some cardiac effects, so there is a potential for tachycardia, cardiac dysrhythmias, hypertension, and palpitations. Side and adverse effects of selective β_2 agonists related to CNS stimulation may include nervousness, anxiety, headache, and insomnia. Sympathetic stimulation also tends to raise the blood glucose, an important consideration in the patient with diabetes.

Inhaled Muscarinics

Inhaled muscarinics are not well absorbed, so they have fewer side effects than sympathomimetics or methylxanthines. These drugs may increase intraocular pressure in patients with narrow-angle glaucoma. Though rare, hypotension may also occur.

NURSING ACTIONS

When patients are receiving bronchodilators, monitor breath sounds, respiratory rate, heart rate, and blood pressure. A positive therapeutic effect is reflected in less wheezing, normal respiratory and heart rates, and decreased patient anxiety. Assess for adverse effects as appropriate, especially cardiac and CNS stimulation.

Patient Teaching

- A metered-dose inhaler with a spacer is preferred (see the Metered-Dose Inhalers box).
- Use only as directed; excessive use may cause bronchospasm.
- Keep appointments for follow-up care as recommended.

Metered-Dose Inhalers

Use: Administration of drugs by inhalation
Equipment: Metered-dose Inhaler: Canister (a) and Spacer (b)

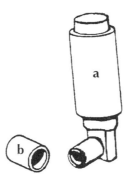

From Monahan (1998). *Medical-Surgical Nursing: Foundations for Clinical Practice*, 2nd ed. Philadelphia: W.B. Saunders, p. 661.

Procedure:

With Spacer	**Without Spacer**
1. Shake canister to mix medication. 2. Holding the canister upside down, place the mouthpiece in the mouth. 3. Exhale. 4. Press the canister to dispense the medication toward the open mouth while inhaling deeply and slowly. 5. Remove the mouthpiece from the mouth, hesitate, then exhale slowly. 6. Wash and dry the mouthpiece.	1. Hold the canister at least two fingerbreadths from the open mouth. 2. Exhale. 3. Press the canister to dispense the medication while inhaling deeply. 4. Close the mouth, hesitate briefly, and exhale.

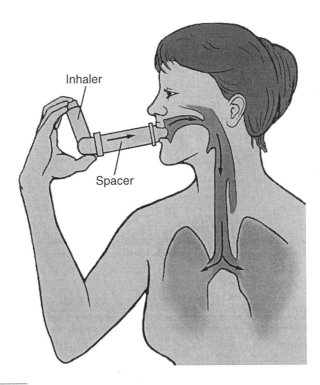

Inhaler

Spacer

From Edmunds (1995). *Introduction to Clinical Pharmacology*, 2nd ed. St. Louis: Mosby, p. 88.

TABLE 24–1

Bronchodilators

Type	Prototype	Specific Considerations
Methylxanthine	theophylline (Theo-Dur)	Periodic blood levels must be assessed to be sure the drug is within the therapeutic range (10–20 mg/mL). For peak levels, draw blood 1 hour after IV dose, 1–2 hours after immediate oral forms, 3–8 hours after extended release forms. Draw specimen for trough level just before next dose. Check lab reports. Effects diminished by cigarette or marijuana smoking. Check for drug-drug interactions.
Sympathomimetic (beta adrenergic agonist)	albuterol (Proventil) and terbutaline (Brethine)	Monitor respiratory, cardiac, and neurologic status. Teach patient proper use of inhaler, not to use more than two inhalations at a time, and to rinse the mouth after inhalation. Explain that overuse can cause bronchospasm.
Inhaled muscarinic agent	ipratropium bromide (Atrovent)	Teach patient proper use of inhaler, not to use more than two inhalations at a time. Monitor respiratory status.

ANTIASTHMATICS

*A*sthma is a condition characterized by recurrent episodes of wheezing (whistling sound in constricted airways) and dyspnea (shortness of breath). Various factors can precipitate asthma attacks, but the basic pathologic process is inflammation with bronchoconstriction. Attacks can be triggered by exposure to allergens (substances to which the person has developed antibodies) or to infectious bacteria or viruses. The allergic response occurs when mast cells release chemical mediators that increase capillary permeability, dilate blood vessels, and cause contraction of smooth muscle in the bronchi. Exercise, emotional stress, and changes in environmental temperature or humidity may also serve as triggers.

Bronchodilators, discussed in the previous chapter, are used to relieve constriction. Other agents are intended to prevent asthmatic attacks. The three primary types of preventive agents are mast cell stabilizers, leukotriene inhibitors, and inhaled corticosteroids.

MAST CELL STABILIZERS

Action and Uses

When a patient is exposed to allergens, mast cell stabilizers prevent the release of chemical mediators that trigger bronchial constriction and increased capillary permeability. Mast cell stabilizers are useful only in preventing acute attacks, not in treating them. The prototype is cromolyn sodium (Intal). Forms include an oral concentrate and capsules for inhalation and a solution for nebulization, an aerosol spray, a nasal spray, oral capsules (intended to be swallowed), and an ophthalmic solution.

Side and Adverse Effects

When inhaled, cromolyn sodium can cause cough, nasal congestion, throat irritation, wheezing, and bronchospasm. The oral preparation can cause pruritus, nausea, diarrhea, and muscle aches.

Patient Teaching

- If the oral inhalation form used, learn how to use the inhaler (see Box).
- Take the drug exactly as prescribed.
- This drug is used to prevent acute attacks, not stop them. In fact, it is ineffective to relieve bronchospasm.
- Capsules that contain the drug for use in the inhaler are not intended for oral ingestion.
- Rinsing the mouth after using the inhaler decreases irritation of the mouth and throat.

LEUKOTRIENE INHIBITORS

Leukotrienes are substances that, like histamine, mediate the inflammatory response. In the asthma patient, the inflammatory response includes edema, mucus secretion, and bronchoconstriction. The two drugs that inhibit leukotrienes are zafirlukast (Accolate) and zileuton (Zyflo).

Actions and Uses

Zafirlukast blocks leukotriene receptors and zileuton interferes with the synthesis of leukotrienes.

Side and Adverse Effects

Zafirlukast may cause headache, nausea, diarrhea, and infection. Side and adverse effects of zileuton are headache, pain, nausea, and elevated liver enzymes.

Patient Teaching

With zafirlukast:
- Take on an empty stomach.
- If also taking inhaled corticosteroids, there is increased risk of upper respiratory infections.

With zileuton:
- Keep follow-up appointments to assess liver function.
- May be taken with or without food.

INHALED CORTICOSTEROIDS

Corticosteroids are very effective in suppressing the inflammation characteristic of asthma. However, long-term use of systemic corticosteroids puts the patient at risk for many serious adverse effects, as described in Chapter 43. Therefore, systemic use is typically limited to short periods of time. Inhaled corticosteroids, on the other hand, can be used safely on a regular basis when taken as prescribed. Examples of corticosteroids for inhalation are beclomethasone (Beclovent, Vanceril), dexamethasone (Dexacort Phosphate), flunisolide (AeroBid), fluticasone (Flovent), and triamcinolone (Azmacort)

Action and Uses

Corticosteroids reduce inflammation and the tendency of the bronchi to constrict with chronic asthma.

Side and Adverse Effects

With inhaled corticosteroids, hoarseness and oral candidiasis are the most common adverse effects. Prolonged use of oral corticosteroids can suppress the normal production of glucocorticoids by the body, lead to glucose intolerance, and cause weight gain, increased blood pressure, loss of bone mass, cataracts, and decreased ability to resist infection.

Nursing Actions

Monitor pulmonary status. Assess response to drug therapy. Instruct patients in proper use of the inhaler and emphasize the value of using a spacer, which improves distribution of the medication in the lungs.

Patient Teaching
• Inhaled glucocorticoids are not effective in stopping an acute asthma attack. • To be effective as a preventive agent, the inhaled medication should be taken regularly rather than PRN. • If both a bronchodilator and a glucocorticoid are ordered, use the bronchodilator first to dilate the airways and permit better distribution of the glucocorticoid in the lungs. • Report pain and lesions in the oral cavity, as this may be a fungal infection (candidiasis) related to steroid inhalation. Rinsing the mouth after using the inhaler will reduce the risk of oral candidiasis.

REVIEW QUESTIONS: UNIT 7

Case Study

Ms. Kellogg has chronic obstructive pulmonary disease (see the Care Plan in Chapter 29 of the textbook) and has been admitted to the hospital because of worsening symptoms. She uses an Atrovent inhaler 2 puffs QID. The following questions relate to this patient.

1. The primary reason Ms. Kellogg is given Atrovent is to _____.

2. True or False? Atrovent is effective in treating acute bronchospasm.

3. Ms. Kellogg complains that her mouth is dry. What could you suggest that might help?

4. Based on her health history, identify one reason Atrovent would be preferred over a sympathomimetic bronchodilator for Ms. Kellogg.

5. Ms. Kellogg's physician changes her bronchodilator to albuterol sulfate (Proventil), a selective B_2 agonist. What is the advantage of a selective B_2 agonist over other sympathomimetics?

6. Ms. Kellogg's hospital roommate, Martha Washington, age 17, is recovering after an acute asthma attack. She has been treating herself with over-the-counter bronchodilators. On admission, she was agitated and her pulse was 120. What could explain this?

7. Martha is started on zafirlukast (Accolate). What is the classification of this drug?

8. On discharge, Martha says "Can I take a zafirlukast tablet whenever I have trouble breathing?" What should you tell her?

9. Martha's brother also has asthma, but he uses an inhaled corticosteroid along with an inhaled bronchodilator. Which should he use first, and why?

10. True or False? Inhaled corticosteroids pose the same risk of serious side effects as oral corticosteroids.

DRUGS THAT AFFECT THE HEMATOLOGIC AND IMMUNOLOGIC SYSTEMS

OBJECTIVES

1. Identify the classifications of drugs that affect hematologic and immunologic function.

2. List the most common uses, side and adverse effects, contraindications, and interactions for hematologic and immunologic agents.

3. Identify nursing actions and patient teaching for people who are taking hematologic and immunologic agents.

CHAPTER 26

HEMATOLOGIC AGENTS

*T*he body has effective mechanisms that protect against excessive bleeding and the formation of potentially dangerous thrombi (clots) in the vascular system. This requires a balance between factors that cause coagulation and factors that inhibit it. An understanding of blood coagulation is basic to understanding the drugs presented in this chapter.

When bleeding occurs, the body prevents excessive blood loss through hemostasis, which involves platelet aggregation and clot formation (Figure 26–1). Affected blood vessels constrict to reduce the amount of bleeding. Platelets (thrombocytes) that are circulating in the blood become sticky, cling together (aggregation), and create plugs to seal the injured vessel. The platelet cell membranes dissolve, spilling chemicals (including thromboplastin) that participate in clot formation. Thromboplastin activates prothrombin which is converted to thrombin. In the presence of calcium ions, thrombin acts on fibrinogen to convert it to fibrin. Fibrin threads form a mesh, which forms clots by trapping blood cells and platelets.

FIGURE 26–1

Hemostasis

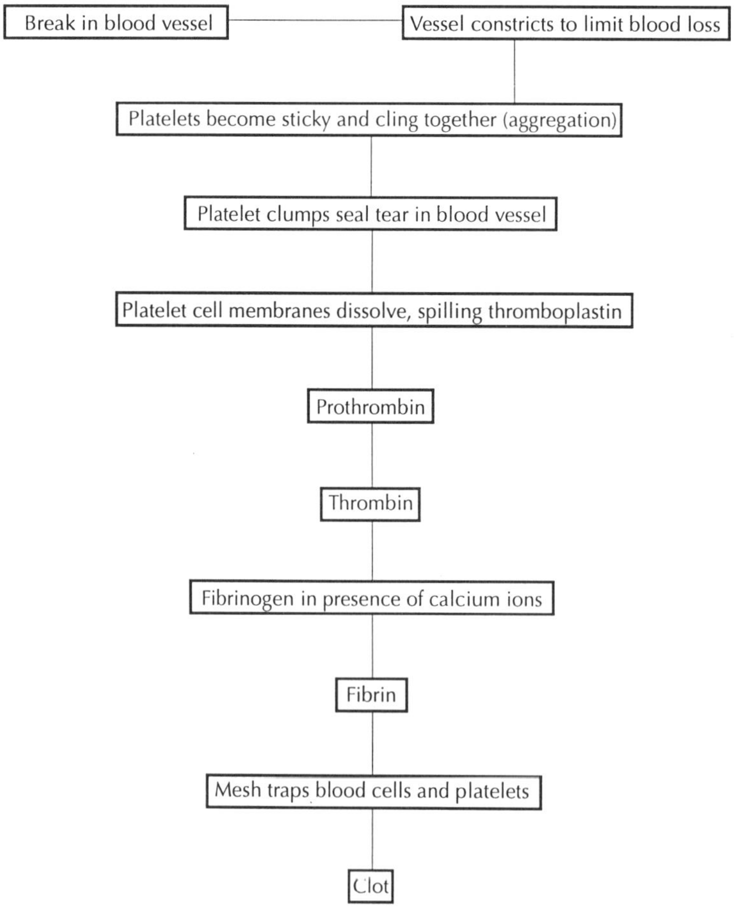

Break in blood vessel — Vessel constricts to limit blood loss

Platelets become sticky and cling together (aggregation)

Platelet clumps seal tear in blood vessel

Platelet cell membranes dissolve, spilling thromboplastin

Prothrombin

Thrombin

Fibrinogen in presence of calcium ions

Fibrin

Mesh traps blood cells and platelets

Clot

Conditions that cause inappropriate clot formation pose a threat because the clots can travel through the bloodstream and lodge in small vessels, obstructing blood flow. Deprived of oxygen and nutrients, tissue beyond the obstruction dies. Factors that increase the risk of undesirable clot formation include atherosclerosis, stasis of blood flow, and venous inflammation (phlebitis). Conditions that interfere with normal coagulation and put the patient at risk for excessive bleeding include thrombocytopenia (platelet deficiency) and conditions like hemophilia in which there are deficiencies of some blood clotting factors. This chapter will introduce drugs used to prevent or treat undesirable clot formation: anticoagulants, thrombolytics, and antiplatelet agents. It will also address some of the agents used in the treatment of blood disorders.

ANTICOAGULANTS

Anticoagulants prevent formation of new clots and extension of existing clots; they do not dissolve existing clots. Commonly used anticoagulants act by preventing the synthesis of certain clotting factors or inactivating them. Clinical conditions that may be treated with these drugs include thrombophlebitis, deep vein thrombosis, and pulmonary embolism. Anticoagulants are used to prevent *venous* thrombosis, whereas prevention of *arterial* thrombosis more appropriately employs antiplatelet agents. The two anticoagulant agents most often used are heparin and warfarin (Coumadin).

Heparin

The most widely used form of heparin is heparin sodium. There is a calcium form as well.

Actions and Uses

Heparin inactivates selected clotting factors, thereby suppressing the formation of fibrin, the substance that provides the framework for clots in the veins. This is the reason it is most effective in preventing venous thrombosis. Other conditions that may be treated with heparin are pulmonary embolism and evolving stroke. It is the drug of choice when rapid anticoagulation is required. Patients having open heart surgery or renal dialysis are given heparin to prevent clot formation as the blood circulates through machines for oxygenation or detoxification. Other surgical patients who are at high risk for venous thrombosis may be given prophylactic (preventive) low-dose heparin. Disseminated intravascular coagulation (DIC), which is characterized by extensive clot formation *and* bleeding tendencies, may also be treated with heparin.

Heparin is given subcutaneously or intravenously and has a rapid onset and a brief duration of action.

Side and Adverse Effects

The principal complication of heparin therapy is bleeding. Other adverse effects are thrombocytopenia and allergic responses. Local tissue irritation may occur at the site of subcutaneous injections.

Interactions and Contraindications

The effects of heparin are increased by a variety of drugs including aspirin, dipyridamole, ticlopidine, and warfarin. Examples of drugs that decrease heparin effects are antihistamines, digitalis, tetracycline, and protamine sulfate. Because of its action, protamine sulfate is used as an antidote for heparin. It is very important to maintain heparin within the therapeutic range to prevent abnormal clot formation while avoiding potentially serious bleeding. Therefore, you must always be aware of ALL drugs the patient is taking and any potential interactions.

Heparin is contraindicated with uncontrolled bleeding, thrombocytopenia, lumbar puncture, and regional anesthesia. Although it may be used postoperatively in some situations, it should not be given during or immediately after surgery of the eye, brain, or spinal cord.

Nursing Actions

Change needles after drawing up the medication. When giving subcutaneous heparin, use a 26 gauge ½ or ⅝ inch needle to minimize trauma, and avoid intramuscular injection. A tuberculin syringe permits accurate dosage measurement. Do not aspirate. To prevent local bleeding, apply gentle pressure to, but do not massage, the injection site. Traditionally, the abdomen (not within 2 inches of the umbilicus) has been used as the site for subcutaneous heparin injection. Some research suggests that the arm or thigh could be used as well, but this is not common practice (Fahs & Kinney, 1991).

Monitor the activated partial thromboplastin time (aPPT), which is measured by laboratory testing of blood samples. When heparin is within the therapeutic range, the aPPT should be 1.5 to 2.5 times normal. Normal aPPT is 30 to 40 seconds. While the dosage is being adjusted, aPPT should be measured every 4 to 6 hours. Once the target aPPT is reached and stabilized, daily measurements will suffice.

Assess for signs of bleeding: bruising, petechiae, increasing pulse, decreasing blood pressure, anxiety, restlessness, and unexplained pain. Excessive anticoagulation with heparin is treated with protamine sulfate.

Patient Teaching

- While on heparin, you will bleed more easily. To prevent serious injury and bleeding:
  - avoid potentially harmful activities such as contact sports.
  - avoid walking barefoot.
  - use an electric razor.
  - use a soft toothbrush.
- If you have any superficial bleeding, apply pressure for 3 to 5 minutes or until bleeding stops.
- Notify your physician if you have any signs of bleeding, including very easy bruising, bleeding gums, black or maroon stools, reddish urine, headache, or pain in the abdomen or back.
- It is important to have periodic blood tests to be sure your heparin is at a safe level.
- Always inform a new physician or dentist that you are on heparin.
- Do not take any over-the-counter drugs without your physician's approval.
- Always wear a medical tag that indicates you are on anticoagulants; also carry an identification card with details about your specific drug and dosage.

Low-Molecular-Weight Heparins

In addition to the standard heparin sodium, there are low-molecular-weight heparins available. Low-molecular-weight (LMW) heparins have several advantages over heparin sodium. They can be used at home because they can be given on a fixed dose schedule and do not require aPPT testing. LMW heparins are much more expensive than standard heparin, but the patient is saved the cost of aPPT monitoring. Two LMW heparins are enoxaparin (Lovenox) and dalteparin (Fragmin).

LMW heparins are primarily used to prevent deep vein thrombosis after hip replacement surgery or high-risk abdominal surgery. Plasma levels are relatively stable with LMW heparins compared to standard heparin. Although bleeding is the most serious adverse effect of LMW heparins, it occurs less often than with standard heparin.

Warfarin

Warfarin (Coumadin) and anisindione (Miradon) are oral anticoagulants. Of the two, warfarin has a much lower incidence of serious side effects and is therefore more widely used.

Actions and Uses

Warfarin inhibits coagulation by antagonizing vitamin K, one of the components needed for synthesis of several clot-ting factors. Warfarin can be used for long-term therapy to prevent venous thrombosis and pulmonary embolism, thromboembolism in people with prosthetic heart valves, and thrombosis associated with atrial fibrillation. Initial effects are not evident until 8 to 12 hours after therapy is begun, and several days are required to achieve peak effects.

Side and Adverse Effects

As one would expect, bleeding is the most serious complication of warfarin therapy. If bleeding occurs, the patient is given vitamin K to counteract the anticoagulation. Other adverse effects are not common but include alopecia (hair loss), gastrointestinal disturbances, dermatitis, and urticaria (hives). Warfarin can impart a red-orange color to the urine, which may be mistaken for blood. Unlike heparin, warfarin crosses the placental barrier and can cause fetal hemorrhage, death, and deformities.

Interactions and Contraindications

The effects of warfarin can be increased by antibiotics, oral hypoglycemics, antineoplastics, heparin, antiplatelet agents including aspirin, allopurinol, anabolic steroids, cimetidine, isoniazid, and tricyclic antidepressants.

The effects of warfarin are decreased by barbiturates, phenytoin, vitamin K, diuretics, and oral contraceptives. Also, absorption is impaired by antacids, cholestyramine, and colestipol.

Warfarin is contraindicated with uncontrolled bleeding and severe thrombocytopenia. Other contraindications are lumbar puncture; surgery of the eye, brain, or spinal cord; and conditions that pose a high risk for bleeding such as gastrointestinal ulcers. The risk of fetal malformation and death contraindicates the use of warfarin during pregnancy. **Pregnancy Category X.**

Nursing Actions

Warfarin is given orally. During the time when the ideal dosage is being determined, blood samples are drawn daily and dosages are based on the prothrombin time (PT). Results are reported in terms of an international normalized ratio (INR). With effective anticoagulation, the target INR is usually between 2 and 3, although it is sometimes as high as 4.5. When the results are obtained, the physician is notified and an order for the next warfarin dose obtained. As with heparin, assess for any abnormal bleeding.

Patient Teaching

- Patient teaching is essentially the same as for heparin.

THROMBOLYTICS

Actions and Uses

Thrombolytics (clot dissolvers) are used to break down clots that have already formed. They work by converting plasminogen to plasmin, which is an enzyme that breaks down fibrin. Thrombolytics are used in the treatment of acute myocardial infarction, deep vein thrombosis, and massive pulmonary emboli.

Side and Adverse Effects

The adverse effect common to all thrombolytics is bleeding. Effects specific to each agent are noted in Table 26–1.

TABLE 26–1

Thrombolytics

Prototype	Specific Considerations
streptokinase (Kabikinase, Streptase)	Can be given IV to treat pulmonary embolism, deep vein thrombosis, and arterial thrombosis or embolism. To treat myocardial infarction, the drug may be infused into the affected coronary artery through a catheter. Adverse effects: Allergic reactions that usually respond to antihistamines. May cause significant hypotension that is not related to bleeding or allergic reactions. Fever is common; is treated with acetaminophen. Is the least expensive thrombolytic.
alteplase (tPA, Activase)	Used for acute myocardial infarction, pulmonary embolism, and ischemic stroke. Adverse effects: Compared with streptokinase, poses greater risk of intracranial bleeding, does not cause allergic reactions or hypotension, is much more expensive. Monitor for changes in neurologic status.
reteplase (Retavase)	Used to treat acute myocardial infarction. Administered IV: bolus dose followed by infusion. Do not infuse through a line that contains heparin.
anistreplase (Eminase)	Used to treat acute myocardial infarction. Administered by slow intravenous injection. Adverse effects: Allergic reactions and hypotension unrelated to allergy or bleeding.
urokinase (Abbokinase)	Used to treat acute myocardial infarction and deep vein thrombosis; to clear IV catheters. Administered per IV infusion.

Interactions and Contraindications

The risk of bleeding is enhanced by anticoagulants and antiplatelet agents. Thrombolytics are contraindicated with active bleeding, aortic dissection, acute pericarditis, cerebral neoplasm, cerebral vascular disease, and a history of intracranial bleeding.

Nursing Actions

Monitor for signs of bleeding: increasing pulse, decreasing blood pressure, restlessness. Note hematocrit, aPPT, PT, fibrinogen level, and platelet count before and after therapy. Handle the patient gently. Avoid invasive procedures, including intramuscular and subcutaneous injections. If bleeding occurs from a superficial wound, apply direct pressure. If severe bleeding occurs, anticipate orders to discontinue the thrombolytics and to administer whole blood or blood products. Intravenous aminocaproic acid (Amicar) may be ordered to block the action of thrombolytics.

Patients who are receiving thrombolytics are acutely ill, and should be given simple explanations of the therapy.

ANTIPLATELET AGENTS

Antiplatelet drugs include aspirin, ticlopidine (Ticlid), dipyridamole (Persantine), and abciximad (ReoPro).

Actions and Uses

Antiplatelet drugs help control clot formation by preventing platelets from clumping. This clumping of platelets, called *platelet aggregation*, is a key factor in the development of arterial thrombi. The primary antiplatelet agent, aspirin, exerts this effect when given in low doses (less than 325 mg/day). The antiplatelet action is achieved by suppression of synthesis of TXA_2, a substance that causes platelet aggregation. Higher doses of aspirin also inhibit the synthesis of prostacyclin, which normally suppresses aggregation. Therefore, higher aspirin doses elicit effects that cancel each other out.

Antiplatelet drugs are used most often to prevent arterial thrombosis. Aspirin is used specifically for the primary prevention of myocardial infarction (MI), to prevent additional infarction after acute myocardial infarction, and to prevent strokes in people who have had transient ischemic attacks (considered an "early warning" of future stroke).

Side and Adverse Effects

Specific adverse effects of the antiplatelet agents vary and are noted in Table 26–2.

TABLE 26–2

Antiplatelet Agents

Prototype	Specific Considerations
aspirin (acetylsalicylic acid, ASA)	Used to prevent initial MI, reinfarction after acute MI, and stroke in high-risk patients. Can take with milk or food if gastrointestinal distress occurs. Risk of ototoxicity, especially if given with other ototoxic drugs. Tell patient to report ringing in the ears (tinnitus) or problems with balance. **Pregnancy Category D** due to potential harm to fetus. ⚠
dipyridamole (Persantine)	Used to prevent thromboembolism after heart valve replacement. Take PO form on empty stomach with full glass of water. Can cause dizziness, headache, nausea, flushing, weakness/syncope, gastrointestinal distress, rash. No significant contraindications.
ticlopidine (Ticlid)	Used to prevent stroke. Give with food or after meals. Commonly causes diarrhea, nausea, heartburn, rash, gastrointestinal distress. Occasionally causes neutropenia and rarely agranulocytosis, so blood count should be monitored every 2 weeks during first 3 months of therapy. Blood cell counts typically return to normal once drug is discontinued.
abciximab (ReoPro)	Used in combination with aspirin and heparin to prevent reocclusion of blood vessels after percutaneous transluminal coronary angioplasty, a procedure done to open blocked coronary arteries. Many contraindications. Can cause hypotension, nausea, vomiting, bradycardia, pain in extremities, and allergic reactions. Handle patient gently. Stop infusion if serious bleeding occurs.

MI, myocardial infarction.

Interactions and Contraindications

In general, antiplatelet agents should not be given with anticoagulants or thrombolytics because of the increased risk of bleeding. Drugs that can cause gastric ulceration (such as nonsteroidal anti-inflammatory drugs and alcohol) may contribute to bleeding when patients are on drugs that affect coagulation.

Contraindications include disorders that predispose the patient to bleeding, and gastrointestinal bleeding or ulceration. Other contraindications specific to each agent are noted in Table 26–2.

Nursing Actions

Monitor for signs of bleeding. Inspect the skin for bruising and petechiae (small purple-red spots caused by hemorrhage into the skin). Note maroon or black stools and reddish or smoky urine, which are all signs of internal bleeding. Document vital signs, watching for increasing pulse and decreasing blood pressure.

Patient Teaching

- This drug can cause bleeding, so notify your physician immediately if that occurs.
- Do not exceed the recommended dosage of aspirin.
- Do not take any other drugs, including over-the-counter drugs, without physician approval.

MISCELLANEOUS HEMATOLOGIC AGENTS

Miscellaneous drugs used for hematologic disorders include hematopoietic growth factors and drugs used for deficiency anemias.

Hematopoietic Growth Factors

The production of blood cells, called *hematopoiesis*, is in part regulated by hematopoietic growth factors. There are three hematopoietic growth factors available.

Hematopoietic growth factors are used to stimulate recovery of bone marrow after transplantation, to stimulate red blood cell production with chronic renal failure, and to stimulate neutrophil production after chemotherapy for cancer. Information about these agents is presented in Table 26–3.

TABLE 26-3

Hematopoietic Growth Factors

Factor	Uses and Adverse Effects	Specific Considerations
epoetin alfa (Epogen, Procrit)	Used to treat anemia associated with chronic renal failure, zidovudine (AZT) therapy, or chemotherapy. Adverse effects: hypertension, headache, arthralgia (joint pain). Patients on AZT often have fever, pulmonary congestion and dyspnea, and skin reactions at injection site.	Comes in single-dose vial; discard unused portion. Do not shake vial. Monitor for increased BP. Explain importance of follow-up blood studies. Monitor respiratory status in patients on AZT.
filgrastim (Neupogen)	Used to treat neutropenia. Adverse effects: bone pain, elevated white blood cell count, and increased serum levels of uric acid, lactate dehydrogenase, and alkaline phosphatase; spleen enlargement with long-term therapy; adult respiratory distress syndrome in patients with sepsis.	Comes in single-dose vial; unused portion must be discarded. Do not shake vial. Monitor respiratory status in patients who have infections. Emphasize to patient the need for frequent blood studies during therapy.
sargramostim (Leukine)	Used after bone marrow transplant to stimulate bone marrow recovery. Enhances actions of neutrophils and during administration, macrophages. Adverse effects: diarrhea, weakness, rash, malaise, fluid retention, bone pain, cardiac dysrhythmias. With very high doses: pleural and pericardial effusion. Can cause excessive elevations in leukocytes and platelets.	Comes in single-dose vial; discard unused portion. Do not shake vial; gently swirl to mix. Monitor for dysrhythmias and dyspnea especially if patient has cardiac or respiratory disease. Assess fluid status.

CHAPTER 27

IMMUNOLOGIC AGENTS

THE IMMUNE SYSTEM

Structures and Components of the Immune System

The immune system protects the body against infection by isolating and destroying pathogens. Structures and components that make up the immune system include the bone marrow, lymph fluid, lymphatic system, lymph nodes, spleen, thymus, stem cells, white blood cells, macrophages, eosinophils, basophils, mast cells, B cells, T cells, cytokines, and eicosanoids.

The bone marrow is the site of manufacture of white blood cells. Lymph fluid is a mixture of white blood cells and plasma that is collected from the tissues and returned to the venous system via tubes that make up the lymphatic system. Lymph nodes are small masses of tissue scattered along the lymphatic pathways. Nodes filter microorganisms. They may become enlarged and tender with infection and with some cancers. The spleen also filters microorganisms and destroys them.

The thymus produces T cells until puberty, when it ceases to be needed for this process. Stem cells, located in the bone marrow and the blood, are precursor cells that can develop into white blood cells, red blood cells, or platelets. White blood cells include neutrophils, lymphocytes, eosinophils, basophils, and monocytes. These cells destroy microorganisms and, in the process, are destroyed themselves. Macrophages are cells that remove the debris left by the dead cells. Mast cells store histamine, which is released in response to foreign protein as part of the inflammatory response. B cells play an important role in the production of antibodies, and T cells secrete hormones, called *cytokines*, that facilitate the immune response. Eicosanoids regulate various aspects of the immune response, including vasodilation, temperature elevation, and activation of white blood cells.

Immunity

Innate (natural) immunity is a generalized response to any foreign substance, including microorganisms. One way innate immunity protects the body is by the inflammatory re-

sponse. Inflammation is characterized by vasodilation and increased capillary permeability, which increase the flow of plasma to the affected tissues and delivers white blood cells.

Whereas innate immunity responds in the same way to any invader, acquired immunity responds only to a specific pathogen or other foreign protein. There are two types of acquired immunity: antibody-mediated and cell-mediated. Antibodies are produced by plasma cells when the body is first exposed to an antigen, usually a pathogenic organism. If the antigen enters the body again, memory B cells produce large amounts of the antibody. Antibodies bind to pathogens, making them recognizable to white blood cells, which move in to destroy them.

Cell-mediated immunity is directed toward viruses and cancer cells rather than pathogens. It is cell-mediated immunity that causes the body to reject transplanted tissue.

DISORDERS OF THE IMMUNOLOGIC SYSTEM

Any disorder of the immunologic system can put the patient at risk for overwhelming infection. Disorders that affect white blood cells include neutropenia and leukemia. Other immunologic disorders include Hodgkin's disease, non-Hodgkin's lymphoma, multiple myeloma, hypersensitivity (allergic) reactions, systemic lupus erythematosus, and human immunodeficiency virus (HIV) infection. After organ transplantation, the recipient's immune response is purposely suppressed to try to prevent rejection of the organ.

DRUGS USED TO TREAT IMMUNOLOGIC DISORDERS

Drugs used to treat immunologic disorders can be classified as immunostimulants or immunosuppressants. Immunostimulants boost immune function and immunosuppressants impede it. This chapter will address selected immunosuppressants and immunostimulants.

Many other drugs that affect the immune response are covered elsewhere. They include the following:

- Corticosteroids: Chapter 43
- Antipurines and antipyramidines: Chapter 14
- Nucleoside reverse transcriptase inhibitors, protease inhibitors, non-nucleoside reverse transcriptase inhibitors: Chapter 5
- Colony-stimulating factors (hematopoietic growth factors): Chapter 26
- Immunizations: Chapter 6

Immunostimulants: Biologic Response Modifiers

Biologic response modifiers (BRMs) alter the host response to cancer. They are used to treat various types of cancer. BRMs act by enhancing the immune response, inhibiting proliferation of cancer cells, or causing cancer cells to change to a form that cannot proliferate. Examples of BRMs are interferon alfa-2a, interferon alfa-2b, interferon alfacon-a, aldesleukin (interleukin-2), levamisole, and bacille Calmett-Guerin vaccine. Specific uses and adverse effects of BRMs vary with the specific agent as detailed in Table 27–1.

TABLE 27–1

Biologic Response Modifiers

Drug	Uses	Side and Adverse Effects	Nursing Considerations
interferon alfa-2a (Roferon-A) and interferon alfa-2b (Intron A)	Hairy cell leukemia, chronic myelogenous leukemia, malignant melanoma, AIDS-related Kaposi's sarcoma; also being studied for treatment of acute leukemias and ovarian, bladder, and kidney cancers	Most common: fever, fatigue, muscle aches, headache, chills. Other effects: anorexia, weight loss, diarrhea, abdominal pain, dizziness, cough. Long-term or high-dose therapy: bone marrow depression, thyroid dysfunction, alopecia, cardiotoxicity, neuro-toxicity, depression.	Tell patient that side effects tend to lessen with continued treatment. Administer acetaminophen as ordered for fever and muscle aches. Monitor blood cell counts. Taking at bedtime may reduce side effects.
interferon alfa-n3 (Alferon N)	Active chronic hepatitis, bladder carcinoma, chronic myelocytic leukemia, laryngeal papillomatosis, non-Hodgkin's lymphoma, malignant melanoma, multiple myeloma, mycosis fungoides, condylomata acuminata (genital warts)	Frequent: fever, chills, fatigue, headache, aches, pain, anorexia. Also, dizziness, pruritus, dry skin, altered taste. Uncommon: confusion, back pain, leg cramps, flushing, tremor, nervousness, eye pain.	Taking at bedtime may reduce side effects. To treat condylomata, is injected at the base of the lesion 3 times a week for up to 8 weeks.
interferon alfacon-1 (Infergen)	Treatment of chronic hepatitis C	Occasionally causes headache, fever, fatigue, depression.	Give SC; at least 48 hours between doses.
aldesleukin, interleukin-2 (Proleukin)	Metastatic renal cell cancer; also being studied for treatment of Kaposi's sarcoma, melanoma, and colorectal cancer	Very toxic: fever, chills, nausea, vomiting, hypotension, anemia, diarrhea, altered mental status, sinus tachycardia, impaired renal and liver function, pulmonary congestion and dyspnea, pruritus. Capillary leak syndrome (CLS) occurs with massive vasodilation and the shift of fluid out of the vascular compartment. It can be fatal.	Monitor for CLS: decreased BP, edema. Monitor blood cell counts, intake, and output. Encourage increased fluid intake to reduce risk of renal damage. Tell patient that nausea usually resolves with continued therapy. Withhold if patient becomes very lethargic. Contraindicated with cardiac, pulmonary, renal, hepatic, or CNS impairment.
levamisole (Ergamisol)	In combination with fluorouracil to treat stage 3 colon cancer	Few adverse effects to levamisole, but when given with fluorouracil can cause bone marrow depression, nausea, vomiting, diarrhea, alopecia, oral and gastrointestinal ulcers, dizziness, joint pain, metallic taste, and flu-like symptoms.	
BCG vaccine (TheraCys, TICE BCG)	Bladder carcinoma in situ (intravesical: instilled in the bladder)	Dysuria, urinary frequency and urgency, hematuria, malaise, fatigue, fever and chills.	Because BCG vaccine is infectious, supplies used in administration must be disposed of according to protocol. All urine voided for 6 hours after the drug has been instilled must be disinfected with 5% hypochlorite.

AIDS, acquired immunodeficiency syndrome; BCG, bacille Calmette-Guerin; BP, blood pressure; CNS, central nervous system.

Immunosuppressants

Immunosuppressants inhibit the body's natural immune responses. This action is useful in preventing rejection of transplanted tissues and in the treatment of some autoimmune disorders. Autoimmune disorders are caused by the production of antibodies produced against the patient's own tissues. Drugs used as immunosuppressants include cyclosporine and tacrolimus, cytotoxic drugs, antibodies, and glucocorticoids. Glucocorticoids are covered in Chapter 43.

Cyclosporine and Tacrolimus

Actions and Uses. Cyclosporine (Sandimmune, Neoral) and tacrolimus (Prograf) are most often used to prevent rejection of transplanted organs. Their possible effectiveness in treating selected autoimmune disorders is under study. These drugs interfere with T cell activity, thereby inhibiting both cell-mediated and antibody-mediated immune responses. They are commonly used in combination with other immunosuppressants.

Side and Adverse Effects. The most serious adverse effects of cyclosporine and tacrolimus are nephrotoxicity and infection. Fortunately, renal function usually recovers when the drug dosage is reduced. They also can cause hypertension, tremor, and hirsutism (excessive hair growth). Other less common adverse effects are hepatotoxicity, malignant lymphomas, leukopenia, sinusitis, hyperkalemia, gynecomastia (breast enlargement), and anaphylaxis.

Contraindications and Interactions. Contraindications include previous allergic response to the drug or to polyoxyethylated castor oil, which is a solvent for the drug. Cyclosporine and tacrolimus are not given together because of the increased risk of toxicity. Cyclosporine may be given with adrenal corticosteroids, but not other immunosuppressants. These drugs interact with many other common drugs. See a drug handbook for specifics.

Nursing Actions. When patients are on cyclosporine or tacrolimus, monitor blood urea nitrogen and creatinine to assess renal function, and liver enzymes to assess for liver damage. Monitor for increase in blood pressure. Assess for

signs of hyperkalemia: muscle weakness; slow, irregular pulse; tingling of hands, feet, and tongue. Be aware that these drugs interact with many other drugs that can either enhance or interfere with the actions of cyclosporine and tacrolimus. During infusion, monitor the patient closely during the first 30 minutes for allergic reaction: itching and wheezing. At the first sign of allergy, discontinued the infusion and notify the physician.

Patient Teaching

- This drug lowers your resistance to infection, so avoid crowds and people with active infections.
- Notify your physician immediately of any signs of infection (fever, sore throat, etc.).
- Avoid becoming pregnant while on this drug. Use condoms or a diaphragm rather than oral contraceptives with this drug. ⚠
- Grapefruit juice prevents your body from breaking down this drug, which could cause serious adverse effects.
- Do not take other drugs unless advised by your physician.
- Oral cyclosporine can be mixed in a glass container with milk, chocolate milk, or orange juice. Be sure you consume all of the medication.

Cytotoxic Drugs

Actions and Uses. Cytotoxic drugs destroy cells that are reproducing. Although they are specifically used for their action against T cells and B cells, they also have toxic effects on the bone marrow, gastrointestinal tract, hair follicles, and reproductive structures. Examples of cytotoxic drugs are azathioprine (Imuran), cyclophosphamide (Cytoxan), methotrexate (Folex, et al.), and mycophenolate mofentil (CellCept). Specific information about each of these drugs is presented in Table 27–2.

TABLE 27-2

Cytoxic Drugs Used for Immunosuppression

Drug	Uses	Side and Adverse Effects	Specific Considerations
azathioprine (Imuran)	Prevention of transplant rejection (in combination with other agents). Under investigation for treatment of myasthenia gravis, systemic lupus erythematosus, Crohn's disease, ulcerative colitis, and type 1 diabetes mellitus.	Neutropenia, thrombocytopenia, teratogenesis (harmful to developing fetus), increased risk of cancer.	Monitor blood cell counts. Counsel patients not to become pregnant while taking this drug.
cyclophosphamide (Cytoxan)	Rheumatoid arthritis, systemic lupus erythematosus, multiple sclerosis. See Chapter 14 for antineoplastic uses.	Neutropenia, hemorrhagic cystitis, sterility.	Monitor blood cell counts. Advise patients to report bladder symptoms or blood in urine. Patients should be counseled about potential for sterility.
methotrexate (Folex, et al.)	Severe rheumatoid arthritis, psoriasis.	In doses used for immunosuppression, liver damage (hepatic fibrosis and cirrhosis) are most serious adverse effects. Bone marrow suppression not expected with this dose range.	Monitor liver enzymes. Assess for jaundice, dark urine.
mycophenolate mofentil (CellCept)	Prevention of transplant rejection (in combination with other agents).	Diarrhea, severe neutropenia, vomiting, sepsis, increased risk of cancer.	Monitor stools. Tell patient to report diarrhea or vomiting. Antiemetics or antidiarrheals agents may be ordered. Monitor blood cell counts. Assess for signs of infection (fever, sore throat, etc.).

Antibodies

Antibodies used for immunosuppression include muromonab-CD3, lymphocyte immune globulin, antithymocyte globulin (ATG), and $Rh_0(D)$ immune globulin. Specific information about each of these agents is presented in Table 27-3.

TABLE 27-3

Antibodies Used For Immunosuppression

Drug	Uses	Side and Adverse Effects	Specific Considerations
muromonab-CD3	Prevention of kidney, liver, heart transplant rejection. Used to deplete bone marrow of T cells before bone marrow transplantation.	Especially with first dose: usually mild fever, chills, dyspnea, chest pain, nausea and vomiting. Potentially life-threatening reactions: anaphylaxis, shock-like condition, pulmonary edema, severe viral infection.	Route: IV. Drawn up with filter. Corticosteroids may be ordered before and after dose to reduce adverse reactions to first dose. Advise patient that side effects usually lessen with continued therapy. Monitor response to drug. Have emergency drugs and equipment available in case anaphylaxis occurs.
lymphocyte immune globulin, antithymocyte globulin (ATG)	Prevention of renal transplant rejection.	Usually mild fever, chills, leukopenia, skin reactions. Anaphylaxis is possible.	Have emergency drugs and equipment on hand in case of anaphylaxis.
$Rh_0(D)$ immune globulin	Prevent Rh negative women from developing Rh antibodies after exposure to Rh positive blood.	Mild fever.	Should be given twice during pregnancy: at 28 weeks gestation and within 72 hours after delivery.

REVIEW QUESTIONS: UNIT 8

Match the action on the right with the drug classification on the left:

1. _____ Anticoagulant
2. _____ Thrombolytic
3. _____ Antiplatelet

A. prevents platelets from clumping

B. prevents formation of new clots

C. dissolves existing clots

Case Studies

Miss Sidney, age 69, has been hospitalized for recurrent pulmonary embolism. She has a history of thrombophlebitis. She has been receiving heparin per continuous IV infusion. The following questions relate to this scenario.

4. What laboratory test should be done to monitor the anticoagulation effects of heparin therapy?

   A. Complete blood cell count
   B. Activated partial thromboplastin time
   C. Prothrombin time
   D. International normalized ratio

5. The most serious adverse effect of heparin therapy is:

   A. alopecia.
   B. vasodilation.
   C. bleeding.
   D. confusion.

6. Miss Sidney's condition has stabilized. She has been changed from heparin to warfarin. She is being discharged on warfarin (Coumadin) 2 mg daily. The laboratory test that will be ordered to assess antico-agulation now is:

   A. complete blood cell count.
   B. activated partial thromboplastin time.
   C. Lee-White clotting time.
   D. international normalized ratio.

7. You should advise Miss Sidney to avoid:

   A. aspirin.
   B. vitamin C.
   C. coffee.
   D. sunlight.

Mrs. Hughes is HIV-positive. She is being treated with interferon alfa-2b for AIDS-related Kaposi's sarcoma. The following questions relate to this scenario.

8. Common side effects of interferon alfa-2b are:

   A. none; this drug is free of adverse effects.
   B. fever, fatigue, chills.
   C. constipation, weight gain.
   D. hypertension, tachycardia.

9. With long-term interferon alfa-2b therapy, the patient may have:

   A. bone marrow depression.
   B. nephrotoxicity.
   C. severe skin rash.
   D. pulmonary fibrosis.

10. Mrs. Hughes says she doesn't think she can tolerate this drug because she feels so badly. What is the most appropriate reply?

   A. "You certainly should refuse this drug."
   B. "You should not feel that way. The drug is helping you."
   C. "Side effects usually lessen with continued treatment."
   D. "Unfortunately, you will probably feel worse before completing the therapy."

Howard Smith, age 32, has had a kidney transplant and is taking cyclosporine (Sandimmune) and corticosteroids. The following questions relate to this scenario.

11. Cyclosporine is prescribed in this situation to:

   A. prevent surgical infection.
   B. stimulate urine production.
   C. treat urinary infection.
   D. prevent rejection of transplanted kidney.

12. What laboratory tests do you anticipate for Mr. Smith?

   A. Blood urea nitrogen, creatinine
   B. Complete blood cell counts
   C. Prothrombin time
   D. Blood glucose

13. What discharge teaching is especially important for Mr. Smith?

   A. "You will probably notice some hair loss."
   B. "Avoid people with active infections."
   C. "Consume a high potassium diet."
   D. "You may have some dizziness caused by low blood pressure."

DRUGS THAT AFFECT THE CARDIOVASCULAR SYSTEM

OBJECTIVES

1. List the drug classifications used to treat cardiovascular disorders.

2. Explain the actions, uses, side and adverse effects, interactions, and contraindications of drugs used to treat cardiovascular disorders.

3. Describe nursing assessment data to be collected when patients are on specific drugs that affect the cardiovascular system.

4. Identify nursing interventions including patient teaching relevant to each major classification of drugs used to treat cardiovascular disorders.

Anatomy and Physiology of the Cardiovascular System

The functions of the cardiovascular system are to provide oxygen and nutrients to the cells and transport carbon dioxide and other wastes from the cells.

The major structures of the cardiovascular system are the heart, the arteries, and the veins. The heart is divided into four chambers, the right and left atria and the right and left ventricles. The right chambers are separated by the tricuspid valve, and the left chambers by the mitral valve. The aortic valve separates the left ventricle from the aorta, and the pulmonic valve separates the right atrium from the pulmonary artery. The heart muscle (myocardium) receives its oxygen supply from the coronary arteries. The heart is innervated by the autonomic nervous system. The cardiac cycle is initiated by the sinoatrial (SA) node in the right atrium. The impulse travels through the right and left atria, causing them to contract. Impulses reach the atrioventricular (AV) node located between the atria and the ventricles and are then conveyed through the ventricles by way of the bundle of His and the Purkinje fibers. When the impulse reaches the Purkinje fibers, the ventricles contract. Muscle contraction occurs as electrolytes shift in and out of myocardial cells.

Normal function of the cardiovascular system depends on adequate blood volume; intact, patent blood vessels; and a pump capable of receiving deoxygenated blood from the venous system, circulating it through the lungs for oxygenation, and sending oxygenated blood through the blood vessels to the cells. Normal pumping action requires adequate blood flow to the myocardium, normal initiation and conduction of electrical impulses, and myocardial cells that are capable of stretching and contracting.

Normal muscle contraction requires normal concentrations of the electrolytes sodium, potassium, and calcium. The physiologic characteristics of cardiac muscle are as follows:

- *Excitability,* the ability to respond to an electrical stimulus
- *Automaticity,* the capacity to generate an impulse without external stimulation
- *Conductivity,* the ability to transmit electric impulses rapidly and efficiently
- *Contractility,* the ability of myocardial fibers to shorten when stimulated, sometimes thought of simply as "elasticity"

Alterations in any of these factors can affect the circulation and oxygenation of body tissues.

Drugs Used to Treat Cardiovascular System Disorders

Drugs used to treat cardiovascular disorders essentially work by affecting one or more of the variables needed for normal cardiac function. For example, drugs can constrict or dilate blood vessels, thereby controlling the flow of blood to body tissues and affecting the blood pressure. Drugs that cause elimination of body water reduce the blood volume, lowering blood pressure and reducing cardiac workload. Other drugs alter the heart rate or cardiac output by affecting the excitability, automaticity, conductivity, and contractility of the myocardium.

Categories of drugs covered in this unit include inotropics, antidysrhythmics, antianginals, antihypertensives, antishock agents, and antilipemics.

CHAPTER 28

INOTROPICS

*T*he terms *inotropic* and *cardiotonic* are used to describe agents that increase the force of myocardial contraction. Inotropic agents include digitalis preparations (sometimes called *cardiac glycosides* or *digitalis glycosides*), phosphodiesterase inhibitors, and adrenergics. Adrenergics are covered in Chapter 15, so only those used to treat heart failure will be discussed here.

DIGITALIS GLYCOSIDES

Actions and Uses

Digitalis has a positive inotropic effect on the myocardium, meaning it increases the force of myocardial contraction resulting in increased cardiac output. It also has a negative chronotropic effect, meaning that it slows the heart rate, and a dromotropic effect, meaning it slows the rate of impulse conduction through the heart.

The most common use of digitalis is in the treatment of congestive heart failure. It is also used to treat cardiac *dysrhythmias,* the term used to describe abnormalities in cardiac rate or rhythm. To rapidly achieve therapeutic blood levels, the adult patient may be given a digitalizing dose. This dose is higher than the usual daily dose and is usually divided into three doses scheduled 9 to12 hours apart. The patient is then given a daily maintenance dose to maintain the blood level. Digitalization is traditional but not always necessary.

Table 28–1 describes two digitalis preparations.

TABLE 28–1

Digitalis Glycosides

Digitalis Preparation	Specific Considerations
digoxin (Lanoxin)	Most commonly used form. Can be given orally or intravenously; intramuscular route is painful. With IV route, continuous cardiac monitoring is essential. Eliminated by the kidneys.
digitoxin (Crystodigin)	Greater risk of toxicity due to longer half-life than digoxin. May produce more stable blood levels. Eliminated by the liver.

Side and Adverse Effects

The most common adverse effects of digitalis therapy are anorexia, nausea, and vomiting. The most serious adverse effects are caused by the effects of digitalis on the heart. It can cause a variety of cardiac dysrhythmias, most commonly heart block and ventricular dysrhythmias associated with bradycardia, slowed conduction of impulses through the AV node, increased automaticity of Purkinje fibers, and the reduced refractory period in the ventricular myocardium. Unfortunately, gastrointestinal and cardiac symptoms may reflect digitalis toxicity. Therefore, when patients have these symptoms, a serum digitalis level is needed to determine whether toxicity is present.

In addition to dysrhythmias and gastrointestinal distress, digitalis toxicity can be manifested by central nervous system (CNS) effects. Effects on the CNS are evident in fatigue, confusion, and visual illusions, which may include halos around dark objects, blurred vision, and a yellowish tint to objects. The risk of digitalis toxicity increases in the presence of low serum potassium (hypokalemia).

Interactions and Contraindications

Digitalis can interact with many drugs; therefore, always consult a drug handbook when giving a patient multiple drugs that include digitalis. For example:

- Thiazide and loop diuretics can lead to hypokalemia, which puts the patient at risk for digitalis toxicity.
- Sympathomimetics enhance the inotropic effects of digitalis but may increase the risk of rapid dysrhythmias.
- Quinidine, used to treat certain cardiac dysrhythmias, increases the serum digitalis level, thereby increasing the risk of toxicity.
- Verapamil is another drug used to treat dysrhythmias that increases the serum digitalis level. It can also counteract the effects of digitalis on myocardial contractility.

Digitalis preparations are contraindicated in ventricular tachycardia and fibrillation and severe myocarditis. They are used with caution in the presence of acute myocardial infarction, heart block, Adams-Stokes syndrome, renal impairment, and electrolyte imbalances (hypokalemia, hypercalcemia, hypomagnesemia).

Nursing Actions

Before each dose of digitalis, count the apical pulse for 1 full minute. If it is less than 60 in an adult, withhold the drug and notify the physician. Depending on what is normal for that patient, the physician may tell you to give the medicine despite the lower heart rate, or may instruct you to omit a dose. A serum digitalis level may be ordered to evaluate for toxicity. Monitor the cardiac rhythm. Report any abnormal rhythm to the physician. Monitor the patient's weight and assess for edema since fluid retention is characteristic of congestive heart failure. If the patient is taking potassium-wasting diuretics, assess for symptoms of hypokalemia: muscle weakness, fatigue, and cardiac dysrhythmias.

Patient Teaching

Patients who take digitalis at home must learn to monitor their pulse. Points to emphasize are the following:

- You should practice assessing and describing the pulse before you are discharged.
- Take your pulse each day before your digitalis. If it is less than 60 or irregular, contact your physician before taking the drug.
- Take this drug at the same time each day. Do not skip doses or take more frequently than prescribed.
- Notify your physician if you have loss of appetite, nausea, or changes in your vision.
- Always take the same brand unless advised to change by your physician because brands vary in their absorption rates.
- Weigh daily and notify your physician if you gain more than 2 lbs in one day.

ADRENERGICS/SYMPATHOMIMETICS

Adrenergic/sympathomimetic drugs used for their inotropic action include dopamine (Intropin) and dobutamine (Dobutrex). Table 28–2 describes the adrenergic agents.

TABLE 28–2

Adrenergic (Sympathomimetic) Inotropic Agents

Adrenergic Agent	Specific Considerations
dopamine (Intropin)	Increases renal blood flow and urine output. Increases afterload (peripheral resistance), which can reduce cardiac output. Should not be given with uncorrected rapid dysrhythmias or ventricular fibrillation.
dobutamine (Dobutrex)	Preferred over dopamine because it does not increase afterload. Used cautiously with hypertension and atrial fibrillation.

Action and Uses

Adrenergics improve cardiac performance by increasing cardiac contractility. They are employed for short-term use only in acute, severe heart failure.

Side and Adverse Effects

Both of these agents can cause tachycardia and palpitations, more commonly with dobutamine than with dopamine. In addition, dopamine can cause headache, hypotension, and nausea and vomiting. Dobutamine increases blood pressure.

Interactions and Contraindications

The drugs' effects may be enhanced by tricyclic antidepressants, monoamine oxidase (MAO) inhibitors, and oxytocics. Effects are antagonized by beta blockers. Digitalis increases the risk of dysrhythmias. These adrenergic agents are contraindicated with sulfite sensitivity.

Nursing Actions

These drugs are given by continuous intravenous infusion, requiring constant monitoring of blood pressure and electrocardiogram. The nurse who administers intravenous medications adjusts the flow rate to maintain pulse and blood pressure within the range (parameters) prescribed by the physician. Assess the infusion site for any signs of extravasation (leakage outside the vein), which can cause tissue necrosis. If infiltration occurs, injection of the affected tissue with phentolamine mesylate (Regitine) per order or protocol can reduce tissue damage. Monitor urine output and peripheral circulation. When adrenergics are discontinued, dosage should be tapered gradually to avoid a sudden drop in blood pressure.

Patient Teaching

- This drug improves your heart function.
- We will be checking your pulse and blood pressure often while you receive this drug.
- Report any pain in your intravenous infusion site.

PHOSPHODIESTERASE INHIBITORS

Phosphodiesterase inhibitors used for their inotropic action include amrinone (Inocor), milrinone (Primacor), and vesnarinone (Arkin Z).

Action and Uses

Phosphodiesterase inhibitors produce vasodilation and increase myocardial contractility.

Side and Adverse Effects

Adverse effects of phosphodiesterase inhibitors include hypotension. Other effects specific to various agents are noted in Table 28–3.

TABLE 28–3

Phosphodiesterase Inhibitors

Phosphodiesterase Inhibitor	Specific Considerations
amrinone (Inocor)	In addition to hypotension, may cause anorexia, nausea, vomiting, abdominal pain, and hepatotoxicity. With prolonged use, which is uncommon, it can cause thrombocytopenia (platelet deficiency).
milrinone (Primacor)	In addition to hypotension, may cause cardiac dysrhythmias.
vesnarinone (Arkin Z)	Less risk of dysrhythmias because it slows the heart rate. Has a narrow margin of safety. Can cause a reversible neutropenia.

Interactions and Contraindications

Phosphodiesterase inhibitors have additive inotropic effects with digitalis glycosides.

Nursing Actions

These drugs are administered by intravenous infusion and require constant monitoring of the electrocardiogram and blood pressure. Assess for indications of improved cardiac function: less edema, easier respirations, clear breath sounds, and improved color.

Patient Teaching

- This drug improves the function of your heart.
- We will closely check your blood pressure and electrocardiogram while you are receiving it.

ANTIDYSRHYTHMICS

A regular heartbeat of 60 to 100 provides the ideal conditions for maintaining normal cardiac output. Significant variations in rate or rhythm can cause cardiac output to fall, possibly to dangerous levels. Abnormalities in cardiac rate or rhythm are called *dysrhythmias* or *arrhythmias*. Dysrhythmias can result from many factors, including heart disease or trauma, fluid and electrolyte imbalances, and the effects of drug therapy. Types of dysrhythmias can be classified by the site of origin.

Sinus dysrhythmias originate in the sinoatrial (SA) node and include:

- Sinus dysrhythmia: irregular rhythm with no other abnormalities; increases and slows with respirations
- Sinus tachycardia: heart rate faster than 100 bpm with no other abnormalities
- Sinus bradycardia: heart rate slower than 60 bpm with no other abnormalities
- Sinus arrest: a pause when the SA node fails to initiate an impulse then resumes normal rhythm

Atrial dysrhythmias originate in the atria and include:

- Premature atrial contraction: an impulse in the atria initiates atrial contraction before the SA node can fire in the normal rhythm
- Paroxysmal atrial tachycardia: very rapid heartbeat that occurs intermittently
- Atrial fibrillation and flutter: abnormal and inefficient contraction of atria, described as quivering or fluttering activity

Nodal dysrhythmias are related to the atrioventricular (AV) node and include:

- Junctional rhythm: an impulse originates in the AV node; can travel upward through the atria and downward through the ventricles
- AV block: impulses from the atria are slowed or blocked from passing through the AV node to the ventricles

Ventricular dysrhythmias originate in the ventricles and include:

- Premature ventricular contractions (PVCs): an impulse initiates contraction of the ventricles out of sequence from the normal cardiac cycle
- Ventricular tachycardia: abnormal contraction of the ventricles without regard to atrial activity
- Ventricular fibrillation: quivering of ventricles; no effective contractions

Drugs used to treat abnormal cardiac rates or rhythms are called *antidysrhythmics* or *antiarrhythmics*. Antidysrhythmics are classified as Class I sodium channel blockers (with subclasses IA, IB, and IC), Class II beta-adrenergic blockers, Class III potassium channel blockers, and Class IV calcium channel blockers. Some additional unclassified agents are used as well.

ACTIONS AND USES

In general, antidysrhythmics work by reducing automaticity. That is, they inhibit the spontaneous electrical activity of myocardial cells. They also tend to slow the conduction of impulses through the myocardium (negative dromotropic effect), and prolong the refractory (resting) period of myocardial contraction. Therefore, you may see them referred to as *cardiac depressants*.

SIDE AND ADVERSE EFFECTS

There are some adverse effects specific to each classification. However, some side and adverse effects are common to most antidysrhythmics. These include new dysrhythmias and hypotension. With excessive depression of impulse initiation or conduction, the patient may develop heart block or other new, sometimes more serious, dysrhythmias. Hypotension can occur because of decreased cardiac output. Other effects specific to each classification are noted in Table 29–1.

INTERACTIONS AND CONTRAINDICATIONS

Drugs that generally enhance the effects of antidysrhythmics include antihypertensives, diuretics, phenothiazine antipsychotic agents, and cimetidine. The effects of antidysrhythmics are diminished by phenytoin (Dilantin), rifampin, and atropine sulfate. Contraindications are specific to each agent.

NURSING ACTIONS

Monitor the patient's heart rate, rhythm, and blood pressure. Notify the physician if dysrhythmias worsen after therapy is initiated.

Patient Teaching

- This drug is intended to improve the rhythm of your heart.
- Report any palpitations or feelings of faintness.
- Take this drug at the same time each day and exactly as prescribed.
- Take your pulse each day to see if the rhythm is regular.
- Alcohol, tobacco, and caffeine may interfere with the effectiveness of this drug.
- Consult with your physician before taking any other drugs.

TABLE 29-1

Antidysrhythmic Classifications and Prototypes

Classification and Prototypes	Specific Adverse Effects	Nursing Considerations
Class I: Sodium channel blockers Class IA prototype: quinidine (Quinaglute)	Adverse effects—CNS: *cinchonism* is toxicity manifested by fever, headache, confusion, and disturbances in hearing, balance, and vision; blood: decreased prothrombin and platelets; gastrointestinal: nausea and vomiting, diarrhea; muscle weakness	Teach patients symptoms of cinchonism to be reported. Assess for easy bruising and bleeding. Contraindicated with myasthenia gravis. Enhances effects of digitalis. Assess for skin rash. Monitor CBC for low red cells, white cells, platelets.
procainamide (Pronestyl)	In addition to above effects, can cause agranulocytosis and a reversible lupus-like syndrome (skin rash, liver enlargement).	
disopyramide (Norpace)	More cardiac depression than quinidine. Lowers blood glucose. Anticholinergic effects: dry mouth, constipation, urinary retention, blurred vision	
Class IB: local anesthetics lidocaine (Xylocaine) mexiletine (Mexitil) tocainide (Tonocard) phenytoin (Dilantin)	CNS depression at therapeutic levels; CNS stimulation with high doses. Tocainide can cause agranulocytosis.	Safety precautions if drowsy. For intravenous administration, use specific lidocaine preparation for that purpose; should not contain epinephrine. When tocainide is used, monitor for anemia (fatigue), leukopenia (signs of infection), and thrombocytopenia (bruising, bleeding).
Class II: Beta adrenergic blockers propranolol (Inderal) acebutolol (Sectral) esmolol (Brevibloc)	Rebound hypertension, possible angina, myocardial infarction with abrupt withdrawal. Can cause bronchial constriction. Decreases blood glucose but obscures signs and symptoms of hypoglycemia. Increases low density lipoproteins.	Monitor pulse and blood pressure; blood glucose in patients with diabetes. Contraindicated with severe chronic pulmonary disease and uncompensated congestive heart failure. Profuse perspiration may be only sign of hypoglycemia.
Class III: Potassium channel blockers amiodarone (Cordarone)	Used for life-threatening dysrhythmias when less toxic drugs fail. Adverse effects of amiodarone: pulmonary inflammation and fibrosis, nausea and vomiting, hepatic necrosis, muscle weakness, peripheral neuropathy, vision impairment, hypothyroidism or hyperthyroidism, blue-gray pigments in skin. Slowly excreted, so effects persist.	Monitor respiratory status, liver enzymes. Assess for nausea and vomiting, muscle weakness, numbness or tingling in extremities, and changes in vision. Inspect skin for color changes.

bretylium (Bretylol) sotalol (Betapace)	Bretylium initially causes increased pulse and blood pressure and worsening of dysrhythmias, then hypotension.	
Class IV: Calcium channel blockers verapamil (Calan) diltiazem (Cardizem)	Side and adverse effects include dizziness, flushing, edema, hypotension. Can cause bradycardia, CHF. Can increase serum digitalis level.	Monitor blood pressure and pulse. Assess for signs and symptoms of CHF: edema, dyspnea.
Miscellaneous dysrhythmics adenosine (Adenocard) ibutilide (Corvert)	Adenosine limited to treatment of paroxysmal supraventricular tachycardia. Given rapidly IV (in 1-2 seconds). May cause flushing, chest pain, headache, new dysrhythmias. Ibutilide used to treat atrial fibrillation or flutter of recent onset. Occasionally causes headache, hypotension, new dysrhythmias.	Electrocardiographic monitoring for 4 hours after administration.

CBC, complete blood count; CHF, congestive heart failure; CNS, central nervous system.

ANTIANGINALS

*A*ngina is the term used to refer to chest pain associated with inadequate oxygenation of the myocardium. Tissue lacking adequate oxygenation is
described as *ischemic*. Antianginals are drugs used to improve blood flow to the myocardium in the presence of heart
disease and arteriosclerosis. Classifications of drugs used
as antianginals are organic nitrates, calcium channel
blockers, and beta adrenergic blockers.

ACTIONS AND USES

Antianginal agents generally work by decreasing myocardial oxygen demand or improving myocardial blood flow.
This can be done by depressing cardiac activity or dilating
blood vessels that supply the heart muscle.

SIDE AND ADVERSE EFFECTS

Antianginals that cause blood vessels to dilate can lower
blood pressure, causing the patient to have episodes of hypotension with position changes. The heart rate may increase
to compensate for the falling blood pressure. Dilation of
blood vessels also causes flushing and headache. Agents
that reduce myocardial oxygen needs by depressing contractility can reduce cardiac output and contribute to congestive heart failure.

INTERACTIONS AND CONTRAINDICATIONS

Interactions and contraindications vary with the specific
agents. In general, vasodilators are contraindicated with
hypotension. Use of alcohol is discouraged because it enhances hypotension. For other precautions, see Table 30–1.

TABLE 30-1

Antianginals

Classification and Prototypes	Specific Adverse Effects	Nursing Considerations
Organic nitrates nitroglycerin (NTG) isosorbide dinitrate (Isordil)	Action is vasodilation, so BP may fall with position changes. Other side and adverse effects: flushing, headache, reflex tachycardia (response to falling BP). Tolerance to nitrates tends to develop over time. Patches may be ordered for 10-12 hr intervals, followed by 10-12 hrs without the patch to reduce development of tolerance. The patch is most often removed at night.	Nitroglycerin available as sublingual or buccal tablets, sustained release tablets, ointment, and transdermal patch. Do not touch ointment or medicated surface of patch with your bare fingers since you may absorb some of the drug through your skin.
Calcium channel blockers amlodipine (Norvasc) diltiazem (Cardizem) nifedipine (Procardia) verapamil (Calan)	Depress myocardial contractility and decrease oxygen needs. Some cause dilation of coronary and peripheral vessels. Extent of each action varies with specific preparations. Can slow heart rate. Alcohol enhances vasodilating effect.	Elderly patients may require lower doses. Teach patients to rise slowly to prevent postural hypotension. Assess for signs and symptoms of CHF: edema, weight gain, dyspnea, fatigue. Note: harmless ankle edema is common. Sublingual nifedipine capsules must be punctured to allow the medication to be dispersed.

| **Beta-adrenergic blockers**
nadolol (Corgard)
propranolol (Inderal)
atenolol (Tenormin)
metoprolol (Lopressor) | Beta blockers depress the conduction of impulses through the myocardium, slowing the heart rate and decreasing BP and cardiac output. If stopped suddenly, BP rises and angina may occur. Can cause bronchial constriction. Decreases blood glucose but obscures usual symptoms of hypoglycemia. Increases low density lipoproteins. | Used cautiously, if at all, with diabetes and chronic pulmonary disease. Monitor for signs and symptoms of CHF: edema, cough, dyspnea, fatigue. Monitor heart rate and BP. Caution patient not to discontinue abruptly. |

BP, blood pressure; CHF, congestive heart failure.

NURSING ACTIONS

Assess heart rate and blood pressure. Document pain location, quality, severity, and radiation as well as response to medication. Monitor for signs and symptoms of congestive heart failure (CHF): edema, weight gain, fatigue, cough, dyspnea.

Patient Teaching

- When you have angina (chest pain), your heart muscle is not getting enough oxygen. Stop what you are doing and sit down.
- If you are taking sublingual nitroglycerin PRN (only when pain occurs):
  — Nitroglycerin will deteriorate if exposed to heat or light.
  — Always keep a small supply of tablets with you, but not close to your body.
  — Place the sublingual tablet or spray the aerosol under your tongue; do not chew or swallow the tablet.
  — If your pain is not relieved within 5 minutes of taking the first tablet, you can take a second tablet. If the pain continues after another 5 minutes, you can take a third tablet. If pain continues after three doses, call for help and transportation for medical care.
  — Once pain is relieved, you can expel any remaining tablet.
  — Tablets should cause a burning sensation under the tongue; if not, they should be replaced.
  — Store tablets in a cool, dark place and replace every 6 months.
- If you take oral nitroglycerin (such as Isordil), do not stop taking it without medical supervision.
- If you use nitroglycerin patches, apply them to hairless areas on the upper arms or trunk; rotate sites to reduce irritation.
- Take your pulse each day and notify your physician if it is less than 60 bpm.
- Smoking aggravates angina.

ANTIHYPERTENSIVES

$\mathcal{H}$ ypertension is a condition in which blood pressure remains abnormally elevated. If sustained, it increases the risk of myocardial infarction, heart failure, stroke, and damage to the kidneys and the eyes. Variables that determine blood pressure include blood volume, cardiac output, peripheral resistance, blood viscosity, and elasticity of peripheral arterial walls. Agents that reduce blood pressure work by affecting one or more of these mechanisms.

Drugs used to treat high blood pressure are called *antihypertensives*. They include diuretics, beta-adrenergic blockers, angiotensin converting enzyme (ACE) inhibitors, calcium channel blockers, angiotensin II receptor antagonists, and alpha-adrenergic blockers.

ACTIONS AND USES

Antihypertensives can work by reducing blood volume, decreasing cardiac output, or decreasing peripheral resistance.

SIDE AND ADVERSE EFFECTS

Antihypertensives can lower blood pressure excessively, causing episodes of dizziness, especially with position changes. When patients move from reclining or sitting to standing positions, they may feel lightheaded. This is called *orthostatic* (or *positional*) *hypotension* and it occurs because the blood vessels in the lower extremities do not constrict promptly to divert blood to the brain.

When blood pressure falls, the body responds with various compensatory mechanisms. The heart rate may increase to improve blood flow and the kidneys may retain sodium and water to increase blood volume. The patient may have tachycardia and palpitations as well as edema. In the case of hypertension, these compensatory mechanisms can defeat the purpose of the antihypertensive agents. Some antihypertensives have been linked to sexual dysfunction, specifically erectile dysfunction and impaired ejaculation. Other adverse effects specific to the agents are noted in Table 31–1. Sometimes combinations of agents are needed to achieve therapeutic actions and control adverse effects.

TABLE 31–1			
Antihypertensives			
Classifications and Prototypes	Action	Side and Adverse Effects	Nursing Considerations
Diuretics hydrochlorothiazide (HCTZ) spironolactone (Aldactone)	Reduce blood volume by increasing urine output. Loss of sodium may make blood vessels less sensitive to sympathetic stimulation.	Most diuretics can cause fluid and electrolyte imbalances: fluid volume deficit, hypokalemia, hyponatremia. Some are potassium sparing like spironolactone and do not cause potassium loss. Long-term therapy may raise blood glucose.	Assess hydration status (moisture of mucous membranes, urine specific gravity, pulse volume, BP). Monitor for hypokalemia manifested by weakness, muscle cramps, numbness and tingling in extremities, cardiac dysrhythmias. Question potassium supplements with spironolactone (can cause hyperkalemia). See Chapter 38.

Classifications and Prototypes	Action	Side and Adverse Effects	Nursing Considerations
Beta-adrenergic blocking agents propranolol (Inderal) atenolol (Tenormin) metoprolol (Lopressor) sotalol (Betapace) Note: these are just a few of many beta blockers	Prevents beta receptors from receiving epinephrine and norepinephrine, thereby reducing cardiac stimulation. Decreases heart rate, myocardial irritability and contractility. Decreases BP and cardiac output.	Can cause orthostatic hypotension, fatigue, weakness, and reflex tachycardia. Serious adverse effects: CHF hypotension, nausea and vomiting, bradycardia, heart block, circulatory failure, bronchial constriction.	Monitor pulse rate and rhythm and BP. Be alert for signs and symptoms of CHF: weight gain, edema, dyspnea, fatigue. Advise patients that stopping these drugs suddenly can result in high BP and chest pain. Activity should be increased slowly because cardiac response to exercise is lessened. Generally contraindicated with asthma because of risk of bronchial constriction. Used cautiously with diabetes because it lowers blood glucose and obscures usual signs and symptoms of hypoglycemia.
Calcium channel blockers verapamil (Calan) amlodipine (Norvasc) nifedipine (Procardia) diltiazem (Cardizem)	Inhibits the flow of calcium ions into myocardial and vascular smooth muscle cells, which dilates blood vessels, depresses impulse formation by SA node, and slows impulse conduction through the AV node.	May cause orthostatic hypotension, constipation, dizziness, nausea, peripheral edema, and headache. More serious adverse effects include severe hypotension, palpitations, bradycardia, heart block, and dyspnea.	Be aware that serious adverse effects are most likely with IV administration of verapamil, nicardipine, and diltiazem. If adequate fluid and fiber intake with increased exercise do not control constipation, ask physician about stool softeners. Advise patients not to discontinue this drug suddenly as it can cause BP to rise sharply.
ACE inhibitors benazepril (Lotensin) enalapril (Vasotec) captopril (Capoten)	Reduces peripheral resistance by preventing the conversion of angiotensin I to angiotensin II. Angiotensin II is a potent vasoconstrictor. Less effective in African-Americans.	Side effects include rash, altered taste sensation, persistent cough, dry mouth, gastrointestinal distress, headache, dizziness. Orthostatic hypotension may occur with initial therapy. Rarely causes hyperkalemia, agranulocytosis, swelling of face and lips (angioedema). Increased risk of renal complications in patients with history of renal disease.	Monitor for hyperkalemia especially if patient receives potassium-sparing diuretics: muscle weakness, tingling sensation, slow irregular heartbeat. Teach patient that stopping this drug suddenly can cause dramatic increase in BP.
Alpha-adrenergic blocking agents *alpha₁ blockers* clonidine (Catapres) guanabenz (Wytensin) guanfacine (Tenex) methyldopa (Aldomet) *alpha₂ blockers* doxazosin (Cardura) prazosin (Minipress) terazosin (Hytrin)	Blocks the effects of norepinephrine which results in dilation of blood vessels. This reduces peripheral resistance and lowers BP.	Adverse effects may include orthostatic hypotension, reflex tachycardia, nasal congestion, inhibited ejaculation, and retention of sodium and water. Especially with alpha₂ blockers, patients may have "first dose syncope:" the blood pressure falls dramatically with the initial dose or the first of an increased dose.	The first dose or any increased dose should be given at bedtime to reduce the risk of injury related to first dose syncope. Caution patients to expect drowsiness and to plan activities accordingly. If taken with CNS depressants, can cause sedation. If taken with NSAIDs, increases fluid retention.
Ganglionic blockers trimethaphan (Arfonad)	Interfere with transmission of impulses through ganglia of the autonomic nervous system; dilate arterioles and veins by blocking sympathetic stimulation of blood vessels.	Adverse effects of trimethaphan include dry mouth, blurred vision, photophobia, urinary retention, constipation, tachycardia, hypotension.	Hypotension can be severe and may occur with or without position changes.
Direct vasodilators hydralazine (Apresoline) minoxidil (Loniten) diazoxide (Hyperstat IV) sodium nitroprusside (Nitropress)	Hydralazine, minoxidil, and diazoxide dilate arterioles, which reduces peripheral resistance causing BP to fall. Sodium nitroprusside dilates arterioles and veins.	With all these drugs, monitor for excessive lowering of BP. All except sodium nitroprusside can cause reflex tachycardia, sodium and water retention, dizziness, and fatigue. Other effects of hydralazine are a lupus-like syndrome characterized by muscle and joint pain, fever, pericarditis, and nephritis. Minoxidil can also cause excessive hair growth, reduced platelets, breast tenderness, and skin rash. Sodium nitroprusside can cause cyanide or thiocyanate poisoning.	Parenteral hydralazine, diazoxide, and nitroprusside are used in hypertensive emergencies to lower BP that is dangerously high. Small doses of diazoxide are given by rapid IV injection, and repeated at 5–15 minute intervals until blood pressure is acceptable. Sodium nitroprusside is diluted and administered in an IV infusion; the rate is adjusted to maintain the desired BP. If a patient receives nitroprusside for more than 3 days, blood levels should be assessed to avoid thiocyanate toxicity.

(continued on p. 150)

Classifications and Prototypes	Action	Side and Adverse Effects	Nursing Considerations
Angiotensin II receptor antagonists losartan (Cozaar) valsartan (Diovan)	Prevent release of aldosterone. Keep angiotensin from engaging with receptors.	Headache, hypotension, dizziness, insomnia, hyperkalemia, diarrhea, heartburn; nasal decongestion	First or increased dose best given at bedtime. Caution about drowsiness, dizziness.

INTERACTIONS AND CONTRAINDICATIONS

The effects of antihypertensives can be enhanced by any other drugs, such as central nervous system depressants, that lower blood pressure. Drugs that tend to increase the blood pressure (central nervous system stimulants, vasoconstrictors) tend to counteract the actions of antihypertensives. Antihypertensives are contraindicated with low blood pressure.

NURSING ACTIONS

Record baseline blood pressure and subsequent readings. Monitor heart rate. Measure blood pressure with patient lying, sitting, then standing. A drop of 20 points or more in pulse or blood pressure with position changes reflects orthostatic hypotension. Assess for peripheral edema.

Patient Teaching

- Hypertension often has no symptoms, so you should continue treatment regardless of how you feel unless your physician discontinues it.
- Take this medication at the same time each day.
- Do not stop the medication unless advised and monitored by your physician. Suddenly discontinuing the drug can cause your blood pressure to rise very high.
- Minimize caffeine intake and avoid over-the-counter allergy, cold, and sinus remedies that can raise blood pressure.
- If you feel lightheaded when arising, change positions slowly, avoid hot baths or showers, and avoid prolonged standing in one place.
- Some medications can make you drowsy. Schedule your medication so that you do not attempt activities requiring alertness when you are most drowsy.

CHAPTER 32

ANTISHOCK AGENTS

Shock is acute circulatory failure that can lead to death. Depending on the cause, shock is classified as hypovolemic, cardiogenic, septic, anaphylactic, or neurogenic. Drugs used to restore or maintain life-sustaining circulation in the treatment of shock are called *antishock agents*. Other treatments vary with the underlying cause of shock. For example, antimicrobials are given for septic shock and inotropics for cardiogenic shock. Antishock agents are described in Table 32–1.

TABLE 32–1

Antishock Agents

Prototypes	Specific Considerations
Alpha-adrenergics	Increase peripheral resistance, which raises BP.
norepinephrine (Levophed)	Used in cardiogenic and septic shock, usually when patients do not respond to dopamine or dobutamine. Violent headache may be first symptom of overdosage. Constricts kidney blood vessels, so monitor urine output. Can cause fetal anoxia due to constriction of uterine blood vessels. **Pregnancy Category D.**
phenylephrine (Neo-Synephrine)	Increased risk of dysrhythmias with digitalis. Overdosage in elderly patients may be manifested as CNS depression, hallucinations, seizures.
Methoxamine (Vasoxyl)	Used occasionally.
Beta-adrenergics	Raise BP by increasing myocardial contractility and heart rate.
dobutamine (Dobutrex)	Short-term use to increase cardiac output in severe, acute heart failure and after cardiac surgery. Less effect on heart rate and BP than other agents.
isoproterenol (Isuprel)	Usefulness limited because it can decrease diastolic BP, increase myocardial oxygen demand, and cause cardiac dysrhythmias.
Alpha- and beta-adrenergics	Increase myocardial contractility and heart rate; increase peripheral resistance and raise BP.
dopamine (Intropin)	Used for cardiogenic and hypovolemic shock. Dilates renal blood vessels, which increases urine output. Beta effects (cardiac stimulation) evident with moderate dosage; more alpha effects (vasoconstriction) with high dosage.
epinephrine (Adrenalin)	Used for anaphylactic shock because it blocks chemical mediators of allergic response. Single dose may be given in cardiac arrest. Low doses have primarily beta effects; higher doses produce alpha effects.
metaraminol (Aramine)	Used occasionally for hypotension.

ACTIONS AND USES

Antishock agents are given to maintain circulation to vital organs. Because they tend to increase the blood pressure, they are called *pressor agents*. They include alpha-adrenergics and beta-adrenergics. Alpha-adrenergics constrict peripheral blood vessels, thereby raising blood pressure. Examples of alpha-adrenergics are norepinephrine (Levophed), phenylephrine (Neo-Synephrine), and methoxamine (Vasoxyl). Beta-adrenergics raise blood pressure by increasing myocardial contractility and heart rate. Examples of beta-adrenergics used to treat shock are dobutamine (Dobutrex) and isoproterenol (Isuprel). Drugs that have both alpha- and beta-adrenergic effects include dopamine (Intropin), epinephrine (Adrenalin), and metaraminol (Aramine). Combinations of drugs are often required.

SIDE AND ADVERSE EFFECTS

All pressor agents can cause angina, dyspnea, and palpitations because they increase the oxygen demands of the heart. Other side and adverse effects vary with the specific agent (Table 32–2).

TABLE 32–2
Side and Adverse Effects of Antishock Agents

Effect	dobutamine (Dobutrex)	dopamine (Intropin)	epinephrine (Adrenalin)	isoproterenol (Isuprel)	metaraminol (Aramine)	methoxamine (Vasoxyl)	norepinephrine (Levophed)	phenylephrine (Neo-Synephrine)
Bradycardia					X	X	X	X
Tachycardia		X	X	X				
Dysrhythmias	X	X	X	X	X	X	X	X
Hypertension					X	X	X	X
Hypotension		X		X				
Angina	X	X	X	X	X	X	X	X
Tissue Necrosis with Extravasation		X			X		X	X

CONTRAINDICATIONS AND INTERACTIONS

Beta-adrenergics may be detrimental after myocardial infarction because cardiac stimulation increases oxygen requirements. Also, when shock is related to cardiac dysrhythmias, beta-adrenergics can aggravate the condition by actually causing additional dysrhythmias.

The effects of pressor agents may be enhanced by halogenated general anesthetics (e.g., halothane) and monoamine oxidase inhibitors. Oxytocics increase the risk of severe hypertension. Anticholinergics increase the risk of tachycardia. Beta-adrenergic blockers oppose the actions of adrenergic agents.

NURSING ACTIONS

Vasopressors are administered intravenously using a large vein. Even though you may not administer these intravenous drugs, you should be aware of the nursing implications when a patient is receiving them. An infusion pump should be used to permit careful rate control. These drugs are most often diluted in 250 to 500 mL of 5% dextrose and titrated (regulated) to maintain the blood pressure within a prescribed range (or parameters). The intravenous infusion should be started slowly, increased as needed, and gradually reduced once the patient is stabilized. Suddenly stopping the drug can cause rebound hypotension. Sometime bolus intravenous injections are given; they too should be diluted according to manufacturer's directions prior to administration. A brownish color or precipitate in the drug indicates that it has deteriorated and should not be used.

Throughout treatment with pressor agents, pulse and blood pressure are monitored every 5 to 15 minutes. It is usually desirable to keep the systolic blood pressure between 80 and 100 mm Hg, and the pulse between 60 and 100. In cardiogenic shock, the goal is to maintain pulmonary-capillary wedge pressure at 15 to 20 mm Hg. Monitor urine output as an indicator of renal blood flow. As the patient's condition improves, increased output is expected. Note peripheral pulses and skin color and warmth, but remember that drugs that constrict peripheral vessels will cause the skin to be pale and cool. Last, assess the infusion site if a peripheral vessel is used. Edema and cool skin around the infusion site suggest that the drug is escaping the vein and entering the tissues (extravasation). Some of these drugs cause profound vasoconstriction that can cause local tissue ischemia and necrosis. If extravasation occurs, phentolamine (Regitine) may be given as ordered or per protocol to reverse the local effects of the pressor agent and prevent tissue destruction.

Patients who are treated with vasopressors are critically ill, but if conscious, they need simple explanations such as follows in the Patient Teaching section.

Patient Teaching

- This drug will help keep your blood pressure normal.
- We will be checking your pulses and blood pressure frequently to help us regulate this medication.
- Tell me if you have any chest pain or shortness of breath.
- If your IV site is painful, tell me immediately.

CHAPTER 33

ANTILIPEMICS

Hyperlipidemia (elevated serum lipids) is a major risk factor for atherosclerosis, which is implicated in cardiovascular, cerebrovascular, and peripheral vascular disease. Serum lipids include cholesterol, triglycerides, and phospholipids. Lipoproteins are specific proteins that transport lipids in the blood. Lipoproteins are described as high density or low density, based on the proportion of lipids to protein. High density lipoproteins (HDLs) have a higher proportion of protein and low density lipoproteins (LDLs) have a higher proportion of lipid. The healthiest serum profile would have high HDLs, low LDLs, low total cholesterol, and low triglycerides.

Various strategies are recommended for people with elevated LDLs, total cholesterol, and triglycerides to lower their lipids. Changes include reduced dietary intake of saturated fats and triglycerides as well as reduced total caloric intake. If dietary interventions fail to lower serum lipids, drug therapy may be employed.

ACTIONS AND USES

Drugs used to treat hyperlipidemia are called *antilipemics*. They lower serum lipids by affecting the production, metabolism, or removal of lipoproteins. Types of antilipemics are bile-acid sequestrants, HMG-CoA reductase inhibitors, niacin, and gemfibrozil. A single drug or multiple drugs may be used depending on which lipids are elevated.

SIDE AND ADVERSE EFFECTS

Nausea, vomiting, flatulence, constipation or diarrhea, and abdominal discomfort are the most common adverse effects of antilipemic drugs. Other adverse effects are specific to the types of drug and are noted in Table 33–1.

INTERACTIONS AND CONTRAINDICATIONS

See Table 33–1.

NURSING ACTIONS

Specific nursing implications are summarized in Table 33–1.

Patient Teaching

- Antilipemic drugs should be used with, not in place of, a low fat diet.
- Constipation can usually be managed with adequate fluids, fiber, and exercise.
- If constipation persists, discuss other options with the physician.
- Keep appointments for blood studies.

TABLE 33–1

Antilipemics

Prototype	Actions	Side and Adverse Effects	Specific Considerations
Bile-acid sequestrants cholestyramine (Questran, Cholybar) colestipol (Colestid)	The liver uses hepatic cholesterol to produce bile acids. Sequestrants bind to bile acids in the intestinal tract so the acids are excreted in the feces. As the liver uses more cholesterol to produce additional bile acids, serum cholesterol falls.	Constipation is common. Though rare, fecal impaction and intestinal obstruction have been reported. May cause rash and irritation of tongue and perianal area. Though not common, can cause gallstones, pancreatitis, peptic ulcers, vitamin K deficiency and bleeding due to calcium excretion and osteoporosis with prolonged use.	Powder must be mixed in 3–6 oz water, milk, fruit juice, or soup. Never take dry powder. Decreases absorption of many other oral drugs. Give 1 hour before or 4 hours after other drugs (especially digoxin, warfarin, propranolol). Advise patient to reduce risk of constipation by increasing fluid and dietary fiber intake (unless contraindicated) and exercise.

(Continued on p. 154)

Prototype	Actions	Side and Adverse Effects	Specific Considerations
HMG-CoA reductase inhibitors atorvastatin (Lipitor) cerivastatin (Baycol) fluvastatin (Lescol) lovastatin (Mevacor) pravastatin (Pravachol) simvastatin (Zocor)	Lowers serum cholesterol by blocking hepatic synthesis	Gastrointestinal symptoms are most common adverse effects. Also, headache, skin rash, blurred vision. Rarely: hepatotoxicity and myopathy. Contraindicated during pregnancy, with liver disease. **Pregnancy Category X.**	Be aware of possible interactions: severe muscle pain if given with erythromycin, itraconazole, or ketoconazole. Risk of acute renal failure and rhabdomyolysis (disintegration of striated muscle fibers) if given with cyclosporine, erythromycin, gemfibrozil, niacin, immunosuppressants. Instruct patient to take with meals. Encourage fluids, fiber, and exercise for constipation. Notify physician of muscle pain or weakness. Note results of liver function tests.
Niacin nicotinic acid (Niaspan, Nicobid, Nico-400, Nicotinex)	Inhibits free fatty acid release, decreases hepatic synthesis of VLDLs and LDLs, increases lipoprotein lipase activity.	Flushing of face and neck caused by vasodilation, itching, hyperuricemia, elevated liver enzymes. Rarely, hyperglycemia. Contraindicated with active peptic ulcer, severe hypotension, liver disease, arterial hemorrhage. **Pregnancy Category C.**	Assess aspirin allergy since that predicts possible niacin allergy. Monitor BP because of vasodilation. Monitor blood glucose in people with diabetes. If given with HMG-CoA reductase inhibitors, risk of rhabdomyolysis. Advise patient to take with meals. Teach management of orthostatic hypotension. Advise that flushing tends to decrease over time.
Fibric acid gemfibrozil (Lopid) clofibrate (Atromid-S)	Decreases serum triglycerides by increasing lipoprotein lipase, which breaks down very low density lipoproteins.	Abdominal pain and diarrhea are most common adverse effects. Nausea, vomiting, dizziness, blurred vision, rash, and pruritus sometimes occur. Rarely causes hypoglycemia (most common in patients taking hypoglycemic agents).	Contraindicated with liver or renal disease. Monitor lab values. Advise patient not to drive if dizziness occurs. Enhances warfarin. With HMG-CoA reductase inhibitors, risk of rhabdomyolysis and renal failure.

REVIEW QUESTIONS: UNIT 9

Case Study

Mrs. Ling is a 73-year-old Chinese-American who has just been admitted to a telemetry unit with a diagnosis of congestive heart failure (CHF). Prior to admission, her only medication was verapamil (Calan) 240 mg daily for hypertension. Her vital signs on admission were as follows: P 104, slightly irregular; R 24; T 98°F; BP 168/96. She is alert and appears anxious. Crackles are heard in the lower lobes of both lungs. She has 3+ edema in both feet and ankles. Medication orders include digoxin 0.25 mg PO daily, and furosemide (Lasix) 20 mg IV now. The following questions apply to this situation.

1. What is the action of digoxin?

2. What three body systems reflect the common adverse effects of digoxin?

3. When preparing to give Mrs. Ling's digoxin, you count an apical heart rate of 88. What should you do?

4. In this situation, which adverse effect of furosemide is especially important?

5. Mrs. Ling is weighed on her third day of hospitalization. She is amazed to see that she has lost 10 lbs. How would you explain this to her?

6. Mrs. Ling's condition has improved and she will be discharged on digoxin soon. Which information would be accurate and appropriate to include in your discharge teaching plan?

   a. If your pulse is less than 80, skip a dose of your digoxin.

   b. Report loss of appetite, nausea, or changes in vision to your physician.

   c. Take your digoxin at the same time each day.

Following discharge from the hospital, Mrs. Ling is being monitored by the home health nurse. The nurse has taught her how to assess her pulse before each dose of digoxin. On the last visit, Mrs. Ling states that her pulse has been irregular. The nurse's assessment confirms this and the physician is notified. Diagnostic studies reveal atrial fibrillation for which quinidine is prescribed. The following questions apply to this situation.

7. In general, antidysrhythmics work by decreasing _____.

8. List two side effects common to most antidysrhythmics.

9. An adverse effect of quinidine that affects the central nervous system is _____.

10. The nurse will inspect Mrs. Ling's skin for bruising and ask about unexplained bleeding because _____.

11. The nurse must be aware of what important drug interaction?

Two months later, Mrs. Ling is being visited at home by a home health nurse. Mrs. Ling is taking digoxin 0.25 mg and verapamil (Calan) 240 mg daily. The nurse's assessment reveals: P 74, R 18, BP 132/76. Mrs. Ling has mild ankle edema that she says resolves overnight. Her lung sounds are clear and her weight remains stable. The following questions apply to this situation.

12. What is the classification of verapamil?

13. What is the effect of verapamil on the blood pressure and heart rate?

14. The nurse asks if Mrs. Ling has any dizziness when she changes positions. What is the rationale for asking this?

15. Mrs. Ling notes that she does feel lightheaded when she rises. What should you advise?

16. Mrs. Ling asks if she could just take the verapamil when she feels like her BP is high. What should you tell her?

17. What might occur if Mrs. Ling were to suddenly stop taking her verapamil?

18. What can she do to reduce ankle edema?

DRUGS THAT AFFECT THE DIGESTIVE SYSTEM

OBJECTIVES

1. List the drug classifications used to treat digestive tract disorders.

2. Explain the actions, side and adverse effects, interactions, and contraindications of antiulcer drugs, emetics and antiemetics, laxatives, and antidiarrheals.

3. Describe nursing assessment data to be collected when patients are on specific drugs that affect the digestive tract.

4. Identify nursing interventions, including patient teaching, relevant to each major classification of drugs used to treat digestive tract disorders.

Anatomy and Physiology of the Digestive Tract

The functions of the digestive tract are digestion, absorption, and elimination. Disorders of the digestive tract can interfere with any or all of these functions, placing the patient at risk for complications such as nutritional deficiencies, fluid and electrolyte deficits, and complications associated with alterations in elimination.

The major structures of the digestive tract are the mouth, pharynx, esophagus, stomach, small intestine, large intestine (colon), and anus. Accessory organs are the salivary glands, liver, gallbladder, and pancreas. The accessory organs secrete enzymes into the digestive tract that are essential for the breakdown or metabolism of foodstuffs.

Normal function of the digestive tract depends on the intake of adequate nutrients and fluid, adequate protective mucus, an intact unobstructed tract, normal smooth muscle tone throughout the tract, adequate blood supply to maintain tissues and to absorb nutrients, secretion of digestive enzymes, hormones that regulate secretion of digestive fluids, and autonomic innervation to regulate neuromuscular activity.

Alterations in any of these factors can create problems affecting ingestion, digestion, absorption, or elimination. For example, anorexia associated with chemotherapy prevents adequate food intake. Lack of adequate mucus or excess acid production, or both, contributes to ulcer formation. Drugs taken to treat pain suppress the sympathetic nervous system and slow peristalsis, resulting in constipation. Thus, a great variety of factors can lead to digestive tract disorders.

Drugs Used to Treat Digestive Tract Disorders

Drugs used to treat digestive tract conditions essentially work by affecting one or more of the variables needed for normal function. For example, they can affect appetite, suppress or stimulate the vomiting center in the brain, influence mucus and acid secretion, replace deficient enzymes, alter rate of peristalsis, and change the consistency of stool. Classifications included in this unit are antiulcer drugs including antacids, emetics and antiemetics, laxatives, and antidiarrheals.

CHAPTER 34

ANTACIDS AND ANTIULCER DRUGS

*D*rugs, including antacids, H_2 receptor antagonists, mucosal barriers, synthetic prostaglandins, anticholinergics, and antibiotics, are used to treat peptic ulcer disease. Combinations of drugs are often employed. The goals of drug therapy with ulcers are to relieve pain and to promote healing by protecting the ulcer from further damage, eliminating causative microorganisms, and reducing gastric acid secretion.

ANTACIDS

Antacids are classified as aluminum, magnesium, calcium, and sodium compounds. They are available "over the counter" (OTC), which means that no prescription is required. Antacids are widely used by the general population for various digestive tract symptoms.

Actions

Antacids are alkaline substances that decrease the acidity of gastric fluids by neutralizing hydrochloric acid in the stomach.

Uses

Antacids are used primarily for peptic ulcer disease and gastroesophageal reflux disease (GERD). In peptic ulcer disease, antacids (1) decrease acidity, which reduces trauma to the ulcerated stomach and duodenal linings, and (2) reduce the activity of pepsin, an enzyme that digests protein, including the exposed ulcer surface. Antacids also may be given to help prevent ulcer formation in susceptible patients by decreasing acidity.

In GERD, acidic gastric contents flow backward into the esophagus, creating pain and a potential for ulceration. Antacids, by reducing gastric acidity, reduce the irritation of the esophagus.

Side and Adverse Effects

Other than sodium bicarbonate, antacids are poorly absorbed and unlikely to have any systemic effects. They do, however, affect bowel function. Antacids containing aluminum or calcium tend to promote constipation, whereas those containing magnesium tend to promote diarrhea. The preparations most often advised are those composed of a combination of aluminum and magnesium to minimize adverse bowel effects. Calcium and sodium preparations release carbon dioxide, which can cause eructation (belching) and flatulence (gas).

Sodium preparations have limited usefulness and are used cautiously, if at all, for people with hypertension, heart failure, and renal disease because the excess sodium may cause fluid retention, which aggravates the cardiac or renal condition. If used excessively, sodium bicarbonate can cause metabolic alkalosis.

Adverse effects specific to each prototype are noted in Table 34–1.

Interactions and Contraindications

Antacids can affect the dissolution, absorption, and elimination of most other drugs if taken simultaneously. For example, iron is best absorbed in an acid environment. If it is given with an antacid, the gastric fluids become less acidic and the iron is not well absorbed. Sucralfate (Carafate) is another drug that is affected by antacids. Since sucralfate is activated in an acid medium, antacids reduce its effectiveness. If the antimicrobial tetracycline is given with an antacid, the two substances form an insoluble complex that cannot be absorbed. Therefore, the patient does not benefit from the antimicrobial. To avoid problems such as these, routinely administer antacids at least 1 hour apart from other drugs.

There are few contraindications to the use of antacids. Patients with renal insufficiency may develop magnesium toxicity with magnesium-based agents. As previously mentioned, hypertensive, cardiac, and renal patients, whose conditions may be adversely affected by fluid retention, should avoid sodium bicarbonate.

Nursing Actions

Assess epigastric pain. Record the frequency and characteristics of stools. Assess for edema in patients who take sodium preparations.

157

Patient Teaching

- Shake liquids before pouring.
- Take antacids at least 1 hour apart from other oral drugs.
- Chew tablets thoroughly before swallowing and follow with a glass of water or milk.
- The preferred schedule is seven doses daily (or as specified by the physician): 1 and 3 hours after each meal and at bedtime.

- Take antacids as directed even if you have no pain.
- Do not skip doses; this allows acidity to increase.
- Report constipation or diarrhea.

TABLE 34–1

Antacids Prototypes

Type	Prototype	Specific Considerations
Aluminum compounds	Aluminum hydroxide (Amphojel)	Causes constipation. Can cause hypophosphatemia (low serum phosphate). Contains significant sodium.
Magnesium compounds	Milk of magnesia	Causes diarrhea. Avoid with undiagnosed abdominal pain because of bowel stimulation. Small doses (5–15 mL) used as antacid; larger doses (30–60 mL) used as laxative. Risk of toxicity with renal impairment.
Calcium compounds	Calcium carbonate	Can cause eructation (belching) and flatulence. Acid production rebounds after initial drug action neutralizes excess acid. RARELY causes milk-alkalai syndrome: hypercalcemia, metabolic alkalosis, impaired renal function, soft tissue calcification.
Sodium compounds	Sodium bicarbonate	Not recommended for peptic ulcer disease. Sodium causes fluid retention. Can cause eructation and flatulence. Excessive use can cause metabolic alkalosis.
Combination agents	Aluminum hydroxide and magnesium hydroxide (Maalox)	Bowel effects minimized. Caution with renal or cardiac disease.

H_2-RECEPTOR ANTAGONISTS

Histamine-2 (H_2)–receptor antagonists include cimetidine (Tagamet), ranitidine (Zantac), famotidine (Pepcid), nizatidine (Axid Pulvules), and roxatidine (Roxin).

Actions

Histamine is a substance secreted by mast cells in the skin and other soft tissues and by basophils in the blood. People usually think about histamine causing symptoms associated with allergies (redness, swelling, itching, bronchoconstriction) because histamine causes such symptoms when it interacts with histamine-1 (H_1) receptors. However, histamine can also interact with other receptors called histamine-2 (H_2) receptors. Stimulation of H_2 receptors causes parietal cells in the stomach to secrete gastric acid. Excess acid can contribute to peptic ulcer disease.

Agents that block H_2 receptors are called H_2 blockers or antagonists. Blocking the receptors reduces the stimulus to produce gastric acid.

Uses

H_2 blockers are used to prevent and to treat peptic ulcer disease by suppressing the secretion of gastric acid.

Side and Adverse Effects

These drugs have a low incidence of serious side effects. Some patients report headache, myalgia (muscle aches), nausea, rash, itching, diarrhea or constipation, and dizziness.

Only cimetidine (Tagamet) has significant central nervous system (CNS) and antiandrogenic effects. Possible CNS effects include confusion, sedation, restlessness, and seizures. Older people seem to be most susceptible to the CNS effects. Antiandrogenic effects prevent androgens from binding to receptors so that male patients may experience gynecomastia (breast enlargement), reduced libido, and erectile dysfunction.

Interactions and Contraindications

Absorption of cimetidine and ranitidine is impaired if given within 1 hour of antacids. Drug interactions are most significant with cimetidine. Because cimetidine inhibits hepatic drug–metabolizing enzymes, drugs normally broken down by the liver remain in the body longer and may reach toxic blood levels. Examples of drugs whose actions may be prolonged or enhanced are warfarin, phenytoin, lidocaine, oral hypoglycemics, and theophylline.

⚠ Although there are no specific contraindications to the use of H₂ blockers, they have not been well studied in pregnant women. They are used with caution in patients with renal or liver dysfunction.

Nursing Actions

Gastric pH may be monitored to assess drug effects. The goal is to keep the pH at 5 or higher. (Remember that a low pH is acidic and a high pH is alkaline.) If antiandrogenic effects occur, reassure the patient that the effects will diminish after the drug is withdrawn. Notify the physician if the patient becomes confused.

Patient Teaching
• Inform your physician if you have dizziness, headache, or confusion. • Do not take cimetidine or ranitidine within 1 hour of taking antacids. • Smoking reduces the effectiveness of cimetidine. • Since cimetidine can affect other drugs you are taking, be sure your physician is aware that you are taking it.

MUCOSAL BARRIER

Actions

Sucralfate (Carafate) is the single member of a category described variously as *mucosal barrier* and *cytoprotective*. In the presence of gastric acids, sucralfate is converted to a thick, sticky gel that adheres to the surface of the ulcer for up to 6 hours. This protects the ulcer from acid and pepsin so that it can heal. The drug is not absorbed.

Uses

Sucralfate is used to treat gastric and duodenal ulcers.

Side and Adverse Effects

About 2% of patients have constipation with sucralfate. Otherwise, there are no known serious side or adverse effects.

Interactions and Contraindications

Antacids can interfere with the action of sucralfate since an acid medium is needed for sucralfate to form a protective gel. Sucralfate can interfere with the absorption of many drugs if they are given close together.

There are no known contraindications to the use of sucralfate.

Nursing Actions

Monitor stool frequency and consistency. Do NOT give sucralfate within 2 hours of phenytoin, warfarin, digoxin, ciproflaxin, or norfloxacin.

Patient Teaching
• Shake suspension. • Do NOT take sucralfate within 30 minutes of antacids. • If you take multiple medications, ask the pharmacist or physician how to schedule doses so that sucralfate does not interfere with absorption of the other drugs.

SYNTHETIC PROSTAGLANDINS

The only approved synthetic prostaglandin in use for the prevention of ulcers is misoprostol (Cytotec).

Actions

Normally occurring prostaglandins are fatty acids that, among other actions, regulate gastric acid secretion. Misoprostol is a synthetic prostaglandin that suppresses gastric acid secretion, promotes bicarbonate and gastric mucus secretion, and improves blood flow to the gastric mucosa.

⚠ The drug is also classified as an abortifacient because it stimulates uterine contractions, which can cause abortion in the pregnant woman.

Uses

In the United States, misoprostol is used primarily to prevent gastric ulcers in patients on long-term therapy with nonsteroidal anti-inflammatory drugs (NSAIDs) including aspirin. In other countries, it is used to treat peptic ulcer disease related to other causes as well. Because of the effects on the uterus, misoprostol may be used to induce abortion.

Side and Adverse Effects

Diarrhea and abdominal pain are fairly common among patients taking misoprostol. Some women report spotting (bleeding between menstrual periods) and menstrual cramps. There have been occasional reports of nausea, flatulence, heartburn, and headache. Symptoms of overdosage include sedation, tremor, convulsions, dyspnea, palpitations, hypotension, and bradycardia.

Interactions and Contraindications

If given with magnesium antacid compounds, the risk of diarrhea increases. The only contraindications to misoprostol are allergy to the drug and pregnancy. Physicians typically require a negative pregnancy test within 2 weeks of prescribing therapy. Therapy is then delayed until the second or third day of the next menstrual cycle. **Pregnancy Category X.**

Nursing Actions

Inquire about pregnancy before first dose. Be sure that patients of childbearing age understand the risk of abortion if pregnancy occurs during misoprostol therapy.

Patient Teaching
• If taken during pregnancy, this drug can cause abortion.

ANTICHOLINERGICS

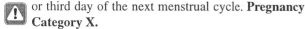

Anticholinergic agents used in the treatment of peptic ulcer disease include atropine (Atropine), glycopyrrolate, (Robinul), clidinium bromide (Quarzan), hyoscyamine sulfate (Anaspaz), and propantheline bromide (Pro-Banthine).

Actions

Acetylcholine is a chemical that conveys messages from nerve endings to body cells. Anticholinergics block the action of acetylcholine, resulting in decreased salivary and gastric secretions, decreased gastrointestinal tone and motility, dilated pupils, increased heart rate, decreased respiratory secretions, bronchodilation, and decreased bladder tone.

Uses

The many clinical uses of anticholinergics include management of peptic ulcer disease.

Side and Adverse Effects

Commonly reported side effects are dry mouth, constipation, blurred vision, urinary retention, and mild tachycardia. Manifestations of toxicity are excitement, nausea and vomiting, elevated temperature, thick respiratory secretions, dyspnea, and erectile dysfunction.
Adverse effects are more common in the elderly.

Interactions and Contraindications

Anticholinergic absorption is impaired by antacids and antidiarrheal agents.

Contraindications include allergy to the specific drug, glaucoma, liver or renal dysfunction, tachycardia, ulcerative colitis, asthma, bladder neck obstruction, paralytic ileus, and myasthenia gravis.

Nursing Actions

Monitor pulse and respirations. Auscultate bowel sounds and record bowel movements. Palpate for bladder distention.

Patient Teaching
• Report difficulty voiding.
• To manage constipation, increase fluid intake (unless contraindicated), dietary fiber, and exercise.
• If you feel drowsy, call for help when getting out of bed and avoid activities that require mental alertness.
• Fluids, mouthwash, gum, and sugar-free hard candy (if permitted) will stimulate salivation and relieve dry mouth.

ANTIBIOTICS

The discovery of a microorganism named *Helicobacter pylori* in the stomachs of many people with ulcers revolutionized treatment of peptic ulcer disease. In patients with documented *H. pylori* infection, treatment includes two or three antibiotics along with an agent that decreases acid secretion. The most commonly used antibiotics are metronidazole, tetracycline, bismuth subsalicylate (Pepto-Bismol), clarithromycin, and amoxicillin. If a single antimicrobial agent is used, there is the likelihood of resistant strains developing. When several antibiotics are used simultaneously, resistance is less common. A package containing bismuth subsalicylate tablets, tetracycline capsules, and metronidazole tablets is marketed as Helidac and is intended to promote compliance by providing the correct combination of drugs in a convenient manner.

Actions

Antimicrobials generally destroy bacteria by disrupting the bacterial cell wall, inhibiting an enzyme that is essential for bacterial growth, or disrupting synthesis of bacterial proteins.

Uses

Antibiotic therapy is used to treat newly diagnosed and recurrent cases of peptic ulcer disease including those in patients whose conditions are associated with NSAID therapy.

Side and Adverse Effects

General adverse effects of antibiotics are allergy, superinfections such as "yeast" infections, and gastrointestinal disturbances. These effects can be mild or very serious. Additional serious problems with some specific antibiotics are nephrotoxicity, neurotoxicity, and blood dyscrasias. Adverse effects of the commonly used antiulcer antibiotics are summarized in Table 34–2.

Interactions and Contraindications

Metronidazole, if taken with alcohol, can cause acute illness referred to as a *disulfiram-like reaction.* A milder reaction is demonstrated by nausea, vomiting, and hypotension. Severe reactions may result in fatal cardiac and respiratory symptoms. Tetracycline binds with calcium in the digestive tract. Therefore, if it is taken with dairy products or antacids, tetracycline will be poorly absorbed.

The most important contraindication for antibiotics is a history of allergic reactions to the specific agent or other agents from the same classification. For example, penicillins and cephalosporins are chemically similar. People who are allergic to one have about a 10% risk of being allergic to the other as well. Other antibiotics may also have specific contraindications.

Nursing Actions

Before giving any antibiotic, always assess known allergies and document them prominently. If the patient reports allergy to the ordered drug, withhold the drug and notify the physician. Allergic reactions can occur following the first or subsequent doses of a drug, so the patient should be observed for rash, itching, edema, and respiratory difficulty when on antibiotics.

To maintain therapeutic blood levels of antibiotics around the clock, schedule doses so they are evenly spaced. If blood levels are not maintained for the period of treatment, resistant strains of the bacteria can develop.

Patient Teaching
• Because many antibiotics can be harmful to the kidneys, you should drink at least eight 8-ounce glasses of liquids daily (unless contraindicated). • It is very important to take the drugs as prescribed and to complete the full course of the drug.

Prototypes

Information about the specific antibiotics used to treat peptic ulcer disease is summarized in Table 34–2.

TABLE 34–2

Antiulcer Antibiotics

Antiulcer Antibiotic	Adverse Effects	Nursing Considerations
Bismuth subsalicylate (Pepto-Bismol)	Grayish-black stools, dark tongue, constipation in debilitated patients.	Contraindicated with bleeding ulcers, renal dysfunction. Can increase risk of bleeding with anticoagulants, heparin, thrombolytics. Increases effects of hypoglycemic agents, so people with diabetes may have low blood glucose. Shake before pouring. Tell patient tablets can be chewed or allowed to dissolve in the mouth. Avoid during pregnancy. ⚠
Metronidazole (Flagyl)	Nausea, headache, dry mouth, anorexia, metallic taste in mouth, vaginitis. Glossitis and peripheral neuropathy (reversible if treatment is stopped promptly).	Avoid during pregnancy. Tell patient urine may be dark or reddish-brown. Avoid alcohol.
Tetracycline (Achromycin, Sumycin, et al.)	Nausea, vomiting, diarrhea, photosensitivity, candidiasis (fungal infection), discoloration of teeth if exposed in utero or up to age 9.	Avoid during pregnancy and before age 9. ⚠
Clarithromycin (Biaxin)	Nausea, vomiting, headache, abnormal taste in mouth, superinfection. Rarely: liver toxicity, low platelet count.	Give with 8 ounces of water. Tell patient to report signs of superinfection: sore mouth, genital or anal itching, severe diarrhea.
Amoxicillin (Augmentin)	Nausea, vomiting, diarrhea, headache, oral and vaginal candidiasis. Possibly serious superinfections, especially severe colitis. Nephritis.	Decreases effects of oral contraceptives. Tell patient to report frequent diarrhea with cramping. Monitor intake and output if hospitalized.

EMETICS AND ANTIEMETICS

ANTIEMETICS

Nausea and vomiting are symptoms associated with many illnesses, severe pain, and stress. They also may represent common adverse drug reactions. Although nausea and vomiting commonly occur together, either can occur alone. Nausea is an unpleasant sensation accompanied by the feeling that vomiting is about to occur. Vomiting is the ejection of stomach contents through the mouth.

When sensors in the stomach, intestines, inner ear, cerebral cortex, or fourth ventricle in the brain (location of the chemoreceptor trigger zone [CTZ]) detect unpleasant physical or psychological stimuli, messages are relayed to the vomiting center in the brain. When the vomiting center is activated, the autonomic nervous system responds with increased salivation, peripheral vasoconstriction, and increased heart rate. The glottis closes, the gastroesophageal sphincter relaxes, and muscles in the stomach, esophagus, and diaphragm contract. Reverse peristalsis propels the gastric contents backward, and vomiting occurs.

Although we tend to think of vomiting as undesirable, it is essentially a protective mechanism to rid the body of potentially harmful substances. Occasional vomiting is unlikely to cause complications in the otherwise healthy patient. However, patients who cannot reposition themselves or are unconscious are at risk for aspiration of gastric contents into the respiratory tract. This could result in obstruction or pneumonia. Further, the loss of fluid and electrolytes with severe or prolonged vomiting can lead to dehydration, electrolyte imbalances, and acid-base imbalances. Young children and the elderly are especially vulnerable to fluid and electrolyte disturbances.

Drugs used to treat nausea and vomiting are called *antiemetics*. Classifications of drugs commonly used as antiemetics include phenothiazines, antihistamines, anticholinergics, and prokinetic agents. Selective serotonin antagonists and cannabinoids are effective antiemetics that are used almost exclusively for patients undergoing chemotherapy for cancer. Other drugs that have antiemetic effects, but are more often used for other purposes, are corticosteroids (covered in Chapter 43) and benzodiazepines (covered in Chapter 51).

Phenothiazines

The phenothiazines that are most effective against vomiting are chlorpromazine (Thorazine), prochlorperazine (Compazine), perphenazine (Trilafon), thiethylperazine (Torecan), and promethazine (Phenergan).

Action

Phenothiazines block dopamine receptors in the chemoreceptor trigger zone and the vomiting center, thereby suppressing the vomiting reflex.

Uses

These drugs are used primarily to treat psychotic symptoms, but many are effective as antiemetics. They are useful in a variety of situations, except treatment of motion sickness.

Side and Adverse Effects

Important adverse effects of phenothiazines include drowsiness, anticholinergic effects, hypotension, and extrapyramidal reactions. Extrapyramidal reactions are abnormal involuntary movements. These effects are more common when the drugs are used long-term for psychosis than when they are used occasionally as antiemetics.

Interactions and Contraindications

If given with other drugs that depress the central nervous system (CNS), excessive sedation and respiratory depression may occur. Combined with vasodilators, phenothiazines may have a marked hypotensive effect. Antacids, tea, coffee, milk, and fruit juice interfere with the absorption of phenothiazines.

Conditions that contraindicate the use of phenothiazines are chronic respiratory disorders such as emphysema and asthma, and Parkinson's disease. They are used with caution in the presence of cardiovascular, liver, or renal disease.

Nursing Actions

Monitor blood pressure and level of alertness. Assess for abnormal movements, although this would be unlikely with only occasional use of phenothiazines. When you give a patient a phenothiazine for nausea and vomiting, anticipate drowsiness and take safety precautions.

Patient Teaching
• You will probably feel drowsy, so call for assistance when getting up.

Antihistamines

Antihistamines that are useful as antiemetics include dimenhydrinate (Dramamine), hydroxyzine (Vistaril), and cyclizine (Marezine).

Actions

Antihistamines block the action of acetylcholine in the brain and interfere with the transmission of impulses from the inner ear to the vomiting center.

Use

Antihistamines are most often used to prevent and treat nausea and vomiting associated with motion sickness.

Side and Adverse Effects

Because antihistamines block acetylcholine, they cause classic anticholinergic side effects, including drowsiness, blurred vision, constipation, and urinary retention.

Interactions and Contraindications

The effects of antihistamines are enhanced by other central nervous system depressants, so the patient may have excessive sedation.

Antihistamines should not be given during an acute asthma attack because they dry secretions, making them more difficult to clear. They must be used cautiously in patients with prostate enlargement, narrow-angle glaucoma, or chronic obstructive pulmonary disease (COPD) because of the respective risks of urinary retention, increased intraocular pressure, and thickened respiratory secretions.

Anticholinergics

Scopolamine is an anticholinergic that is especially effective in preventing motion sickness. It is available as a tablet and as a transdermal patch that is applied to the skin behind the ear. Like antihistamines, this drug causes drowsiness, dry mouth, and blurred vision. Urinary retention is an uncommon adverse effect. The drug is contraindicated with glaucoma.

Prokinetic Agents

The prokinetic agent that is used as an antiemetic drug is metoclopramide (Reglan).

Action

Metoclopramide increases the release of acetylcholine in the gastrointestinal tract, resulting in increased gastrointestinal motility, which causes the stomach to empty more rapidly. It also blocks dopamine and serotonin receptors in the CTZ to suppress nausea and vomiting.

Uses

Metoclopramide is useful in treating gastroparesis (a condition in which the movement of food from the stomach to the intestines is delayed) and esophageal reflux, and to prevent nausea related to chemotherapy.

Side and Adverse Effects

The most common adverse effects of metoclopramide are drowsiness, dizziness, insomnia, and headache. Extrapyramidal symptoms may occur in children and young adults who receive high doses with chemotherapy.

Interactions and Contraindications

Expect increased sedation if metoclopramide is given with other CNS depressants. Other drugs that cause extrapyramidal symptoms increase the risk of that adverse effect with metoclopramide.

Because it stimulates the gastrointestinal tract, metoclopramide should not be given in the presence of gastrointestinal perforation, hemorrhage, or obstruction. It is also contraindicated with seizure disorders.

Nursing Actions

Take safety precautions for drowsiness (side rails up, call bell in reach, advise patient to call for help to get out of bed). Assess for motor restlessness. Document effect of drug.

Patient Teaching
• This drug may make you drowsy, so avoid activities requiring alertness.
• Report any abnormal movements or difficulty sleeping.

Selective Serotonin Antagonists

Ondansetron (Zofran) and granisetron (Kytril) are selective serotonin antagonists.

Action

These drugs control nausea by blocking serotonin receptors in the CTZ.

Uses

The primary use for selective serotonin antagonists is to suppress nausea and vomiting in patients who are receiving chemotherapeutic agents.

Side and Adverse Effects

Headache, diarrhea, and dizziness are the most common side effects of ondansetron. Granisetron may cause headache, weakness, and diarrhea or constipation.

Interactions and Contraindications

There are no significant drug interactions with ondansetron. However, drugs that stimulate liver enzymes can decrease the effectiveness of granisetron.

There are no contraindications for either of these drugs.

Nursing Implications

Administer as ordered 30 minutes prior to the beginning of chemotherapy. This will permit the drug to take effect before the patient receives the chemotherapeutic drug that tends to be emetogenic (causing nausea and vomiting). Document the patient's response.

Cannabinoids

The two cannabinoids available as antiemetics are dronabinol (Marinol) and nabilone (Cesamet). Although these drugs are effective antiemetics, their use is limited because of the potential for abuse.

Action

The mechanism by which cannabinoids exert antiemetic effects is not known.

Uses

The primary use of dronabinol and nabilone is to treat nausea and vomiting associated with chemotherapy. Dronabinol is also used as an appetite stimulant in people with acquired immunodeficiency syndrome (AIDS).

Side and Adverse Effects

The effect of taking cannabinoids is like that experienced when smoking marijuana: feelings of elation, mood changes, distorted perceptions, and hallucinations. In addition to CNS effects, the drugs can cause tachycardia and hypotension.

Interactions and Contraindications

There is a risk of excessive CNS depression if cannabinoids are taken with alcohol or barbiturates.

Patients with psychiatric disorders should not take cannabinoids because of the CNS effects. Cannabinoids must be used cautiously in people with cardiovascular disease because of the effects on the heart rate and blood pressure.

Nursing Actions

Observe the patient's response to the drug. If the patient has a psychotic episode after receiving the drug, withhold further doses and notify the physician. Provide a quiet environment and supervise the patient. Dronabinol and nabilone are classified under Schedule II of the Controlled Substances Act.

Patient Teaching
• The side and adverse effects of cannabinoids preclude activities requiring mental alertness.

Glucocorticoids

Methylprednisolone (Solu-Medrol) and dexamethasone (Decadron) are used to prevent nausea and vomiting with chemotherapy, even though they are not approved by the Food and Drug Administration (FDA) for that purpose. Glucocorticoids are discussed in detail in Chapter 43. However, when they are used short-term with chemotherapy, serious adverse effects are unlikely.

DRUGS USED TO TREAT POISONING

Drugs used to treat poisoning include emetics, absorptive agents, and antidotes and antagonists. It is very important to remember that treatment must be specific to the type of substance ingested. Therefore, when poisoning occurs in the home setting, the first action should be to collect the substance container and call the local Poison Control Center. Some poisons need prompt dilution, others can be neutralized, and still others should be removed from the system as promptly as possible.

Emetics

We have given considerable attention to antiemetics, since it is usually desirable to prevent or treat nausea and vomiting. However, in situations such as ingestion of drug overdoses or poisons, vomiting may be therapeutic. Drugs that induce vomiting are called emetics. The most commonly used emetic is syrup of ipecac.

Action

Syrup of ipecac irritates the gastric mucosa and stimulates the vomiting center. The drug is usually effective in 5 to 30 minutes.

Uses

Ipecac should be administered as directed by the Poison Control Center or according to product label information.

Side and Adverse Effects

After ipecac is given, the patient's heart rate may increase and blood pressure decrease before vomiting occurs. After vomiting, diarrhea and mild CNS depression are common. If a patient does not vomit after taking ipecac, there is a risk of potentially fatal cardiotoxicity with cardiac dysrhythmias and dyspnea.

People who abuse the drug by taking it regularly can develop toxicity manifested by generalized weakness and aching, muscular incoordination, slurred speech, and changes in cardiac function.

Contraindications

Vomiting should NOT be induced by any means in the patient who

- is not fully alert.
- is having seizure activity.
- has consumed caustic substances.
- has consumed petroleum products.

There is a risk of aspiration if the patient is not alert, is having seizures, or has ingested petroleum products. Caustic substances can cause additional damage to the esophagus during vomiting.

Nursing Actions

Once vomiting occurs, document the characteristics of the emesis and monitor pulse, blood pressure, and respirations for CNS depression. Be aware of the risk for abuse of ipecac by people with eating disorders. In addition, in rare cases, parents have been known to induce "illness" in children by administering it unnecessarily.

Patient Teaching
• Syrup of ipecac should be readily available in the home, **but it is not appropriate in all circumstances**. Call Poison Control before taking action.
• Follow a dose of ipecac with three or four 8-ounce glasses of water for an adult.
• If an initial dose of ipecac does not result in vomiting, it can be repeated one time. If the second dose is ineffective, the patient should be taken to an emergency room for care.
• Syrup of ipecac can be toxic if used regularly.

Absorptive Agents

Activated charcoal is an absorptive agent. It is available as a liquid or a powder.

Uses

Activated charcoal absorbs and inactivates toxic substances so that they pass harmlessly through the digestive tract.

Side and Adverse Effects

Activated charcoal has few side effects except occasional diarrhea, gastrointestinal distress, and intestinal gas.

Contraindications

There are no significant contraindications.

Nursing Actions

Typically, activated charcoal is used after vomiting has been induced with ipecac. The dosage is based on the amount of poison ingested and the patient's weight. The powder is mixed with tap water or fruit juice (a minimum of 250 mL) to form a thick syrup. It should not be mixed with diary products, which would reduce the absorptive capacity of the agent. It may be given orally or through a nasogastric tube.

Antidotes and Antagonists

Emetics and activated charcoal are generally nonspecific and aimed at removing or inactivating whatever substance is present. For some drugs, specific agents are available. An example is naloxone (Narcan), which antagonizes narcotics, meaning it blocks the action of narcotics. Other specific examples are mentioned with specific drugs throughout this book.

CHAPTER 36

LAXATIVES AND CATHARTICS

$\mathcal{M}$any factors contribute to constipation, including inadequate fluids or fiber, immobility, and drugs such as anticholinergics, antidepressants, and analgesics. Laxatives and cathartics are used to treat constipation. Both stimulate bowel elimination, but cathartics act more quickly and are more likely to produce a watery stool. Laxatives can be classified as bulk-forming, surfactant, stimulant, osmotic, and miscellaneous.

Laxatives are appropriately used for treatment of occasional constipation. They are also used to prevent constipation in conditions in which it might be harmful, such as rectal surgery, heart conditions, and hemorrhoids. Lastly, they are given to empty the bowel before diagnostic and surgical procedures.

Laxatives are contraindicated when the patient has undiagnosed abdominal pain. There is always a possibility that such pain is associated with appendicitis, other bowel inflammation, or obstruction. In those cases, stimulation could result in rupture of the bowel.

An important problem with laxatives is the potential for abuse leading to dependency. Many people have the misconception that a daily bowel movement is necessary, when, in fact, healthy people may have as few as three bowel movements each week.

People who abuse laxatives fall into a pattern of using cathartics to empty the bowel on a regular basis. A common scenario is as follows. A patient has not had a bowel movement for 2 days. Concerned, he takes a laxative that empties the bowel. Since it takes 2 to 5 days for the bowel contents to be restored, he has no additional bowel movements for several days. Once again, he takes a cathartic to induce bowel emptying and a cycle of laxative abuse becomes established.

Nurses must educate the public that the frequency of bowel elimination is less important that the consistency of the stool. As long as stools are soft and passed without difficulty, the patient is not constipated. People who often report hard, infrequent stools passed with straining should be taught to increase fluid and fiber intake, increase physical activity, and respond promptly to the defecation urge.

General nursing actions when administering laxatives and cathartics are listed here and are not repeated with each classification.

- Monitor stool frequency and characteristics.
- Assess for bowel sounds and abdominal pain and distention.
- Do not administer laxatives if appendicitis or obstruction is suspected.
- Monitor fluid and electrolyte status when using cathartics, especially with elderly patients.
- Encourage increased exercise and fluid and fiber intake to prevent constipation.
- Do not give laxatives with other drugs, as they may affect absorption of the other drugs.
- Evaluate and document effects.

BULK-FORMING LAXATIVES

Bulk-forming laxatives include methylcellulose (Citrucel), psyllium (Metamucil), and calcium polycarbophil (FiberCon).

Action

Bulk-forming laxatives are indigestible substances that absorb water in the colon and swell, increasing and softening the fecal mass. The increased bulk of fecal material stretches the colon wall, which stimulates peristalsis. The softening action allows the passage of softer stool without straining.

Uses

Bulk-forming laxatives are widely used for treatment of temporary constipation as well as for long-term management of diverticulosis and irritable bowel syndrome. Because of the way they alter the stool characteristics, they are sometimes used to produce a more formed stool in people with fecal diversions. Bulk-forming agents require several days to take effect, so they are not effective for relieving acute constipation.

Side and Adverse Effects

Most people tolerate bulk-forming laxatives well, although some report flatulence and bloating. The most dangerous adverse effect is esophageal or bowel obstruction, which can occur when the patient's fluid intake is inadequate. Without adequate fluids, the agent forms a hard mass that cannot be moved through the gastrointestinal tract.

Interactions and Contraindications

Bulk-forming laxatives may decrease absorption of warfarin, digoxin, and salicylates. They may interfere with the effects of potassium-sparing diuretics and potassium supplements.

Because of the risk of intestinal obstruction, bulk-forming laxatives are contraindicated with conditions in which the intestinal lumen is narrowed. Diabetic patients should avoid preparations containing sugar, and people with heart failure or hypertension should avoid the preparations that contain sodium.

Patient Teaching
• Take each dose with a full glass of water or juice to prevent esophageal obstruction.   • Good hydration is essential to prevent intestinal obstruction; drink eight 8-ounce glasses of fluids each day with your physician's approval.

SURFACTANT LAXATIVES

Examples of surfactant laxatives are docusate sodium (Colace) and docusate calcium (Surfak).

Action

Surfactants reduce surface tension in the fecal mass so that more water is retained in the feces. This results in a softer stool that is easily passed. It takes several days for the drug effect to be evident. Because of the mechanism of action and low risk of dependency, surfactants are called *stool softeners* and are sometimes not included in laxative classifications.

Uses

Surfactants are used to prevent constipation. Because of the delayed effects on the stool, they are not useful for immediate relief of constipation.

Side and Adverse Effects

Serious side effects are rare. Some patients report mild cramping. Throat irritation has been reported with the liquid preparation.

Interactions and Contraindications

Docusate increases absorption of digoxin, salicylates, quinidine, and mineral oil. Surfactant laxatives should not be given when the patient has abdominal symptoms that may be caused by inflammation or obstruction.

Patient Teaching
• Take a full glass of water with each dose.

STIMULANT LAXATIVES

Examples of stimulant laxatives are bisacodyl (Dulcolax), phenolphthalein (Ex-Lax), anthraquinone of cascara (Senokot), and castor oil.

Action

Stimulant laxatives, as the name implies, stimulate intestinal motility to promote bowel evacuation. They also draw water and electrolytes into the intestinal lumen, producing a more liquid stool. A semiliquid stool usually results within 6 to 12 hours after oral administration of the medication. Rectal suppositories act within 60 minutes.

Castor oil is different in that it stimulates the small intestine, causing more rapid results and more watery stools.

Uses

Stimulants are used to treat acute constipation.

Side and Adverse Effects

The primary adverse effect of stimulant laxatives is abdominal cramping. With excessive use, the patient can lose excess water, potassium, and sodium.

Interactions and Contraindications

Stimulants may affect the absorption of other oral drugs. Also, if the patient develops fluid and electrolyte disturbances, this will affect the actions of some drugs. Antacids and milk can interfere with the action of stimulants. Like all laxatives, stimulants are contraindicated with symptoms that may indicate intestinal inflammation or obstruction.

Patient Teaching
• Do not chew enteric-coated tablets.   • Take tablets at least 1 hour apart from antacids and milk.   • Phenolphthalein can cause the urine to appear pink, but that effect is harmless.

OSMOTIC LAXATIVES

Examples of osmotic laxatives are magnesium hydroxide (milk of magnesia), sodium phosphate (Fleet Phospho-Soda), and magnesium citrate.

Action

Osmotic laxatives are salts that are poorly absorbed. By osmosis, they draw fluid into the lumen of the intestinal tract. The fluid increases the volume of the fecal mass, which stretches the intestinal wall and triggers propulsive movement. The onset of action and liquidity of the stool vary with the different salts and the dosage.

Uses

Osmotic laxatives should be used only to treat acute constipation or for prompt bowel evacuation in preparation for diagnostic studies. They should not be used for long-term management.

Side and Adverse Effects

The most common side effect is abdominal cramping. If excessive diarrhea results, the patient is at risk for fluid deficits and electrolyte imbalances.

Interactions and Contraindications

Magnesium salts can decrease the effects of oral anticoagulants, digoxin, phenothiazines, and tetracycline. Agents containing phosphates have a number of potential interactions.

Even though little magnesium is absorbed, patients with renal disease are at risk for hypermagnesemia. Therefore, another laxative should be selected for those patients.

Nursing Actions

In patients at risk for hypermagnesemia, assess for signs of neuromuscular depression: muscle weakness, cardiac arrhythmias, and hypotension.

Patient Teaching

- Avoid frequent use of magnesium laxatives because of the risk of dependence.
- Report weakness, palpitations, and dizziness.
- If dizziness occurs, change positions slowly and avoid hazardous activities.

BOWEL LAVAGE AGENTS

Polyethylene glycol-electrolyte solution (GoLYTELY, Colyte) is an isosmotic solution that quickly purges the bowel, beginning as soon as 1 hour after ingestion. It may be used for severe constipation but is most often used to cleanse the bowel before diagnostic or surgical procedures. This agent comes in powder form and is dissolved in 4 liters of water. The large volume of fluid distends the bowel and stimulates peristalsis. Because the solution is isosmotic, it does not draw fluids and electrolytes from the intestinal walls. Often patients take GoLYTELY at home before coming in for medical tests or procedures, so correct instructions are essential.

Patient Teaching

- Chill the solution beforehand to make it more palatable.
- Drink 230 to 300 mL every 10 minutes until all the solution is taken.
- Do not eat or take any medications within 1 hour of taking the solution.
- You may have some cramping and a feeling of fullness.

CHAPTER 37

ANTIDIARRHEALS

*D*iarrhea is defined as the passage of frequent, watery stools. Among the many causes of diarrhea are bowel infection or inflammation, malabsorption, dumping syndrome, and adverse effects of drugs. Diarrhea of short duration is tolerated by most people, but there is a risk of fluid and electrolyte and acid-base imbalances with severe or prolonged diarrhea. In addition, irritation of the perianal area can lead to skin breakdown.

Antidiarrheal agents can be classified as nonspecific or specific. Nonspecific agents provide symptomatic relief regardless of the cause. Specific agents relieve diarrhea by treating the underlying problem.

NONSPECIFIC AGENTS

Nonspecific antidiarrheal agents include opioids, adsorbents, bulk-forming agents, and anticholinergic antispasmodics. Bulk-forming agents, covered in Chapter 36, are generally thought of as stool softeners. However, by absorbing water and holding it in a hydrophilic mass, these agents can be useful in treating diarrhea as well.

Opioids

Examples of opioids used to treat diarrhea are diphenoxylate HCl and atropine sulfate (Lomotil), loperamide HCl (Imodium A-D), and camphorated opium tincture (paregoric). Diphenoxylate HCl is classified as a Schedule V controlled substance, and camphorated opium tincture as a Schedule III controlled substance. Loperamide is considered to have low potential for abuse and is not controlled. It is available without a prescription.

Action

Opioids decrease intestinal motility, which allows time for increased absorption of water and electrolytes. They also decrease the secretion of fluid into the small intestine.

Uses

Opioids are used in the short-term treatment of acute diarrhea.

Side and Adverse Effects

Unless taken in excess, opioid antidiarrheals have minimal side effects. With large or frequent dosages, however, the patient may develop central nervous system (CNS) depression with mental depression, confusion, euphoria, sedation, and headache.

Interactions and Contraindications

If given with other CNS depressants, patients are more likely to exhibit evidence of CNS effects of the opioids. Opioids can cause a very serious condition called *toxic megacolon* in patients with inflammatory bowel disease.

Nursing Actions

When giving opioids, monitor the patient for signs of adverse CNS effects.

Specific Opioids

In addition to the general effects just covered, specific agents may require additional cautions and nursing interventions, as shown in Table 37–1.

	TABLE 37–1	
	Opioid Antidiarrheals	
Opioid Antidiarrheal	Adverse Effects	Nursing Considerations
Diphenoxylate HCl and atropine sulfate (Lomotil)	Drug contains atropine sulfate, so assess for anticholinergic effects: dry mouth, urinary retention, tachycardia, hyperthermia.	Offer oral hygiene. Assess for urinary retention: bladder distention, lower abdominal discomfort, low urine output. Monitor pulse and temperature.
Loperamide HCl (Imodium A-D)	May cause dry mouth, drowsiness, and abdominal discomfort.	Assist with oral hygiene. Institute safety precautions if drowsy. Note pain, which should be transient.
Camphorated opium tincture (paregoric)	May cause euphoria, but only with very high doses.	Assess response to drug. Maintain drug security due to potential for abuse.

Adsorbents

Adsorbents are substances that attract and retain other substances, such as toxins, poisons, and bacteria. Although its effectiveness has not been proven, Kaopectate is an adsorbent that is often used to treat diarrhea. Kaopectate generally results in more formed stools, but the patient may continue to lose excess fluid and electrolytes. Other antidiarrheal products are preferred.

Bismuth subsalicylate (Pepto-Bismol) also has adsorbent action that inactivates some bacterial toxins. In addition, it has an anti-inflammatory effect that inhibits motility in the large intestine. Large doses can cause tinnitus and other neurologic symptoms associated with salicylate or bismuth toxicity. Pepto-Bismol is contraindicated in patients who are allergic to aspirin and in children with Reye's syndrome.

SPECIFIC ANTIDIARRHEAL AGENTS

Specific agents are those employed to treat diarrhea caused by infections or associated with inflammatory bowel disease (IBD). Agents used to decrease inflammation in IBD may include aminosalicylate antibiotics, other anti-inflammatory agents, glucocorticoids, and immunosuppressants.

Antibiotics

Antibiotic therapy is indicated when diarrhea is caused by *Salmonella, Shigella, Campylobacter,* or *Clostridium.* "Traveler's diarrhea" is usually caused by *Escherichia coli.* It will usually resolve without treatment in a few days. When it persists, however, a fluoroquinolone such as ciprofloxacin (Cipro) may be prescribed.

Sulfasalazine (Azulfidine) is a sulfonamide that is used specifically for its anti-inflammatory action in IBD. Common adverse effects are nausea, fever, rash, and muscle aches. Less common, but more dangerous, is the risk of agranulocytosis and anemia in patients taking sulfasalazine.

Anti-Inflammatory Agents

In addition to sulfasalazine, the anti-inflammatory agents mesalamine (Asacol) and olsalazine (Dipentum) may be used to treat IBD. Mesalamine can be given orally, by retention enema, or by rectal suppository. Adverse effects, including headache, nausea, and abdominal discomfort, are generally mild and transient. Patients who are sensitive to sulfites experience cramping, diarrhea, fever, rash, and urticaria. If these symptoms occur, the drug should be stopped immediately. The most common adverse effect of olsalazine is watery diarrhea. Additional information about anti-inflammatory agents is given in Chapter 4.

Glucocorticoids

Glucocorticoids are discussed in Chapter 43. In IBD, benefits are attributed to the anti-inflammatory effects of glucocorticoids. Because of the serious adverse effects associated with glucocorticoids, they are usually employed only for short-term therapy in the treatment of IBD.

Immunosuppressants

Immunosuppressants are discussed in Chapter 27. Specific ones used to treat IBD are azathioprine, mercaptopurine, cyclosporine, and methotrexate.

REVIEW QUESTIONS: UNIT 10

Case Study

Mr. Kennon has been diagnosed with peptic ulcer disease, and the presence of *Helicobacter pylori* has been confirmed. (See Care Plan, Chapter 35 in the textbook). His physician prescribes Helidac QID for 14 days and famitidine (Pepcid) 40 mg HS. Complete the following statements and answer the questions related to these drugs.

1. Helidac is a package containing _____, _____, and _____.

2. Why are multiple antimicrobial agents used to treat peptic ulcer disease?

3. Mr. Kennon complains he has a sore mouth and a tingling sensation in the fingers. These symptoms are most likely adverse effects of

_____.

4. The action of famotidine is to _____

_____.

5. Famotidine is preferred over cimetidine because of the adverse effects of cimetidine, which include _____ , _____, and _____.

6. Mr. Kennon takes warfarin (Coumadin) for atrial fibrillation. How will the famotidine affect his metabolism of the warfarin?

DRUGS THAT AFFECT THE UROLOGICAL SYSTEM

OBJECTIVES

1. Explain the actions and uses, side and adverse effects, interactions, and contraindications of osmotic, thiazide, carbonic anhydrase inhibitor, potassium-sparing, and loop diuretics.

2. Discuss general and class-specific patient education guidelines and appropriate nursing actions for patients receiving diuretics.

3. Identify actions, side and adverse effects, interactions, and contraindications for common urinary tract analgesics and antiseptics.

4. Discuss patient education guidelines and appropriate nursing actions for patients receiving urinary tract analgesics and antiseptics.

The kidney is the principal organ of the body involved with water balance. It consists of more than one million functional units called *nephrons*. The nephron is composed of four distinct regions: (1) the glomerulus, (2) the proximal convoluted tubule, (3) the loop of Henle, and (4) the distal convoluted tubule. The glomerulus is a tuft of capillaries enclosed in a cup-like structure called *Bowman's capsule*. Water, electrolytes, and waste products can filter through the thin walls of the capillaries into the Bowman's capsule and through the convoluted tubule to the renal pelvis. The renal pelvis opens into the ureter, the ureter leads to the bladder, and from the bladder excretion is accomplished via the urethra.

The proximal convoluted tubule is closest to Bowman's capsule; next is the loop of Henle, so named because of its shape. Last comes the distal convoluted tubule, farthest from Bowman's capsule. Along this convoluted tubule selective reabsorption occurs, influenced by the hormone aldosterone and antidiuretic hormone from the posterior pituitary gland, resulting in retention of required body substances. Approximately 1 quart of blood flows through the kidneys each minute. Although the kidneys actually filter out about 50 liters of liquid a day, only about 1 liter (or 1 quart) is excreted by the body. The rest of the filtrate is reabsorbed along the convoluted tubule.

The kidneys are responsible for the excretion of water and nitrogenous waste (the products of protein metabolism). These nitrogenous wastes are mainly uric acid, urea, ammonia, and creatinine. The kidneys also help maintain fluid and electrolyte balance, especially for potassium, chloride, sodium, and bicarbonate. Other functions of the kidneys include assisting in the regulation of the acid-base balance in the body, the production of the enzyme renin, which acts to raise the blood pressure, and the production of erythropoietin, which acts to stimulate the bone marrow to produce more red blood cells.

Details of a Nephron

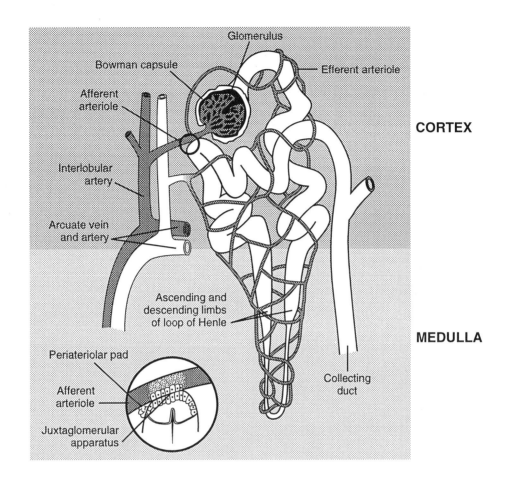

From Linton, Matteson, and Maebius (2000). *Introductory Nursing Care of Adults*, 2nd ed. Philadelphia: W.B. Saunders, p. 772.

DIURETICS

A *diuretic* is a drug that acts primarily on the kidneys to enhance or promote the excretion of sodium and water by increasing urine formation and output. Diuretics are generally used to help treat diseases associated with fluid retention, such as hypertension, diseases of the heart, kidney, and liver, and certain types of toxic drug effects. Diuretics are classified under the following major groups: (1) thiazides, (2) loop diuretics, (3) carbonic anhydrase inhibitors, (4) osmotics, and (5) potassium-sparing,

Many diuretics can cause electrolyte imbalances. For this reason, the nurse administering diuretics must be familiar with symptoms of electrolyte disturbances (see Chapter 7) and must monitor serum electrolyte results. Nursing actions whenever a patient is prescribed a diuretic include the following:

- automatically initiating intake and output monitoring
- weighing daily at the same time of day, in the same type of clothing, on the same scale
- assessing for signs of dehydration and electrolyte imbalances
- teaching patients how to identify drug effectiveness and adverse reactions

Additional nursing actions and patient education specific to each major diuretic group will be discussed where appropriate.

FIGURE 38–1

The Nephron and Diuretic Sites of Action

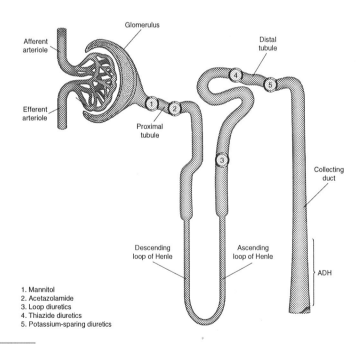

1. Mannitol
2. Acetazolamide
3. Loop diuretics
4. Thiazide diuretics
5. Potassium-sparing diuretics

From Lilley & Aucker (1998). *Pharmacology and the Nursing Process*, 2nd ed. St. Louis: Mosby, p. 321.

THIAZIDE DIURETICS

Actions

Thiazide diuretics are chemical derivatives of sulfonamides. Although acting in part to inhibit carbonic anhydrase, their diuretic effect arises mainly from their ability to promote the excretion of sodium and water primarily from the ascending loop of Henle and the distal convoluted tubule. Potassium, chloride, and bicarbonate are also excreted. By dilating arterioles, these drugs also lower peripheral vascular resistance, thus lowering blood pressure. The two most commonly prescribed thiazide diuretics are chlorothiazide, or CTZ, (Diuril) and hydrochlorothiazide, or HCTZ (HydroDIURIL, Esidrix, Oretic). A small alteration in the chemical structure of CTZ increases the potency of HCTZ, so that smaller doses of this drug give diuretic effects comparable to CTZ.

Uses

Because the combined effects of sodium and water depletion and decreased peripheral vascular resistance produce an antihypertensive effect, the thiazide diuretics are one of the most prescribed group of drugs for the treatment of hypertension, either as the sole drug or in combination with other drugs. In addition to hypertension, these drugs may also be useful as adjunct agents in the treatment of edema related to congestive heart failure (CHF), hepatic cirrhosis, and corticosteroid or estrogen therapy.

Side and Adverse Effects

- **Hematologic**: hypokalemia, hypercalcemia, hypomagnesemia, hyperglycemia, hyperlipidemia, hyperuricemia, thrombocytopenia, dehydration
- **Gastrointestinal**: nausea, vomiting, anorexia, abdominal cramps, cholecystitis, pancreatitis
- **Other**: photosensitivity, skin rashes, headache, impotence, and decreased libido

Interactions and Contraindications

Concomitant use of corticosteroids and thiazide diuretics have an additive effect, which may produce significant hypokalemia. Thiazides antagonize the action of oral hypoglycemic drugs, increasing the risk of hyperglycemia. Thiazides decrease clearance of lithium, which increases the potential for lithium toxicity. The use of nonsteroidal anti-inflammatory drugs (NSAIDs) with thiazides may reduce the effectiveness of the diuretic therapy.

Thiazides are contraindicated for persons with known hypersensitivity to sulfonamides, as well as those suffering from anuria or altered renal function.

Nursing Actions

Be aware of patient's medical history, as patients with chronic obstructive pulmonary disease (COPD) are more likely to be sensitive to the effects of thiazide diuretics. Check for drug and food allergies, especially to sulfonamides. Monitor serum electrolyte and glucose levels. Assess for signs and symptoms of dehydration and electrolyte imbalances (see Chapter 7). These are potassium-wasting drugs, so encourage patients to increase intake of potassium-rich foods.

LOOP DIURETICS

Actions

The loop diuretics are the strongest acting of the oral diuretics. Loop diuretics act directly on the ascending loop of Henle to inhibit sodium, chloride, and water reabsorption. They are also believed to activate the renal prostaglandins, resulting in the dilation of blood vessels in the kidneys, lungs, and possibly the entire body. This reduction in peripheral vascular resistance may account for their antihypertensive effects. Loop diuretics include bumetanide (Bumex), ethacrynic acid (Edecrin), furosemide (Lasix), and torsemide (Demadex). The most commonly prescribed drug in this category is furosemide (Lasix).

Uses

Loop diuretics are used to manage the edema associated with CHF and liver or kidney disease, to control hypertension, and to increase renal excretion of calcium in patients with hypercalcemia. Because these drugs are also very fast acting, they are often used in emergency situations, such as severe pulmonary or cerebral edema.

Side and Adverse Effects

- **Hematologic**: hypokalemia, hyponatremia, hyperglycemia, dehydration
- **Central nervous system**: dizziness, weakness
- **Gastrointestinal**: nausea, vomiting, anorexia, jaundice
- **Other**: photosensitivity, leg cramps, blurred vision, orthostatic hypotension

Loop diuretics are *ototoxic*, which may cause tinnitus and hearing loss.

Interactions and Contraindications

Concurrent use of corticosteroids and digitalis with loop diuretics may cause significant hypokalemia. With aminoglycoside antibiotics, there is increased risk for ototoxicity. Antihypertensive drugs and loop diuretics potentiate each other, increasing the risk for orthostatic hypotension. NSAIDs decrease the effects of loop diuretics. Because furosemide (Lasix) and bumetanide (Bumex) are chemically related to the sulfonamides, patients with sulfonamide hypersensitivity should avoid use of those drugs. Loop diuretics are contraindicated for persons with severe renal failure. Cautious use is indicated for patients with liver disease and diabetes mellitus, infants, the elderly, and patients taking digitalis or potassium-wasting steroids.

Nursing Actions

Check for drug and food allergies, especially to sulfonamides. Be alert for signs of dehydration. Monitor serum electrolyte, glucose, urea nitrogen, and creatinine levels. Assess for signs and symptoms of electrolyte disturbances and dehydration. This group of drugs is potassium-wasting, so teach patients to include potassium-rich foods in their diets. Close observation of elderly patients during the initial period of increased diuresis is important, as sudden change in fluid and electrolyte status could cause adverse reactions.

CARBONIC ANHYDRASE INHIBITORS

Actions

Carbonic anhydrase in an enzyme located in the proximal tubule of the kidney that assists in the maintenance of sodium and water balance. For sodium and water to be reabsorbed back into the blood, hydrogen must be exchanged for sodium. Carbonic anhydrase helps make the hydrogen ions available for this exchange. When carbonic anhydrase inhibitors (CAIs) block this action, little sodium and water can be reabsorbed into the blood and they are eliminated with the urine. Potassium and bicarbonate will also be excreted. Carbonic anhydrase is also located in the eye, where it functions in the formation of intraocular aqueous humor.

Uses

The CAIs include dichlorphenamide (Daranide), methazolamide (Neptazane), and acetazolamide (Diamox). Acetazolamide is the most widely prescribed of the three drugs. It is used principally as an adjunct agent in the management of glaucoma because it increases the outflow of aqueous humor. It is also useful in treating edema resulting from CHF that has become resistant to other diuretics.

Side and Adverse Effects

- **Central nervous system**: paresthesias (numbness, tingling, burning), drowsiness, depression, fatigue, muscle weakness, blurred vision
- **Gastrointestinal**: nausea, vomiting, diarrhea, anorexia, weight loss, dry mouth, thirst
- **Hematologic**: hyperglycemia, hypokalemia, hyponatremia, hypocalcemia, and hypomagnesemia, agranulocytosis, aplastic anemia, hemolytic anemia, leukopenia, and metabolic acidosis
- **Renal**: glycosuria, urinary frequency, dysuria, hematuria

Interactions and Contraindications

Because CAIs may induce hypokalemia, there may be an increase in digitalis toxicity. Their concomitant use with corticosteroids may cause hypokalemia and their use with oral antidiabetic agents and quinidine may induce toxicity of these drugs.

Carbonic anhydrase inhibitors are sulfonamide derivatives, so persons with sulfonamide hypersensitivity should avoid their use. In addition, the drugs are contraindicated for persons with marked renal and hepatic dysfunction, Addison's disease, hypokalemia, and hyponatremia. These drugs should be used cautiously in persons with diabetes mellitus or obstructive respiratory disorders and in those receiving digitalis therapy.

Nursing Actions

Carbonic anhydrase inhibitors are for adult use only. Check for allergies to sulfonamides. Alert the physician if the patient has diabetes mellitus or COPD. Because these drugs are potassium-wasting, teach patients to include potassium-rich foods in their diets. Teach patients to force fluids to 1.5 to 2.5 L/day to prevent kidney stones.

OSMOTIC DIURETICS

Actions

The major site of action of the osmotic diuretics is the proximal convoluted tubule. These drugs exert their effect by pulling water into the blood vessels and nephrons from the surrounding tissues. They will also induce the rapid excretion of water, sodium, and other electrolytes as well as rapid excretion of toxic substances from the kidney. The osmotics may cause vasodilation, which increases glomerular filtration rate and renal blood flow. Osmotic diuretics will reduce intracranial pressure and cerebral edema, as well as intraocular pressure. Mannitol (Osmitrol) is the osmotic drug of choice.

Uses

Mannitol is sometimes used to prevent kidney damage during the early, oliguric phase of acute renal failure. It can also be used to reduce intracranial pressure, treat cerebral edema, and promote excretion of toxic substances. It may be used as adjunct therapy for patients with edema from other conditions. Mannitol is only administered intravenously in an inpatient setting.

Side and Adverse Effects

Severe adverse effects include convulsions, thrombophlebitis, and pulmonary edema. Less significant side effects include headache, chest pain, tachycardia, blurred vision, chills, and fever.

Interactions and Contraindications

There are no known significant drug interactions.

These drugs should not be used in patients with anuria, severe dehydration, pulmonary edema, or cerebral hemorrhage.

Nursing Actions

Mannitol may crystallize at low temperatures, so the drug is always administered intravenously through a filter. Maintain strict intake and output monitoring and monitor for anuria. Assess lung sounds. Monitor vital signs. Assess for improvement in neurologic status (i.e., level of consciousness). Monitor status of edema. Perform Homan's sign to check for thrombophlebitis.

POTASSIUM-SPARING DIURETICS

Actions

The most commonly prescribed potassium-sparing diuretics are amiloride (Midamor), triamterene (Dyrenium), and spironolactone (Aldactone). Spironolactone is an antagonist of aldosterone, the steroid that promotes sodium reabsorption and potassium excretion. Thus, spironolactone causes sodium and water excretion and potassium retention. Amiloride and triamterene act directly on the distal convoluted tubule to inhibit reabsorption of sodium and water and excretion of potassium and hydrogen. Therefore, the body will lose sodium and water and retain potassium and hydrogen.

Uses

Spironolactone may be used to treat ascites associated with cirrhosis of the liver, hypokalemia, hyperaldosteronism,

CHF, and hypertension. It may also be used in conjunction with potassium-wasting diuretics to prevent drug-induced hypokalemia.

Amiloride and triamterene are generally used in combination with a thiazide or loop diuretic in the management of CHF. Since both of these drugs have little or no antihypertensive effect, they must be used with other antihypertensive agents.

Side and Adverse Effects

Potassium-sparing diuretics have several side effects in common. These include hyperkalemia, headache, dizziness, gastrointestinal upset, urinary frequency, and weakness. Spironolactone can cause gynecomastia (breast enlargement in males), impotence, amenorrhea, irregular menses, and postmenopausal bleeding. Triamterene may reduce folic acid levels, cause formation of kidney stones, and raise serum glucose levels.

Interactions and Contraindications

Indomethacin (Indocin) with spironolactone may cause more severe hyperkalemia; indomethacin with triamterene may cause acute renal failure. Triamterene with lithium may precipitate lithium toxicity. Concurrent use of potassium supplements, other medications containing potassium (e.g., penicillin G), or salt substitutes have an additive effect, which may lead to hyperkalemia. Use of chlorpropamide (Diabinese) and triamterene increases the risk of hyponatremia.

These drugs should not be used in patients with anuria, liver or kidney disease, and hyperkalemia. Spironolactone and triamterene are **pregnancy category D**.

Nursing Actions

Assess the patient's ability to produce urine. Monitor serum sodium, potassium, and glucose levels. Teach patients not to take potassium supplements, other potassium-sparing diuretics, or salt substitutes or low-salt products. Persons with diabetes mellitus should be especially alert for signs and symptoms of hyperglycemia. Teach patients the signs and symptoms of hyperkalemia (see Chapter 7).

Patient Teaching for Diuretic Therapy

- Potassium-rich foods include citrus fruits, bananas, dates, raisins, plums, fresh vegetables, potatoes (especially the skins), and fish.
- Diuretics should be taken early in the day to prevent nocturia.
- Report signs and symptoms of hypokalemia (weakness, constipation, irregular pulse rate, and lethargy) to health care provider immediately.
- Change positions or rise from a sitting or lying position slowly to prevent dizziness or faintness from orthostatic hypotension.
- Weigh yourself daily at the same time of day in the same type of clothes on the same scale. Keeping a record of weights will be useful for health care provider to assess the effectiveness of the therapy.
- Unless specifically contraindicated, the drug may be taken with food or milk to decrease gastrointestinal upset.
- If you are also taking digitalis, you and your family should learn how to monitor pulse rate and be prepared to call the health care provider if signs of toxicity occur. These symptoms include anorexia, nausea, vomiting, and bradycardia (pulse rate less than 60 bpm).
- If you have diabetes mellitus, you should closely monitor your blood sugar levels because of the increased risk of hyperglycemia.
- Illness associated with nausea, vomiting, and/or diarrhea should be reported to the health care provider because of the potential for electrolyte imbalance and fluid loss.
- Notify the health care provider immediately if tachycardia or syncope occurs, as this may be the result of hypotension or excessive fluid volume loss.
- Report to the health care provider any weight gain of 2 or more pounds (1 kg) per day or 5 or more pounds (2.25 kg) in 1 week (because of the possibility of CHF).
- Consult with a health care provider before using over-the-counter preparations (because many contain sodium and/or potassium).

URINARY ANTISEPTICS

*C*ystitis, *pyelitis*, and *pyelonephritis* are terms indicating an infection in the urinary tract, known collectively as *urinary tract infection (UTI)*. Symptoms include pain and burning on urination and urinary frequency and urgency. A urine culture should be taken prior to the start of any anti-infective or antiseptic therapy. This chapter covers *urinary analgesics*, which relieve the symptoms of UTI, and *urinary antiseptics*, which specifically treat the cause.

Additional anti-infective agents used to treat UTIs are discussed in Chapter 5.

URINARY ANALGESICS

Phenazopyridine Hydrochloride (Pyridium)

Actions

Phenazopyridine HCl (Pyridium) is a form of azo dye that acts within 30 minutes of oral administration to relieve the symptoms of pain, burning, urgency, and frequency associated with UTIs. It does not decrease the bacterial count, so cannot be used alone to treat an infection. The precise mechanism of action is unknown.

Uses

In addition to treatment of UTIs, urinary analgesics may also be prescribed after urinary tract surgery or cystoscopy, trauma, or following removal of an indwelling catheter. Phenazopyridine HCl is often prescribed with antibacterial (anti-infective) agents, especially sulfa drugs, but its use is recommended for only 3 to 5 days, the time period before the antibacterial drugs begin to control the infection and symptoms.

Side and Adverse Effects

Side effects are usually mild and may include headache, gastrointestinal upset, and red-orange urine.

Interactions and Contraindications

There are no known drug interactions.

Renal insufficiency is a contraindication to the use of azo dyes.

Nuring Actions

Warn patients regarding the occurrence of orange-red urine and other body fluids. This drug can stain fabrics, so protection should be worn in the perineal area. Azo dyes may stain contact lenses; glasses should be worn during therapy. Observe the patient's skin for a yellow cast, as this may mean the drug is not being excreted. Notify the laboratory if the patient is to have a urinalysis done, as the drug can alter results of certain urine tests that are based on color readings.

URINARY ANTISEPTICS

Methenamine Mandelate (Mandelamine)

Actions and Uses

Methenamine mandelate (Mandelamine) is an antibacterial agent that is effective against both gram-negative and gram-positive organisms. It is particularly useful for chronic, resistant, or recurrent UTIs and may be effective even against strains resistant to sulfonamides or other anti-infectives. It may be given alone or in combination with other drugs. Azo-Mandelamine combines the analgesic qualities of azo dye and the antiseptic properties of methenamine mandelate.

Side and Adverse Effects

Adverse reactions are unusual and mild. These may include gastrointestinal upset, rash, and (rarely) hematuria. Large doses may cause dysuria. Elderly and debilitated patients are at risk for lipid pneumonia with use of the oral suspension. Rare allergic reactions may occur.

Interactions and Contraindications

Concurrent use with sulfonamides increases the chances of crystalluria (the excretion of crystals in the urine, causing irritation of the kidney).

Severe hepatitis or renal insufficiency are contraindications to use of methenamine mandelate.

Nursing Actions

This drug works best in acidic urine with pH of 5.5 or less, so encourage foods known to acidify urine, such as cranberries, plums, prunes, nuts, and cereals. Meats, eggs, and cheese also acidify urine, but may be contraindicated for patients with high cholesterol. Mix granules, one packet in 2 to 4 oz water, just before administration. The solution will be cloudy. Shake well before administration.

Nitrofurantoin (Furadantin)

Actions and Uses

This broad-spectrum synthetic urinary antiseptic is useful against the majority of urinary tract infective organisms. Once sterility of the urine has been achieved, the drug should be continued for at least 3 days to minimize the possibility of recurrent infections.

Side and Adverse Effects

- **Central nervous system**: headache, drowsiness, nystagmus, dizziness, peripheral neuropathy
- **Gastrointestinal**: nausea, vomiting, anorexia, diarrhea, abdominal pain
- **Other**: transient alopecia, genitourinary superinfections, tooth staining from direct contact with oral suspension or crushed tablets, crystalluria (elderly patients), asthmatic attacks (in patients with history of asthma)

Nursing Actions and Patient Teaching

- Monitor intake and output. Report to health care provider if oliguria or anuria develops.
- Be alert for signs of urinary tract superinfections: milky, foul-smelling urine, perineal irritation, dysuria. Report occurrence to health care provider.
- Be aware that urine will turn brown.
- Take the drug with food or milk to minimize gastrointestinal symptoms.
- Avoid crushing the tablets, dilute the oral suspension in milk, water, or fruit juice, and rinse mouth thoroughly after taking the drug because of the possibility of tooth staining.
- Assess for and report muscle weakness, numbness, tingling, or burning sensations (signs of potentially irreversible peripheral neuropathy). Discontinue drug immediately.

Trimethoprim and Sulfamethoxazole (Bactrim, Septra)

Actions and Uses

This combination drug is effective against chronic UTIs, primarily pyelonephritis, pyelitis, and cystitis.

Side and Adverse Effects

- **Gastrointestinal**: nausea, vomiting, diarrhea, anorexia, abdominal pain
- **Blood dyscrasias**: agranulocytosis, aplastic anemia, hemolytic anemia, hypoprothrombinemia, thrombocytopenia.
- **Other**: weakness, joint or muscle pain, photosensitivity, mild to moderate skin rashes

Interactions and Contraindications

Concurrent use with oral anticoagulants may increase risk for hypoprothrombinemia.

This drug should not be used in patients with sulfonamide allergy, folate deficiency anemia, or impaired renal or liver function. It is not recommended for infants less than 2 months old.

Nursing Actions and Patient Teaching

- Report immediately to the health care provider sore throat, fever, pallor, purpura, jaundice, or rashes (these may be signs of blood dyscrasias).
- Have adequate fluid intake to prevent renal calculi (at least 1500 mL/day).
- Take the drug with a full glass of desired fluid.
- Report continuation of UTI symptoms to the health care provider.

REVIEW QUESTIONS: UNIT 11

1. Thiazide and loop diuretics are contraindicated for persons allergic or hypersensitive to which of the following groups of drugs?

    A. Aminoglycosides

    B. Estrogens

    C. Sulfonamides

    D. Nonsteroidal anti-inflammatory drugs

2. Patient teaching for a person taking triamterene with an antihypertensive agent should include which of the following points?

   A. Avoid use of salt substitutes.

   B. Increase intake of potassium-rich foods.

   C. Drug must be taken on an empty stomach.

   D. Take drug at bedtime.

3. A patient with insulin-dependent diabetes mellitus is taking hydrochlorothiazide. Patient teaching includes information that:

   A. insulin requirements will not change.

   B. insulin dose may need to be increased.

   C. insulin dose may need to be decreased.

   D. there will be no need for additional monitoring of blood glucose.

4. A patient who is taking Pyridium tells the nurse that his urine is an orange-red color. The most appropriate response is:

   A. "That is the first sign of drug toxicity and you must stop taking the drug."

   B. "This is an indication that the drug is killing the bacteria."

   C. "The drug dose is too high and will have to be reduced."

   D. "This is a harmless occurrence, but your clothing could become stained if any urine gets on the fabric."

5. A contraindication to the use of Bactrim is:

   A. concurrent use of Pyridium.

   B. sulfonamide allergy.

   C. penicillin hypersensitivity.

   D. diabetes mellitus.

6. Why should the oral suspension of nitrofurantoin be diluted in milk, water, or juice?

   A. Because the drug is not effective unless diluted.

   B. To minimize the occurrence of brown urine.

   C. To make the taste more palatable and to ensure that patient will take the drug.

   D. To prevent tooth discoloration.

DRUGS THAT AFFECT THE SKELETAL SYSTEM

OBJECTIVES

1. Identify classifications of drugs used to treat skeletal disorders.

2. Explain the actions, side and adverse effects, interactions, and contraindications of drugs used to treat skeletal disorders.

3. Identify nursing implications relevant to each major classification of drugs used to treat skeletal disorders.

BONE RESORPTION INHIBITORS, BONE-FORMING AGENTS, ANTIRHEUMATICS

*B*one and joint disorders have a variety of pathologic origins, such as inflammation, degeneration, and metabolic alterations. Therefore, a wide range of drug classifications are employed in their treatments. These include disease-modifying antirheumatic drugs, antigout agents, bone resorption inhibitors, and bone-forming agents.

Antirheumatic drugs are used to treat arthritis, a variety of joint disorders characterized by pain and stiffness. Types of arthritis include osteoarthritis, which is commonly associated with aging and wear on the joints, rheumatoid arthritis, which is an autoimmune disorder, and gouty arthritis, which is caused by urate crystals deposited in the joints of people with gout.

DISEASE-MODIFYING ANTIRHEUMATIC DRUGS

The three types of drugs used to treat arthritis are nonsteroidal anti-inflammatory drugs, glucocorticoids, and disease-modifying antirheumatic drugs (DMARDs). Nonsteroidal anti-inflammatory drugs are covered in detail in Chapter 4, so that information will not be repeated here. Methotrexate, hydroxychloroquine, and sulfasalazine are first choice DMARDs. Other DMARDs most often used for rheumatoid arthritis are leflunomide, gold salts, and azathioprine. Penicillamine is an effective DMARD, but it is reserved for patients with severe disease who do not respond to less toxic drugs, since it can cause bone marrow depression and autoimmune disorders.

Methotrexate (Folex)

Action and Uses

Methotrexate (Folex) is an antiarthritic and an antineoplastic drug. For the treatment of rheumatoid arthritis, its benefits seem to derive from mild immunosuppressant activity.

Side and Adverse Effects

Patients treated with methotrexate frequently report anorexia, nausea, vomiting, and diarrhea as side effects of the drug. Adverse effects can be severe and reflect toxic effects on the gastrointestinal tract, lungs, bone marrow, skin, liver, nerve tissue, and kidneys. Inflammation may be manifested throughout the gastrointestinal tract and the lungs. Bone marrow activity may be depressed, causing production of red and white blood cells and platelets to fall to dangerously low levels. Liver and renal function may decline and progress to failure.

Interactions and Contraindications

Any drug that is potentially toxic to the gastrointestinal tract, liver, kidneys, nerve tissue, bone marrow, and skin can increase the risk of those toxic effects with methotrexate. One drug that may decrease the effectiveness of methotrexate is asparaginase.

Methotrexate is contraindicated with impaired renal function. It is not used during pregnancy because it may cause fetal deformities. Since methotrexate is secreted in breast milk, women should not breastfeed while taking it. **Pregnancy Category X.**

Nursing Implications

Monitor periodic blood and urine studies to detect abnormalities caused by toxicity. Assess the skin for rashes, bruises, and petechiae. Inspect the oral cavity for lesions and inflammation. Monitor respiratory status.

Patient Teaching
• Drink at least eight 8-ounce glasses of fluids every day unless advised otherwise by your physician.
• Your resistance to infection may be low, so avoid crowds and people with infections.
• Your skin will be more sensitive to sunlight, so use sunscreens and clothing to avoid sun exposure.
• Immediately report any signs of infection (fever, sore throat) or abnormal bleeding to your physician.
• You may have hair loss while taking methotrexate. Your hair will grow back after therapy is completed, but it may be a different color or texture.

Hydroxychloroquine (Plaquenil)

Action and Uses

Hydroxychloroquine (Plaquenil) is used to treat rheumatoid arthritis, malaria, and lupus erythematosus. The mechanism by which it relieves symptoms of arthritis is unknown, but it may suppress hypersensitivity reactions.

Side and Adverse Effects

Headache, nausea, vomiting, and anorexia are frequent side effects of hydroxychloroquine therapy. Some patients experience visual disturbances, nervousness, and irritability. The most serious adverse effect is ocular toxicity manifested as retinopathy. With long-term therapy, there is a risk of neuropathy, hypotension, agranulocytosis, convulsions, and psychosis. Overdose can lead to neurotoxicity, cardiovascular collapse, and death.

Interactions and Contraindications

If given with penicillamine, there is increased risk of hematologic, renal, and skin toxicities. Hydroxychloroquine is contraindicated in patients with retinal changes, psoriasis, and porphyria. Risks of toxicities are greater in children.

Nursing Actions

Assess vision and hearing. Monitor blood pressure. Monitor blood cell counts and liver function tests.

Patient Teaching

- Immediately notify your physician if you have problems with vision or hearing, abnormal bruising or bleeding, or any signs of infection.
- Taking the drug with meals will reduce gastrointestinal effects.
- It is important to keep follow-up appointments for blood studies.

Sulfasalazine (Azulfidine)

Actions and Uses

Sulfasalazine (Azulfidine) is most recognized as an antimicrobial. However, it is also used in the treatment of rheumatoid arthritis and inflammatory bowel disease because of its anti-inflammatory properties.

Side and Adverse Effects

Frequent side effects of sulfasalazine are anorexia, nausea, vomiting, headache, and oligospermia. Potential adverse effects include anaphylaxis and hematologic (bone marrow) toxicity. Liver and renal toxicity may occur, but are relatively rare.

Interactions and Contraindications

The risk of liver toxicity increases if sulfasalazine is given with other drugs that are hepatotoxic. Sulfasalazine enhances the effects of many other drugs, including anticoagulants, anticonvulsants, oral hypoglycemics, and methotrexate.

Patients who are allergic to any of the following should not take sulfasalazine: salicylates, sulfonamides, sulfonylureas, thiazide or loop diuretics, carbonic anhydrase inhibitors, sunscreens containing PABA, and local anesthetics. Sulfasalazine is also contraindicated in severely impaired liver or renal function and in patients with intestinal or urinary obstructions. It should not be given to children under age 2.

Leflunomide (Arava)

Action and Uses

Leflunomide (Arava) reduces signs and symptoms of rheumatoid arthritis and appears to actually slow the progression of the disease.

Side and Adverse Effects

Leflunomide can cause diarrhea, respiratory tract infection, hypertension, tachycardia, peripheral edema, headache, nausea, gastrointestinal disturbances, back pain, hair loss, liver toxicity, and a number of other adverse effects. Because of its long half-life, adverse effects may persist for a while, even after dosage is decreased or the drug is discontinued. Leflunomide is teratogenic. **Pregnancy Category X.**

Interactions and Contraindications

Nonsteroidal anti-inflammatory drugs may increase the risk of toxicity with leflunomide. Methotrexate increases the risk of hepatotoxicity. Patients with immune deficiency may be at increased risk for malignancy. Because of adverse effects on the fetus, this drug should not be used during pregnancy.

Nursing Actions

Monitor liver function studies, pulse and blood pressure, serum potassium, blood glucose, urinalysis, and pulmonary status for abnormalities related to adverse effects of leflunomide. Assess improvement in joint function and reduction in pain.

Patient Teaching

- Notify the physician if you have severe diarrhea, palpitations, headache, gastrointestinal disturbances, painful urination, back or new joint pain, cough, sore throat, or blurred vision.
- You will need periodic blood tests to check your liver function while taking this drug.
- Avoid conception while taking this drug.

Patient Teaching

- It may be as long as 6 months before therapeutic effects are evident.
- Exposure to sunlight may cause your skin to appear bluish.
- Notify your physician if you have sores or a metallic taste in your mouth, skin rash, or bruises.
- Keep follow-up appointments for blood and urine studies.

Gold Salts

Gold preparations for intramuscular injection include aurothioglucose (Solganal) and gold sodium thiomalate (Myochrysine). The oral preparation which is more convenient but less effective is auranofin (Ridaura). See Table 40–1 for prototypes.

Action and Uses

Gold preparations may prevent joint degeneration but cannot reverse existing damage. Although most patients report symptomatic improvement, the exact mechanism of action is unknown.

Side and Adverse Effects

Unfortunately, adverse reactions to gold salts are common. They include intense pruritus, rashes, stomatitis, renal toxicity, severe blood dyscrasias, hepatitis, peripheral neuritis, pulmonary infiltrates, and profound hypotension. Oral preparations have fewer renal, skin, and mucous membrane adverse effects, but more gastrointestinal side effects.

Interactions and Contraindications

The risk of toxic effects of gold salts increases if given with other hepatotoxic or nephrotoxic drugs or drugs that depress the bone marrow. Concurrent penicillamine increases the risk of renal toxicity and blood dyscrasias.

Gold salts are contraindicated in patients with a history of bone marrow aplasia, severe blood dyscrasias, or other severe adverse effects associated with gold therapy.

Nursing Actions

Give intramuscular preparations in the upper outer quadrant of the gluteus maximus while the patient is lying down. Assess skin for rash or bruises, and mucous membranes for lesions. Monitor urinalysis results for hematuria and proteinuria. Monitor blood cell counts and liver enzymes for abnormalities. Assess joint stiffness, pain, and swelling.

TABLE 40–1

Gold Salts

Prototype	Specific Considerations
gold sodium thiomalate (Myochrysine)	Diarrhea, rash, pruritus, nausea, and abdominal pain are common. Some patients have vomiting, anorexia, flatulence, dyspepsia, conjunctivitis, and photosensitivity.
aurothioglucose (Solganal)	The following adverse effects have been reported occasionally: rash, pruritus, gingivitis, metallic taste in mouth, and stomatitis.
auranofin (Ridaura)	Diarrhea, nausea, abdominal pain, rash, and pruritus are common side effects. Oral medication can be given with or without food.

Azathioprine (Imuran)

Actions and Uses

Azathioprine inhibits RNA, DNA, and protein synthesis; it antagonizes metabolism. It is an immunosuppressant that is used to treat a variety of inflammatory conditions including rheumatoid arthritis and inflammatory bowel disease. It is also used to prevent rejection following kidney transplantation.

Side and Adverse Effects

Azathioprine often causes nausea, vomiting, and anorexia. Patients may develop leukopenia and thrombocytopenia. This drug is associated with increased risk of tumors. Though rare, hepatotoxicity can occur.

Interactions and Contraindications

The bone marrow depressant effects of azathioprine are enhanced by other bone marrow depressants. The risk of infection increases if azathioprine is given in combination with other immunosuppressants.

⚠ Azathioprine is not recommended during pregnancy or lactation. It is contraindicated in patients who have previously been treated for rheumatoid arthritis with cyclophosphamide, chlorambucil, or melphalan.

Nursing Actions

Monitor results of CBC, platelet counts, and liver function studies. Assess for signs of infection: sore throat, fatigue, fever. Assess joints for pain, tenderness, and swelling.

Patient Teaching

- Notify your physician if you have sores in your mouth, unusual bleeding, or bruising.
- Since this drug can reduce your resistance to infection, protect yourself from sick people; report fever, sore throat, or other signs and symptoms of infection.
- It may take as long as 3 months before you notice improvement in your symptoms.
- You should avoid pregnancy while on this drug.
- Since this drug can affect your blood cells, it is very important to keep follow-up appointments for blood studies.

ANTIGOUT AGENTS

Gout is a systemic disease in which excess uric acid in the blood is caused by excessive production or decreased excretion of the acid. Urate crystals are deposited in the joints and other body tissues. Effects can include painful joint inflammation and deformities and renal damage incurred by the urate crystals in fragile kidney structures.

Drugs used to treat gout either decrease the synthesis of uric acid, increase the urinary excretion of uric acid, or reduce inflammation.

Allopurinol (Zyloprim)

Actions and Uses

Allopurinol is effective in the treatment of gout because it decreases uric acid production. It is also used to prevent recurrent calcium stones in the urinary tract.

Side and Adverse Effects

Drowsiness is an occasional side effect. Toxic effects include a maculopapular rash, fever, chills, and joint pain. Although rare, bone marrow depression, renal failure, hepatotoxicity, and peripheral neuritis have been reported.

Interactions and Contraindications

Allopurinol enhances the effects of oral anticoagulants, azathioprine, and mercaptopurine. Effects of allopurinol are decreased by thiazide diuretics.

Allopurinol is contraindicated with asymptomatic hyperuricemia and used with caution in patients with impaired renal or hepatic function.

Nursing Actions

Inspect urine for abnormalities. Assess joint pain, swelling, and mobility.

Patient Teaching

- Unless your physician advises otherwise, drink enough fluids (10 to 12 8-ounce glasses) to produce 2000 mL of urine daily.
- Give with (or immediately after) meals or milk.
- Avoid dangerous activities if drowsiness occurs.
- Notify physician of rash or irritation of the oral tissues or the eyes.
- It may take several weeks before you notice improvement in your symptoms.

Probenecid (Benemid)

Action and Uses

Probenecid (Benemid) is used to prevent acute gout attacks by increasing the urinary excretion of uric acid. However, it is not used during an acute attack. It is also given with penicillins and cephalosporins because it reduces excretion of those drugs, thereby elevating blood levels.

Side and Adverse Effects

Side effects of probenecid include headache, urinary frequency, and gastrointestinal distress. Increased uric acid in the urine poses a risk of urinary calculi. Anaphylaxis, though rare, has occurred. Toxicity is manifested by maculopapular rash, fever, joint pain, and leukopenia.

Interactions and Contraindications

Probenecid increases serum levels of penicillins, cephalosporins, methotrexate, NSAIDs, nitrofurantoin, and zidovudine. It may also prolong the action of heparin. Salicylates may interfere with the action of probenecid.

Probenecid is contraindicated with blood dyscrasias and uric acid kidney stones, and it is used cautiously with renal impairment or peptic ulcer disease. Do not give with penicillin if the patient has impaired renal function.

Nursing Actions

Monitor blood cell counts and liver and renal function tests. Assess joints for pain and swelling. Note abnormal urine characteristics.

Patient Teaching
• Unless advised otherwise by your physician, drink 10 to 12 8-ounce glasses of fluid daily to prevent urinary stones. • It may take several weeks before drug effects are evident. • If drowsiness occurs, avoid dangerous activities or tasks requiring alertness. • Report rash or irritation of the eyes or mouth to your physician.

Colchicine

Action and Uses

Colchicine is the drug of choice for treatment of the first acute gouty attack. Even though it is an anti-inflammatory agent, it is not effective for conditions other than gout. The exact mechanism by which it relieves symptoms of gout is unclear. Once the acute attack has been resolved, it may be ordered in small doses to reduce the frequency and intensity of acute attacks. If the patient has early symptoms of an impending acute attack, larger doses of colchicine may avert the attack.

Side and Adverse Effects

When colchicine is given orally, the patient may have nausea, vomiting, diarrhea, and abdominal pain. With intravenous administration, gastrointestinal effects are lessened, but there is a risk of neuritis in the injected arm and the injection site may be painful. Extravasation can cause tissue necrosis. Patients with impaired renal function may have generalized weakness. With long-term therapy, bone marrow depression may occur.

Early signs of toxicity include a burning feeling in the throat and skin, severe diarrhea, and abdominal pain. This is followed by fever, seizures, delirium, and renal damage. The last stage is marked by loss of hair, leukocytosis, and inflammation of the oral cavity.

Interactions and Contraindications

The risk of bone marrow depression increases if colchicine is given with NSAIDs.

Colchicine is contraindicated with severe gastrointestinal, renal, hepatic, or cardiac disorders, and blood dyscrasias. For the oral route: **Pregnancy Category C.**

 For the intravenous route: **Pregnancy Category D.**

Nursing Actions

Monitor the complete blood cell count in patients on long-term therapy. To minimize irritation to the vein, follow the manufacturer's directions to dilute the intravenous drug and infuse slowly.

Patient Teaching
• Discontinue colchicine and notify your physician if you develop nausea, vomiting, and abdominal pain. • You need to drink 10 to 12 8-ounce glasses of fluids each day. • If your physician instructs you to use colchicine to avert an impending attack, be sure to keep some tablets with you at all times.

BONE RESORPTION INHIBITORS AND BONE-FORMING AGENTS

Although it may appear inert, bone is living tissue. Old cells are constantly dying and being absorbed (a process called *resorption*) while new cells are produced to create a matrix for the deposition of minerals that create bone mass and strength. The three types of cells involved in bone development are osteoclasts, osteocytes, and osteoblasts. *Osteoblasts* form bone cells. *Osteoclasts* are responsible for the breakdown and resorption of old bone. Mature bone cells are called *osteocytes*.

During periods of bone growth, the deposition of new bone exceeds bone resorption. During the young adult years, resorption and deposition are balanced so bones remain strong. However, in the fifth decade, resorption of old bone begins to exceed the deposition of new bone. Loss of bone mass creates fragile bones that are easily fractured. *Osteoporosis* is the term used to describe low bone mass. It affects more women than men and results in over 1 million fractures each year in the United States.

Drugs that may be used to prevent or treat osteoporosis are calcium, vitamin D, bone resorption inhibitors, and bone-forming agents. For prevention of osteoporosis before age 50, the recommended daily intake of calcium is 1000 mg and 200 IU of vitamin D. After age 50, 1200 mg of calcium and 600 IU of vitamin D are recommended. Some sources recommend 1500 mg of calcium daily for postmenopausal women.

Bone Resorption Inhibitors

Drugs used to inhibit bone resorption are estrogen, bisphosphonates, and calcitonin. These agents slow the loss of bone mass but cannot restore mass already lost.

Estrogen

When natural estrogen production declines during menopause, bone resorption increases sharply. Estrogen replacement therapy reduces this bone loss, thereby reducing the risk of fractures as well as cardiovascular disease. However, replacement estrogen increases the risk of endometrial cancer in women who still have a uterus. This adverse effect is minimized by giving progestins in addition to estrogen. There is controversy about other potential adverse effects of estrogen, and each woman's situation must be considered individually before a decision is made to recommend estrogen. Estrogen therapy is covered in detail in Chapter 45.

Bisphosphonates

Action and Uses

The only bisphosphonate approved for use in the treatment of osteoporosis is alendronate (Fosamax). Alendronate inhibits the resorption of bone by osteoclasts. An adequate intake of calcium and vitamin D is essential for alendronate to be effective. For women who cannot take estrogen, alendronate is the best alternative to reduce loss of bone mass.

Side and Adverse Effects

Abdominal pain is a common side effect of alendronate. Some patients report muscle pain, nausea, constipation or diarrhea, flatulence, headache, and heartburn. Other, potentially serious, adverse effects include hypocalcemia, hypophosphatemia, and severe gastrointestinal disturbances.

Interactions and Contraindications

Food and many beverages interfere with absorption of alendronate. Aspirin increases the likelihood of gastrointestinal distress. Intravenous ranitidine increases the blood level of alendronate.

Alendronate should be used cautiously in patients with gastrointestinal disorders. It is contraindicated with a creatinine clearance of 5 mg/dL or less and in the patient who is taking estrogen replacement therapy.

Nursing Actions

Assess for hypocalcemia, characterized by muscle cramps, tingling sensations in the hands and face, and slow reflexes.

Patient Teaching

- Take alendronate first thing in the morning with 8 ounces of plain water. Wait at least 30 minutes before taking anything else by mouth.
- To decrease heartburn, do not lie down for at least 30 minutes after taking this drug.
- Withhold the drug and notify your physician if you have chest pain.
- Notify your physician if you have muscle cramps, which may indicate low calcium in your blood.
- Keep appointments for follow-up blood studies of your calcium and phosphate.

Calcitonin

Action and Uses

Calcitonin-salmon (Calcimar, Miacalcin) is used to treat osteoporosis by decreasing the number and activity of osteoclasts. One form is available as a nasal spray; another form is available for subcutaneous or intramuscular injection.

Side and Adverse Effects

Regardless of route of administration, the two major adverse effects of calcitonin are severe hypocalcemia and anaphylaxis.

Intramuscular or Subcutaneous Route. Within 30 minutes of injection, the patient may experience nausea. Fortunately, this effect usually diminishes as the therapy is continued. Other side effects of parenteral therapy may be anorexia, vomiting, diarrhea, and flushing of the face, ears, hands, and feet.

Nasal Route. Side effects reported with the nasal spray include rhinitis, rhinorrhea, nasal dryness, epistaxis, headache, muscle aches, and facial flushing.

Interactions and Contraindications

There are no significant drug interactions with calcitonin. People who are allergic to fish or calcitonin should not take this drug.

Nursing Actions

An intradermal skin test should be done as ordered to assess for allergy before administering this drug. Redness and swelling indicate allergy, in which case the patient should not be given the medication.

If the drug is given by injection, you must teach the patient and/or a family member proper procedure. Emphasize the need to rotate sites.

Patient Teaching

- You may have some nausea and flushing with initial therapy; this usually decreases with continued therapy.
- Consult with your physician before taking any other medications while on calcitonin.
- If you have shortness of breath or urticaria (hives) after taking this drug, notify the physician immediately.
- It is important for you to keep regular appointments for your blood calcium level to be monitored.
- This drug can only be effective if you continue to take in adequate amounts of calcium and vitamin D.

Raloxifene (Evista)

Actions and Uses

Raloxifene (Evista) is used in postmenopausal women to prevent osteoporosis by increasing bone density. Advantages to this drug are that it does not stimulate the endometrium and it lowers cholesterol.

Side and Adverse Effects

The most common side effects of raloxifene are infection, flu-like symptoms, hot flashes, nausea, weight gain, joint pain, and sinusitis. Less common adverse effects include migraine, edema, chest pain, insomnia, depression, thrombosis, and pneumonia.

Interactions and Contraindications

Raloxifene absorption is reduced by ampicillin and cholestyramine. It may cause toxicity of drugs that are highly bound to plasma proteins such as warfarin, ibuprofen, and phenytoin if taken concurrently. Raloxifene is contraindicated during pregnancy, and during periods of immobility. **Pregnancy Category X.**

Nursing Actions

Check Homan's sign for pain associated with vascular inflammation.

Patient Teaching

- Report edema in the legs or chest pain to the physician.

Bone-Forming Therapy: Slow-Release Sodium Fluoride

A *bone-forming agent* is one that promotes bone growth by stimulating the proliferation of osteoblasts. The only drug currently available that has this action is slow-release sodium fluoride (Slow Fluoride). Unlike the resorption inhibitors, it can actually rebuild bone in the patient with osteoporosis. It must be noted that the drug has not been approved for this use.

REVIEW QUESTIONS: UNIT 12

Case Study

Minnie Smith, 74 years old, is recovering from a total hip replacement. (See the Care Plan in Chapter 38 of the textbook). She has osteoporosis. Her physician orders alendronate sodium (Fosamax). The following questions apply to this situation.

1. What is the action of Fosamax in relation to osteoporosis?

2. Which directions should you give Mrs. Smith?

   a. Take this medication at bedtime.

   b. Always take Fosamax after meals.

   c. Lie flat for 30 minutes after taking Fosamax.

   d. Take this medication with a glass of plain water.

3. On a follow-up visit, Mrs. Smith complains of muscle cramps. In this situation, you should suspect:

   a. hypocalcemia.

   b. hypermagnesemia.

   c. hyponatremia.

   d. hypokalemia.

4. List two other drugs that inhibit bone resorption.

5. If the physician considers prescribing estrogen for Mrs. Smith, what information would be critical to making that decision? Why?

DRUGS THAT AFFECT THE ENDOCRINE SYSTEM

OBJECTIVES

1. Name the endocrine glands and their respective hormones.

2. Identify conditions caused by abnormal functioning of each endocrine gland.

3. Discuss the regulatory mechanisms of the endocrine system, particularly negative feedback.

4. State the actions, uses, side and adverse effects, and contraindications of various endocrine drugs.

5. Identify appropriate nursing actions and patient teaching for patients receiving various endocrine drugs.

Homeostasis, the mechanisms whereby the body processes are kept in a state of balance, are regulated by two major control systems, the nervous system and the endocrine system. The nervous system has the primary responsibility for promoting rapid adjustments of organs, glands, and musculature to changes occurring both within and outside of the body, often on a moment-by-moment basis (see Unit 6).

The primary responsibility of the endocrine system is regulation of body processes for relatively long periods of time. Although some endocrine responses may occur in seconds (e.g., action of epinephrine from the adrenal glands), most are slow in onset (requiring hours or days) and long in duration.

Hormones are secretions formed by body tissue and carried in the blood to act on some other organ or tissue. Although separated physically, the organs of the endocrine system are unified and well integrated. The primary organs of this system are the pituitary, the thyroid, the parathyroids, the adrenals, the gonads, and the pancreatic islets of Langerhans. The primary connecting link between the nervous system and the endocrine system is the hypothalamus, which responds to neural stimuli by producing hormones, called

releasing factors and *inhibitory factors*, which in turn control secretion of almost all hormones from the pituitary gland. The endocrine glands, as well as the mammary glands and growth of the body's skeletal system, are under control of the anterior pituitary gland. Specific pituitary hormones are discussed in the following chapters.

Regulation of Hormone Release and Activity

Hormones are regulated by one of the four following mechanisms:

1. *Neural stimuli:* nerve fibers stimulate hormone-producing cells. For example, stimulation of the adrenal medulla by nerves during times of stress causes the release of epinephrine and norepinephrine.

2. *Hormonal stimuli* (this is also known as the *negative feedback system*): a decrease in available (or circulating) hormone signals the hypothalamus to produce the appropriate hormone-releasing factor, which causes the anterior pituitary gland to release the corresponding tropic (regulating) hormone, which in turn signals the target endocrine gland to secrete its hormone. When circulating hormone levels reach normal, the hypothalamus releases hormone-inhibiting factors that "shut off" tropic hormone release from the anterior pituitary gland.

   Because there is such a wide range in onset and duration of action among the various hormones, the precise control necessary for blood concentrations is accomplished by this negative feedback system. (See figure on p. 191.)

3. *Humoral stimuli:* chemicals other than hormones can trigger hormone release. For example, a decrease in serum calcium triggers the release of parathormone (or parathyroid hormone, PTH) from the parathyroid gland, which causes metabolic changes in bone, small intestine, and

Negative Feedback Regulation of the Hypothalamus and Anterior Pituitary

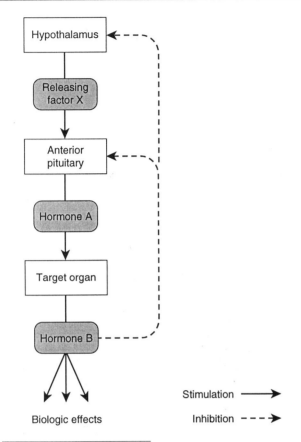

Stimulation ⟶

Inhibition - - - ⟶

From Lehne (1998). *Pharmacology for Nursing Care*, 3rd ed. Philadelphia: W.B. Saunders, p. 610.

kidney tubule cells, thus releasing calcium into circulation. When serum calcium levels reach normal, parathormone release is inhibited.

4. *Other factors:* a decrease in renal blood flow triggers the release of aldosterone from the adrenal cortex, which reduces excretion of water, thus maintaining or increasing blood volume.

General Characteristics of Hormones

- Hormones are either natural (human/animal) or synthetic. The synthetic forms may have more potent and prolonged effects than endogenous (naturally occurring) hormones.
- Physiologic effects: replacement doses to bring hormone levels to normal (e.g., insulin or thyroid).

- Pharmacologic effects: larger than replacement doses for greater than physiologic effects (e.g., corticosteroids to treat inflammatory disorders).
- Hormones cannot initiate nonexistent functions (e.g., therapeutic insulin administration will not cause nonfunctional pancreatic beta cells to begin producing insulin again).
- Hormones produce widespread therapeutic and adverse effects.
- Administration of one hormone may alter the effects of other hormones (e.g., corticosteroids raise blood glucose, which affects insulin production and release).
- Hormones produce their effects by altering cellular activity, either by increasing or decreasing the rate of certain biochemical processes.

Clinical Uses for Hormones (or Synthetic Preparations)

Most endocrine abnormalities are related to hyposecretion, hypersecretion, or inappropriate secretion of an endocrine organ. Problems may also occur with deficiencies or abnormalities of specific hormone receptors on target cells. Clinical indications for use of hormones include the following:

- Replacement therapy for hormone deficiencies.
- Inhibition of the action of other hormones (e.g., birth control pills suppress hypothalamic and anterior pituitary function to prevent ovulation).
- Treatment for certain nonendocrine disorders (e.g., rheumatoid arthritis, asthma, cancer, organ transplants).
- As diagnostic agents (e.g., administration of thyroid-stimulating hormone to assess thyroid gland function).

Hormonal regulation, characteristics, and clinical uses are discussed in more detail in the chapters of this unit and in Unit 14.

CHAPTER 41

PITUITARY HORMONES

PITUITARY GLAND

The anterior pituitary is composed of various types of glandular cells, which synthesize and secrete different hormones. These hormones include *tropic* (or regulating) hormones, which cause endocrine glands to secrete their respective hormones into the bloodstream; prolactin, which promotes milk production by the mammary glands; and growth hormone, which promotes growth of all body tissue, except the brain and eye. The posterior pituitary is an extension of the hypothalamus and is composed mainly of nerve fibers. It stores and releases hormones synthesized in the hypothalamus. These hormones include vasopressin (antidiuretic hormone, ADH), which acts mainly on renal distal tubules to reduce excretion of water; and oxytocin, which stimulates uterine contractions during pregnancy and promotes milk ejection during lactation.

A variety of drugs can affect the pituitary gland. The mechanism of action of these agents differs depending on the drug, but overall they either augment or antagonize the natural effects of pituitary hormones. The anterior pituitary drugs discussed in this chapter include corticotropin (Acthar), somatropin (Humatrope), and somatrem (Protropin); the posterior pituitary drugs discussed are vasopressin (Pitressin), desmopressin (DDAVP), and lypressin (Diapid). Other drugs that affect the pituitary are covered in other chapters.

CORTICOTROPIN (ACTHAR)

Actions and Uses

The exogenous (drug) form of corticotropin produces all the same physiologic responses as that of endogenous (naturally occurring) corticotropin (ACTH): stimulation of the adrenal glands to secrete cortisol (hydrocortisone and other substances) (see Chapter 43).

Uses of corticotropin are as follows:

- To aid in the diagnosis of adrenocortical insufficiency.
- As part of the treatment plan for multiple sclerosis.
- For corticotropin insufficiency due to long-term corticosteroid use.
- As anti-inflammatory and immunosuppressive agents.

Side and Adverse Effects

Corticotropin causes sodium and water retention, resulting in edema and hypertension, as well as hypokalemia. It also produces the following effects:

- **Central nervous system:** headache, dizziness, insomnia, depression, psychosis, and convulsions.
- **Gastrointestinal:** nausea and vomiting, peptic ulcer perforation, and pancreatitis.
- **Other:** sweating, muscle atrophy and weakness, acne and hyperpigmentation, impaired wound healing, hyperglycemia, and joint and muscle pain.

Interactions and Contraindications

Corticotropin with diuretics and amphotericin B has an additive hypokalemic effect. Concurrent use with aspirin and other nonsteroidal anti-inflammatory drugs increases potential for hypoprothrombinemia and gastric ulcers.

Corticotropin is contraindicated for patients with pork allergy, scleroderma, osteoporosis, congestive heart failure, peptic ulcer disease, hypertension, primary adrenocortical insufficiency, adrenal hyperfunction, or recent surgery.

Nursing Actions

Perform a thorough nursing assessment including baseline vital signs and weight. Determine drug and food allergies, especially to pork. Monitor and report abnormal complete blood count results, serum electrolytes, and blood glucose levels. Check for possible contraindications to therapy. Assess for and report occurrence of side and adverse effects.

Patient Teaching

- Maintain adequate hydration, up to 2000 mL/ day, unless contraindicated.
- If you have diabetes mellitus, monitor your blood glucose closely until your response to the drug stabilizes.
- Do not take over-the-counter drugs without consulting the health care provider (many over-the-counter preparations contain sodium).
- Monitor your weight and report steady gain, especially if it is accompanied by edema.
- You may have to limit your dietary sodium and take potassium supplements to minimize edema and prevent hypertension and hypokalemia.
- Do not discontinue the drug abruptly, because of the potential for adverse reactions.
- Avoid live vaccine immunizations during therapy.
- Report infection, fever, sore throat, and joint or muscle pain to the health care provider immediately.

SOMATROPIN (HUMATROPE) AND SOMATREM (PROTROPIN)

Actions and Uses

When a child's body is deficient in growth hormone (GH), a condition known as *pituitary dwarfism* results and the child fails to develop normally. Somatropin (Humatrope) and somatrem (Protropin) mimic GH by stimulating the processes that cause growth of bones and tissues. Natural sources of GH are difficult to obtain and are very expensive. Recent technology has made somatropin and somatrem more readily available through recombinant DNA techniques.

Side and Adverse Effects

Somatropin and somatrem may cause headache, hypercalciuria and kidney stones, hyperglycemia, and hypothyroidism. Other reactions may include rash, urticaria, and inflammation at the injection site.

Interactions and Contraindications

There are no known interactions with these drugs.

These drugs are contraindicated for anyone whose bones have stopped growing, as well as for any patient with evidence of an active intracranial tumor.

Nursing Actions

Obtain baseline height, weight, and head circumference; plot the measurements on the appropriate boy's or girl's growth chart. Monitor serum GH, ACTH, and thyroid-stimulating hormone (TSH) levels. Report abnormal findings to the health care provider.

Do not use a cloudy or discolored solution. When mixing the drug, do not shake the solution. Teach the patient and parents how to perform fingerstick blood glucose assessments. Teach the patient and parents how to perform injection techniques (the drug is administered intramuscularly or subcutaneously several times a week).

Patient (Parent) Teaching

- Discuss the importance of monitoring growth measurements.
- Encourage emotional care: emphasize interests, hobbies, and sports for which size is not important (e.g., swimming, golf, tennis).
- Report signs and symptoms of hyperglycemia; obtain periodic blood glucose levels as recommended by the health care provider.
- Report hip pain and limping (which may indicate a slipped epiphyses) to the health care provider.

VASOPRESSIN (PITRESSIN), DESMOPRESSIN (DDAVP), LYPRESSIN (DIAPID)

Actions and Uses

Vasopressin, desmopressin, and lypressin mimic the actions of endogenous antidiuretic hormone (ADH). They increase sodium and water absorption in the renal distal tubules and collecting ducts of the nephrons, concentrate urine, and are potent vasoconstrictors. Desmopressin causes a dose-dependent increase in plasma levels of factor VIII (antihemophilic factor or von Willebrand's factor).

These drugs are used to treat hyposecretion of endogenous ADH, known as *neurogenic diabetes insipidus*. The symptoms of neurogenic diabetes insipidus include excessive thirst, urination of large amounts of very dilute urine, and dehydration. Because of their vasoconstrictive effects, these drugs are also useful for treatment of various types of bleeding, especially gastrointestinal hemorrhage. Owing to its ability to increase plasma levels of factor VIII, desmopressin is particularly useful in the treatment of hemophilia and type I von Willebrand's disease.

Side and Adverse Effects

Side effects include headache, lethargy, flushing, drowsiness, hypertension, uterine cramping, nasal irritation and congestion, tremors, sweating, and dizziness. Gastrointestinal effects include nausea, heartburn, and abdominal cramps.

Interactions and Contraindications

Desmopressin with carbamazepine (Tegretol) and chlorpropamide (Diabinese) increase the effect of desmopressin. Desmopressin with lithium, alcohol, demeclocycline (Declomycin), and heparin decrease the response to desmopressin.

These drugs are contraindicated for patients with *nephrogenic* diabetes insipidus and chronic nephritis.

Nursing Actions

Assess for and report signs and symptoms of dehydration. Monitor vital signs, especially blood pressure. Carefully monitor intake and output. Monitor for and report abnormal serum electrolyte values and urine specific gravity. Weigh the patient daily. Observe for symptoms of excessive drug dose: blanching skin, nausea, and abdominal cramps; notify the health care provider, as the next dose may need to be reduced. One or two glasses of water will help relieve the symptoms, which last only a few minutes. Teach the patient injection technique if an intramuscular or a subcutaneous form of the drug is being used.

Patient Teaching
• Nasal spray should be used exactly as prescribed, after nasal passages have been cleared, and should not be inhaled.
• Carry the medication with you at all times, especially while traveling, as the drug may not be readily available at all pharmacies.
• Continue home monitoring of intake and output and urine specific gravity.
• Avoid over-the-counter cold, cough, and allergy preparations (because epinephrine or ephedrine can increase blood pressure).
• All patients who are taking a pituitary drug should wear a Medic-Alert tag identifying the specific medication.

THYROID AND PARATHYROID HORMONES

THYROID HORMONES

The anterior pituitary gland secretes a tropic (regulating) hormone called *thyrotropin* (or thyroid-stimulating hormone, TSH) which controls activity of the thyroid gland. Thyroid gland hormones are known as *thyroxin* (T_4), *triiodothyronine* (T_3), and *calcitonin*.

Thyroxine (T_4) and triiodothyronine (T_3) are secreted by the thyroid gland to regulate the metabolic rate and activity of nearly all body tissues and organs and are controlled by the negative feedback system. When there is a thyroid deficiency (hypothyroidism), synthetic T_4 and T_3 may be prescribed, either alone or in combination. When there is secretion of too much thyroid hormone (hyperthyroidism), antithyroid drugs may be indicated.

Calcitonin plays a role in calcium regulation and is discussed with parathyroid hormone.

Hypothyroidism

Primary hypothyroidism (thyroid gland dysfunction) is more common than *secondary hypothyroidism* (lack of TSH secretion from the pituitary). Causes for primary hypothyroidism include acute or chronic inflammation of the thyroid gland, excess intake of antithyroid drugs, radioiodine therapy, and surgery. Symptoms include lethargy, weight gain, memory impairment, apathy, slow speech and hoarse voice, facial edema, especially of the eyelids, thickened and dry skin, cold intolerance, slow pulse, constipation, and abnormal menses. Adult-onset hypothyroidism is known as *myxedema*; the condition in children can be congenital (*cretinism*) or prepubertal (*juvenile hypothyroidism*). If the condition is not recognized and treatment begun early, cretinism can lead to mental and growth retardation. The drugs used to treat hypothyroidism include levothyroxine sodium (Synthroid), liothyronine sodium (Cytomel), liotrix (Euthyroid), thyroglobulin (Proloid), and thyroid extract (Armour Thyroid). The major difference between these drugs is onset and duration of action. Thyroglobulin (Proloid) is derived from hog thyroid and is rarely used. These drugs are all **Pregnancy Category A.**

Actions and Uses

These drugs are used as replacement therapy and produce the same effects as endogenous thyroid hormone to increase metabolic rate, cardiac output, protein synthesis, and glucose utilization. They are mostly excreted in bile and feces.

Side and Adverse Effects

Side effects include nausea, vomiting, diarrhea, abdominal cramps, headache, weight loss, tremors, nervousness, and insomnia. More serious adverse effects are tachycardia, hypertension, and palpitations; life-threatening reactions are angina pectoris, cardiac arrhythmias, cardiovascular collapse, and *thyroid storm* or *thyroid crisis* (symptoms include tachycardia, cardiac arrhythmias, fever, heart failure, flushed skin, apathy, behavioral changes, confusion, hypotension, and vascular collapse).

Interactions and Contraindications

These drugs increase the effect of oral anticoagulants, tricyclic antidepressants, vasopressors, and decongestants. They antagonize the effects of insulin and oral antidiabetic drugs, and digitalis preparations. Estrogen can increase the effect of liothyronine (Cytomel), and phenytoin and aspirin can increase the action of all forms of thyroid hormone replacements.

Contraindications include *thyrotoxicosis* (hyperthyroidism), myocardial infarction, and severe renal disease. These drugs should be used with caution for patients with cardiovascular disease, hypertension, and angina pectoris.

Nursing Actions

Determine drug and food allergies. Obtain baseline vital signs. Check serum T_4, T_3, and TSH levels periodically and report abnormalities to the health care provider. Assess for and report signs and symptoms of side and adverse effects. Monitor the patient's weight.

<table>
<tr><td>

Patient Teaching

- Clinical response (symptom relief) may take 1 to 2 weeks. Do not change the drug dose without consulting the health care provider.
- Take the drug at the same time every day, preferably before breakfast (food decreases absorption).
- Avoid over-the-counter drugs that caution against use by people with heart or thyroid disease and hypertension.
- Report symptoms of hyperthyroidism (tachycardia, chest pain, palpitations, excessive sweating).
- Learn and demonstrate how to take your own pulse and report marked increases or decreases to the health care provider.
- Avoid foods that inhibit thyroid secretion: peas, cauliflower, radishes, spinach, cabbage, Brussels sprouts, turnips, kale, peaches, pears, and strawberries.

</td></tr>
</table>

Hyperthyroidism

Hyperthyroidism is a result of an overactive thyroid gland with excessive output of thyroxine and triiodothyronine. Symptoms may be mild or severe, as in thyroid storm in which death may result from vascular collapse. The most common type of hyperthyroidism is *Graves' disease*, or *thyrotoxicosis*. Symptoms include tachycardia, palpitations, excessive sweating, nervousness, heat intolerance, irritability, and weight loss. A characteristic sign is *exophthalmos* (bulging eyes). Treatment may include subtotal thyroidectomy (removal of part of the thyroid gland), radioactive iodine, or antithyroid drugs. Any of these treatments may cause hypothyroidism. Antithyroid drugs include methimazole (Tapazole), propylthiouracil (PTU), and iodine (Lugol solution or potassium iodide solution). Propranolol (Inderal), a beta-adrenergic blocker, is used to control the cardiac symptoms due to hyperthyroidism.

Actions and Uses

Antithyroid drugs act to inhibit either the synthesis or release of thyroid hormone and are used to treat hyperthyroid conditions.

Side and Adverse Effects

Side effects include rash, urticaria, headache, gastrointestinal upset, petechiae or bruising, weakness, and loss of hair and hair pigment. A serious adverse effect is agranulocytosis (decreased white blood cells). Symptoms of hypothyroidism may occur. Symptoms of thyroid storm can result from thyroidectomy (release of excess thyroid hormone),

abrupt withdrawal of antithyroid drug, excess ingestion of thyroid drug, or failure to give antithyroid drug before surgery.

Interactions and Contraindications

Antithyroid drugs can increase the effects of oral anticoagulants. They decrease the effects of insulin and oral hypoglycemic drugs. Digoxin and lithium increase the action of antithyroid agents, and phenytoin (Dilantin) increases serum thyroxine levels.

Use of these drugs is contraindicated in pregnancy and for nursing mothers because of the potential for hypothyroidism in the fetus or infant. Use cautiously in persons with bone marrow depression, impaired hepatic function, agranulocytosis, or infection. **Pregnancy Category D.**

Nursing Actions

Obtain baseline vital signs. Check serum T_4, T_3, and TSH levels periodically. Report abnormal findings. Assess for and report signs of thyroid storm.

<table>
<tr><td>

Patient Teaching

- It may take 1 to 2 weeks to see a therapeutic response. Do not alter the drug dose without consulting the health care provider.
- Take the drug with meals (to decrease gastrointestinal upset).
- Dilute and take iodine solutions after meals; use a straw to prevent tooth discoloration.
- Avoid iodized salt, shellfish, and over-the-counter cough preparations.
- Do not abruptly discontinue the drug (because of the possibility of thyroid storm).
- Report symptoms of hypothyroidism or adverse effects to the health care provider.
- Learn and demonstrate how to take your own pulse and report marked increases or decreases to the health care provider.
- Report sore throat or fever (because of the possibility of decreased white blood cells, which may precipitate a serious infection) to the health care provider.
- Report the possibility of pregnancy to the health care provider as soon as possible.

</td></tr>
</table>

PARATHYROID HORMONES

The parathyroid glands secrete parathormone, or parathyroid hormone (PTH), which regulates serum calcium levels. A decrease in serum calcium stimulates release of PTH, which acts by causing calcium to be released from bone, promoting calcium absorption in the intestine, and increasing calcium reabsorption from renal tubules. Calcitonin, a hormone produced primarily by the thyroid gland, antagonizes the effects of PTH on bone and kidneys.

Hypoparathyroidism

Hypoparathyroidism, and its associated hypocalcemia, can be caused by PTH deficiency, vitamin D deficiency, renal dysfunction, or diuretic therapy. Drugs used as replacement and supplement therapy include calcifediol (Calderol), calcitriol (Rocaltrol), and ergocalciferol (Drisdol Drops).

Actions and Uses

These drugs are vitamin D analogues (similar in structure) that promote calcium absorption from the gastrointestinal tract and renal tubules and movement of calcium from bone to serum. They are readily absorbed from the gastrointestinal tract and mostly excreted in the feces.

In addition to management of hypocalcemia associated with chronic renal dialysis and hypoparathyroidism, unlabeled uses for these drugs include treatment for vitamin D–resistant and –dependent rickets and hypocalcemia in preterm infants.

Side and Adverse Effects

Side effects include anorexia, nausea, vomiting, diarrhea, abdominal cramps, headache, lethargy and drowsiness, dizziness, and photophobia. More serious adverse effects may be hypercalciuria (increased calcium in urine), hyperphosphatemia, and hematuria. Symptoms of hypercalcemia may occur (see Chapter 7).

Interactions and Contraindications

Concurrent use with digoxin and verapamil increases the potential for cardiac arrhythmias. Cholestyramine (Questran) decreases absorption of these drugs. If given with thiazide diuretics or calcium supplements, hypercalcemia may occur.

These drugs are contraindicated for persons with hypercalcemia, hyperphosphatemia, hypervitaminosis D, and malabsorption syndrome. Use cautiously in the presence of cardiovascular disease and kidney stones.

Nursing Actions

Monitor serum calcium (and other electrolyte) levels; report abnormal findings to the health care provider. Assess for and report symptoms of hypocalcemic tetany: numbness and tingling of fingers and lips, muscle spasms, and abdominal cramping (see Chapter 7). Assess for and report signs and symptoms of hypercalcemia (bone pain, anorexia, nausea and vomiting, thirst, constipation, lethargy, bradycardia, and polyuria).

Patient Teaching

- The drug may be taken with food or milk to minimize gastrointestinal upset.
- If symptoms of hypercalcemia occur, stop the drug and notify the health care provider.
- Reduction of dietary calcium may need to be considered during therapy.
- Avoid all sources of vitamin D during therapy to prevent hypercalcemia.
- Consult the health care provider before taking an over-the-counter medication (many over-the-counter products contain calcium, vitamin D, phosphates, or magnesium, which can increase the potential for adverse effects).

Hyperparathyroidism

Hyperparathyroidism, and hypercalcemia, may be caused by parathyroid tumors, abnormal PTH secretion from lung cancer, hyperthyroidism, prolonged immobility (calcium is released from bone), or anticancer therapy. Drugs used in the management of hyperparathyroidism include calcitonin human (Cibacalcin), calcitonin salmon (Calcimar), and etidronate (Didronel).

Actions and Uses

These drugs decrease serum calcium by binding at receptor sites on the osteoclasts of bone, thus decreasing release of calcium from bone. They also promote renal excretion of calcium and phosphorus. Calcitonin salmon is more potent and has a longer duration of action than calcitonin human.

Uses for these drugs include symptomatic Paget's disease and postmenopausal osteoporosis. Calcitonin human is a short-term adjunctive treatment for severe hypercalcemic emergencies. Unlabeled uses include diagnosis and management of thyroid cancer and as treatment for osteogenesis imperfecta.

Side and Adverse Effects

Side effects include transient nausea, vomiting and diarrhea, anorexia, unusual taste sensation, and abdominal pain. Skin effects may include flushing of hands and feet, itching of ear lobes, edema of feet, and rashes. Calcitonin human may cause urinary frequency, chills, chest pressure, tender palms and soles, and nasal congestion.

Interactions and Contraindications

Concurrent use with over-the-counter vitamins and antacids containing calcium or vitamin D may decrease the effects of these drugs.

Persons who are hypersensitive to fish protein should not take calcitonin salmon. Use cautiously in persons with renal disease and osteoporosis.

Nursing Actions

Monitor serum calcium (and other electrolyte) levels; report abnormal findings to the health care provider. Monitor for and report symptoms of hypocalcemia and hypercalcemia. If the nasal spray form of the drug is used, assess for nasal irritation, ulceration, or heavy bleeding. Administer calcitonin human by subcutaneous route only; calcitonin salmon may be administered subcutaneously, intramuscularly, or intranasally. Teach the patient to self-administer the subcutaneous injection.

Patient Teaching
• Report signs and symptoms of hypocalcemia and hypercalcemia to the health care provider.   • Contact the health care provider before taking prescribed or over-the-counter drugs containing calcium or vitamin D.

CHAPTER 43

ADRENAL HORMONES

*T*he paired adrenal glands, located above the kidneys, are composed of the outer portion, or adrenal cortex, and the inner portion, or adrenal medulla. The adrenal medulla secretes epinephrine and norephineprine (see Chapter 15). This chapter focuses on the hormones produced by the adrenal cortex, which may be referred to as *steroids, corticosteroids*, or *adrenocorticosteroids*, but which all refer to the same thing: *glucocorticoids* and *mineralocorticoids*. Cortisol is the endogenous glucocorticoid and aldosterone the endogenous mineralocorticoid. The adrenal cortex also produces sex steroids, which are discussed in Chapters 45 and 46.

GLUCOCORTICOIDS

Based on the negative feedback system of hormonal control, the anterior pituitary gland secretes corticotropin, or adrenocorticotropic hormone (ACTH), which regulates adrenal gland activity. A decrease in serum cortisol levels causes the release of ACTH from the pituitary gland, which stimulates the adrenals to secrete cortisol. An increased serum cortisol level produces the negative feedback mechanism, which inhibits release of cortisol.

When steroids are taken as medications, they initiate the process of negative feedback. The pituitary gland is unable to distinguish between endogenous hormones and those taken as medications. Therefore, therapeutic administration of steroids may cause the anterior pituitary to decrease secretion and release of ACTH and the adrenal glands to stop producing cortisol. Because of this decrease in ACTH and cortisol release, when the steroid medications are stopped, it may take several days to weeks for the anterior pituitary to begin to stimulate the adrenal cortex and several weeks to months to get endogenous hormone secretion back up to normal levels. Long-term treatment of nonendocrine disorders (e.g., organ transplants, certain malignancies, severe asthma, or obstructive lung disease) with pharmacologic doses of glucocorticoids may produce pituitary ACTH suppression for up to 1 year after drug therapy has been discontinued. Therefore, abrupt discontinuation of corticosteroid drugs may produce a life-threatening condition known as *Addisonian*, or *adrenal, crisis* (hypoadrenalism), which is characterized by cyanosis, fever, and symptoms of shock (increased pulse and respirations and decreased blood pressure). Other symptoms may include headache, nausea, vomiting, abdominal pain, diarrhea, confusion, and restlessness. To prevent the occurrence of this serious complication, steroid drugs are discontinued gradually, over a number of weeks. Specific measures to reduce the risk of adrenal crisis and weaning patients off the drugs are discussed under Nursing Actions.

There are numerous corticosteroid drugs that can be administered by a number of routes. Some of the more commonly used drugs include cortisone acetate (Cortistan, Cortone), hydrocortisone (cortisol, Cortef), and hydrocortisone sodium succinate (Solu-Cortef), prednisolone (Cortalone), methylprednisolone (Medrol) and methylprednisolone sodium succinate (Solu-Medrol), betamethasone (Celestone), dexamethasone sodium phosphate (Decadron), prednisone (Deltasone, Colisone), and triamcinolone (Aristocort, Kenacort). Most of these drugs also have mineralocorticoid activity (sodium and water retention, potassium and hydrogen excretion). Betamethasone and dexamethasone have minimal mineralocorticoid activity, so are particularly useful for persons for whom sodium and water retention and potassium loss could be a problem (e.g., hypertension, congestive heart failure, pulmonary edema). Routes of administration include intravenous, intramuscular, oral, intra-articular (into joints), topical to skin and mucous membranes, and rectal. Ophthalmic, otic, and intranasal preparations are also available. These drugs may be ordered in "physiologic doses," or doses comparable to normal serum cortisol levels, or "pharmacologic doses," in which increased, or greater than normal, doses are given. Physiologic doses are usually ordered as replacement therapy for patients with low functioning or nonfunctioning adrenal glands to return serum cortisol levels to normal. The pharmacologic doses are generally used to treat nonendocrine disorders.

Actions and Uses

The major actions of cortisol and exogenous steroids are to suppress acute inflammation and for immunosuppression. Other functions are to maintain normal blood pressure, carbohydrate, protein, and fat metabolism, and stress response.

However, cortisol has widespread physiologic effects, as follows:

- Metabolism:
  — proteins: increased breakdown of protein to amino acids and decreased rate of protein synthesis
  — carbohydrates: increased production and decreased use of glucose
  — lipids: increased breakdown of adipose tissue to fatty acids
- Nervous system:
  — physiologic doses: maintenance of normal nerve excitability
  — pharmacologic doses: decrease nerve excitability, slow cerebral cortex activity, alter brain wave patterns
- Musculoskeletal system:
  — physiologic doses: maintenance of muscle strength
  — pharmacologic doses: muscle atrophy, inhibition of bone formation, and increased bone breakdown
- Respiratory system: maintain open airways and inhibit release of bronchoconstrictive and inflammatory substances
- Gastrointestinal system: decreased gastric mucus viscosity, increased potential for ulcers
- Fluids and electrolytes: sodium and water retention, potassium and calcium depletion
- Immune system: suppression
- Inflammatory response: suppression

Corticosteroids are used to treat many diseases and health problems. These may include the following:

- Allergic disorders such as drug reactions, dermatitis, rhinitis
- Replacement therapy for chronic adrenocortical hyposecretion (Addison's disease) or acute-onset adrenal crisis
- Malignancies
- Inflammatory disorders such as autoimmune diseases (e.g., multiple sclerosis, rheumatoid arthritis, myasthenia gravis), ulcerative colitis, glomerulonephritis, ocular and vascular inflammation, cirrhosis of the liver, and hepatitis
- Suppression of organ graft/transplant rejection process
- Respiratory disorders such as asthma or chronic obstructive pulmonary disease
- Emergency situations for anaphylaxis, cerebral edema, increased intracranial pressure, septic and other types of shock (to stabilize and maintain blood pressure)

Side and Adverse Effects

Side and adverse effects are virtually nonexistent with replacement (physiologic) doses or short-term therapy but are common with long-term use of pharmacologic doses.

These effects may occur during therapy or upon discontinuation of the drug. Those that occur during therapy are usually exaggerations of normal hormonal actions, producing a condition known as iatrogenic (medically induced) *Cushing's syndrome*. The signs and symptoms of Cushing's syndrome are numerous and result from hypersecretion of the adrenal glands or excess cortisol. These effects include abnormal fat deposits in face, posterior neck, and torso (moon face, buffalo hump, and protruding abdomen), muscle wasting and decreased extremity size and strength, sodium and water retention with potassium excretion (with possible edema, hypernatremia, and hypokalemia), hyperglycemia, hypertension, thinned skin with easy bruising, increased intraocular pressure (glaucoma) or cataracts, peptic ulcers, growth retardation in children, and euphoria or psychosis. Additional adverse effects may include poor wound healing, aggravation or masking of infections, convulsions, congestive heart failure, and osteoporosis. Increased appetite, weight gain, and menstrual irregularities may also occur. Because of pituitary ACTH and adrenal gland suppression, long-term use of corticosteroids can cause loss of adrenal gland function. Abrupt withdrawal of the drug could result in acute adrenal crisis. Side and adverse effects that may occur on discontinuation of the drug are caused by adrenal suppression during therapy and are characterized by signs and symptoms of acute adrenal crisis.

MINERALOCORTICOIDS

The only physiologically important mineralocorticoid in humans is aldosterone. Its primary role is to maintain sodium homeostasis by causing sodium to be reabsorbed from the renal tubules in exchange for potassium and hydrogen ions. Because sodium attracts water, water retention also occurs. In this way, aldosterone not only regulates serum sodium levels but also influences serum potassium and pH, as well as blood volume and blood pressure.

Actions and Uses

The mechanism that regulates aldosterone is related to hypovolemia and hyponatremia: a decrease in blood volume, blood pressure, and serum sodium with rising serum potassium leads to secretion of aldosterone. When homeostasis is reached, secretion of aldosterone ceases. Aldosterone also contributes to sodium reabsorption from other body sites such as sweat and salivary glands, and gastrointestinal mucosa. The primary drug in this category is fludrocortisone (Florinef), a synthetic mineralocorticoid with weak glucocorticoid but very potent mineralocorticoid activity.

Fludrocortisone is used for replacement therapy (in conjunction with a glucocorticoid) in patients with adrenocortical insufficiency such as Addison's disease. It has also been used to increase blood pressure in patients with chronic severe postural hypotension. It is only available in oral form.

Side and Adverse Effects

Side and adverse effects are dependent on dose and duration of treatment. Fludrocortisone may cause a negative nitrogen balance, so a high-protein diet is usually indicated. Hypernatremia, hypokalemia, and hypertension may occur. In addition, all of the side and adverse effects related to glucocorticoids are possible.

INTERACTIONS AND CONTRAINDICATIONS

The greatest risk of drug interactions are with long-term therapy. Alcohol, aspirin, and nonsteroidal anti-inflammatory drugs increase the risk of gastrointestinal bleeding and ulcers. Concurrent use of potassium-wasting diuretics increases the potential for hypokalemia. Glucocorticoids antagonize the effects of insulin and oral hypoglycemics, as well as diuretics, antihypertensive drugs, digitalis, and oral anticoagulants. Phenytoin, theophylline, rifampin, and barbiturates decrease the effects of glucocorticoids. Antacids will decrease the effects of oral glucocorticoids but may be recommended to reduce occurrence of gastrointestinal side effects.

Aldosterone is antagonized by the potassium-sparing diuretic spironolactone (Aldactone).

Corticosteroids are contraindicated in persons with fungal or bacterial infections, severe glaucoma, and history of tuberculosis. Because of the risk for steroid-induced psychosis, cautious use of these drugs is advised in patients with pre-existing psychiatric disorders.

NURSING ACTIONS

Monitor vital signs, intake and output, and weight (an increase in blood pressure and gain in weight may indicate water retention; fever may mean infection). Administer drug only as ordered. Check labels carefully, as drug strength may vary according to route of administration. Drug dose may require several adjustments based on therapeutic effect, individual responses, or occurrence of side or adverse effects. Observe for and report the occurrence of side and adverse effects. Administer intramuscular forms only into a deep muscle mass such as the gluteal area. Assess wounds for healing or infection. Once-daily dosing should be administered between 6 and 9 AM (to minimize adrenal suppression and more closely mimic natural cortisol secretion). Monitor blood glucose in patients with diabetes mellitus or who are

at risk for developing the disease (potential for hyperglycemia). To reduce the risk of adrenal gland suppression:

- Alternate-day therapy (not useful for all steroids), whereby the dose changes every other day (e.g., BID on Monday, Wednesday, Friday, Sunday and QD [or none] on Tuesday, Thursday, and Saturday).
- Inhaled or topical forms if possible.
- Use less than 10 to 14 days.

Following prolonged systemic use, corticosteroids must be discontinued gradually: dose is reduced by a specified amount every 4 to 10 days; if withdrawal symptoms occur (fever, muscle or joint pain, depression, fatigue, nausea and vomiting, anorexia), previous dose is reinstituted for 7 days before continuing drug weaning.

Patient Teaching

- Take the drug exactly as prescribed. Do NOT abruptly stop taking the drug. The drug may be tapered even if taken for less than 10 days.
- Avoid persons with infections and report any fever, sore throat, or malaise.
- Learn the correct use of the aerosol nebulizer. Do not overuse to avoid possible rebound effect.
- You may take the drug with food to avoid gastrointestinal irritation.
- Consume a potassium- and calcium-rich diet (fresh and dried fruits, especially bananas and oranges, vegetables, meats, nuts, and dairy products).
- Avoid foods high in sodium.
- Alcohol enhances the tendency of steroids to cause ulcers.
- Nicotine increases steroid effects.
- To minimize the occurrence of systemic effects, apply topical preparations sparingly and only to affected areas. Do not use an occlusive dressing without instructions from the health care provider.
- Report signs of side or adverse effects:
  — Gastrointestinal: abdominal distention, tarry stools, nausea, hematemesis
  — Skin: bruising, petechiae, rash, acne
  — Muscle/bone: decreased muscle mass and weakness
  — Central nervous system: headache, dizziness, paresthesias (numbness and tingling), mental changes (anxiety, depression, euphoria). Seizures may also occur.

(Continued on p. 202)

- Perform careful blood glucose monitoring. Report signs and symptoms of hyperglycemia (polyuria [excess urine], polydipsia [excess thirst], polyphagia [increased hunger], weight loss).
- Maintain (or establish) routine eye examinations.
- Consult the health care provider before receiving immunizations.
- Report signs of Cushing's syndrome (moon face, puffy eyelids, pedal edema, increased bruising, etc.), but do NOT stop taking the drug if symptoms occur.
- Wear a Medic-Alert tag at all times.

ANTIADRENALS

Actions and Uses

Aminoglutethimide (Cytadren) is the primary drug used in this category. It inhibits the normal actions of the adrenal cortex by inhibiting the conversion of cholesterol into corticosteroids.

Aminoglutethimide is primarily used for Cushing's syndrome associated with adrenal cancer. Unlabeled uses include metastatic prostate cancer and advanced breast cancer in postmenopausal women. (Unlabeled uses do not appear on the drug label or in the manufacturer's literature. These are clinical indications other than those for which the drug was originally intended, but which now have accepted use supported by medical literature).

Side and Adverse Effects

The most common side effects are nausea, anorexia, dizziness, drowsiness, lethargy, headache, and skin rash. Dose-dependent reversible masculinization may occur. This drug is hepatotoxic.

Interactions and Contraindications

Aminoglutethimide may decrease the therapeutic effects of dexamethasone, digitoxin, medroxyprogesterone, theophyllin, and warfarin.

Contraindications include hypothyroidism and infection. Safe use in children has not been established. Cautious use is indicated in the elderly. **Pregnancy Category X.**

Nursing Actions

Obtain baseline and periodic cortisol and electrolyte levels, as well as liver and thyroid function studies as ordered by the health care provider. Obtain baseline and regularly scheduled blood pressure readings (potential for orthostatic hypotension). Administer drug exactly as ordered. Monitor nutritional status. Assess for improvement in condition (decrease in signs and symptoms of Cushing's syndrome). Observe for and report rash, jaundice, fever, or skin lesions. Observe for and report symptoms of hypoadrenalism. Drug may have to be discontinued if this occurs. Because the elderly are especially susceptible to drug-related drowsiness and dizziness, provide appropriate assistance with ambulation.

Patient Teaching
• Change from sitting or lying positions slowly.
• Drowsiness, nausea, anorexia usually last only 1 to 2 weeks. If symptoms persist, notify the health care provider but continue taking the drug.
• Contact the health care provider immediately in times of stress (e.g., surgery, dental work, acute illness, acute emotional distress). Steroid supplements may be indicated.
• Notify the health care provider immediately if pregnancy is suspected.
• If masculinization occurs, this will disappear when treatment is stopped.
• Always carry a Medic-Alert tag.

INSULIN AND ORAL HYPOGLYCEMIC AGENTS

*T*he regulation of blood glucose is tightly controlled to prevent excess loss of glucose in urine and to ensure availability of energy to glucose-dependent tissue such as the brain, kidneys, retina, blood cells, and germinal epithelium in the gonads.

In the pancreas, clusters of specialized cells known as *islets of Langerhans* secrete two hormones called *insulin* and *glucagon*, which antagonize each other. Insulin, the primary hormone, is secreted by the beta cells, while glucagon comes from the alpha cells. When insulin and glucagon are in balance, glucose is properly utilized and homeostasis is maintained. When inadequate insulin is secreted or there is a resistance to insulin, or both, there is not enough glucose available for cell metabolism, even though there is glucose in the bloodstream. This produces a condition known as *diabetes mellitus*, a disease characterized by abnormal breakdown of fats and proteins. Incomplete fat metabolism produces acetone and leads to a condition known as *diabetic ketoacidosis*. Blood glucose levels rise, resulting in hyperglycemia. If there is too much insulin secreted, or too little glucagon, available glucose is used up by the cells, blood glucose falls, and hypoglycemia (or "insulin shock") occurs. Normal ranges for blood glucose levels vary with each laboratory and must be indicated on the lab report, but, in general, normal fasting blood glucose is considered 80 to 120 mg/dL.

Signs and symptoms of *hyperglycemia* include the "three Ps," which characterize diabetes mellitus: polyuria (increased urine output), polydipsia (increased thirst), and polyphagia (increased appetite). Additional signs and symptoms are weight loss, fruity breath (from acetone), flushed, dry skin, Kussmaul respirations (rapid, deep, labored breathing), headache, abdominal pain, numbness of fingers and toes, full, bounding pulse, dry mucous membranes with poor skin turgor, and glycosuria (glucose in the urine). If untreated, the condition will progress to unconsciousness, coma, and death. When these signs and symptoms become evident, blood glucose levels are usually greater than 250 mg/dL.

Hypoglycemia is characterized by predictable sets of symptoms. *Cluster one* symptoms (associated with epinephrine release) include tremors, faintness, cold, clammy skin, rapid, thready pulse, hunger, and excess perspiration. *Cluster two* symptoms (neurologic signs related to decreased glucose in the brain) include headache, confusion, visual disturbances, weakness, slurred speech, memory lapse, and seizures. If untreated, coma and death may result. When these signs and symptoms occur, blood glucose levels are usually less than 60 mg/dL.

Drugs used to lower blood glucose are known as *hypoglycemic agents* or *antidiabetic drugs*. The oldest hypoglycemic is insulin and is required by persons who are unable to produce adequate amounts of that hormone. These persons have a condition known as *insulin-dependent diabetes mellitus* (IDDM or type 1 diabetes). Oral hypoglycemics may be used by persons with *non-insulin-dependent diabetes mellitus* (NIDDM or type 2 diabetes) whose disease is not controlled by diet and exercise alone.

INSULIN

Insulin is the primary treatment for persons with type 1 diabetes mellitus (IDDM). Sources of exogenous insulin include extraction from cattle and pigs and laboratory synthesis using recombinant DNA technology.

Actions and Uses

Insulin (1) promotes glucose storage from carbohydrates, fats, and protein metabolism and also from amino acids, fatty acids, potassium, and magnesium; (2) stimulates hepatic cells to form glycogen, the major storage form of glucose; and (3) lowers blood glucose levels.

Exogenously administered insulin produces all the same effects on the body as insulin normally produced endogenously. Insulin functions on the negative feedback system: when blood glucose levels rise, insulin is secreted, and when blood glucose levels decrease, insulin secretion is reduced.

The primary therapeutic use of insulin is to restore or maintain glucose homeostasis. Exogenous insulin is replacement therapy for insufficient or defective natural hormone and causes the same appropriate utilization, mobilization, and storage of glucose.

There are three general types of insulin: rapid-acting, intermediate-acting, and long-acting. Each of these types is based on three pharmacokinetic properties: (1) onset of action (when insulin begins to act in the body), (2) peak (when insulin exerts its maximum action and blood glucose is at its lowest), (3) duration of action (length of time the insulin dose acts in the body). These properties may be modified or altered by the addition of zinc or protamine (a protein), which slow absorption from the injection site, thus prolonging onset and duration of action.

Rapid-Acting Insulins

Products include Regular, Semilente, Novolin R, and Humulin R. *Unmodified* regular insulin is a clear solution and is the only type safe for both intravenous and subcutaneous administration. All other forms of insulin are administered subcutaneously or intramuscularly.

Regular, Novolin R, Humulin R

Intravenous: Onset: 10–20 min
                 Peak: 15–30 min
                 Duration: 1–2 hr

Subcutaneous: Onset: 0.5–1 hr
                 Peak: 2–4 hr
                 Duration: 4–8 hr

Insulin lispro (Humalog) is a very rapid acting regular insulin of recombinant DNA origin. It has the same glucose-lowering ability of human regular insulin, but the effect is more rapid and of shorter duration. Although lispro is also a clear solution, it is **only** given **subcutaneously.**

Onset: <15 min
Peak: 0.5–1 hr
Duration: 3–4 hr

Semilente is a modified rapid-acting drug with slightly longer pharmacokinetics.

Onset: 0.5–1 hr
Peak: 5–10 hr
Duration: 12–16 hr

Intermediate-Acting Insulins

Products include *NPH, Lente, Novolin N*, and *Humulin N.* All of these products are modified.

Onset: 1–2 hr
Peak: 8–12 hr
Duration: 18–24 hr

Long-Acting Insulins

Long-acting insulins are seldom ordered because their peak occurs during the night or early morning hours. Products include Ultralente and Humulin U. These products are also modified.

Onset: 4–8 hr
Peak: 14–20 hr
Duration: 36+ hr

Fixed-Combination Insulins

Insulin levels are normally variable in nondiabetic persons. Fixed-combination insulins were developed for persons with type 1 diabetes mellitus to more closely simulate this variability. Some insulin regimens call for a combination of a rapid-acting insulin to cover glucose surges after meals and an intermediate-acting insulin to cover in between meals when glucose levels are lower. Fixed-combination insulins may eliminate the need for mixing different types of insulin and can more closely mimic the body's own varying insulin levels. Fixed-combination products include the following:

Humulin 50/50:   50 U (units) intermediate and 50 U regular insulin
Humulin 70/30:   70 U intermediate and 30 U regular insulin
Novolin 70/30:   70 U intermediate and 30 U regular insulin
Mixtard 70/30:   70 U intermediate and 30 U regular insulin

Side and Adverse Effects

Hypoglycemia is the most serious adverse effect of insulin. In addition to the symptoms of hypoglycemia, other side effects may include irritation, redness, or swelling at the injection site. Allergic (or anaphylactic) symptoms (hives, edema, rash, itching, difficulty breathing) are usually related to an allergy to pork, beef, or the modifier used (zinc or protamine).

Interactions and Contraindications

Drugs that antagonize the effect of insulin (and increase potential for hyperglycemia) include corticosteroids, diazoxide (Proglycem), epinephrine, estrogens, ethacrynic acid (Edecrin), furosemide (Lasix), phenytoin (Dilantin), thiazide diuretics, and thyroid hormones. Drugs that increase the effect of insulin (and increase the potential for hypoglycemia) include alcohol, anabolic steroids, guanethidine, monoamine oxidase inhibitors, beta-adrenergic blockers, salicylates, oral anticoagulants, tricyclic antidepressants, and tetracycline.

Because persons with type 1 diabetes mellitus have an absolute need for insulin, there are no contraindications to its use. Use of human insulin should prevent the occurrence of allergic reactions.

Nursing Actions

Insulin is always ordered and measured in units. It is most commonly available in U-100 concentrations, which means that each milliliter contains 100 units (U). Insulin should be administered with an insulin syringe calibrated in units. The calibration on the syringe must match the concentration on the insulin bottle (i.e., insulin bottle U-100, syringe marked U-100; insulin bottle U-500, syringe marked U-500). Failure to match the insulin concentration with the correct syringe could result in a serious medication error. Do not use insulin that has changed color. Regular insulins are clear, all others have a cloudy, milky appearance. Modified insulins are suspensions and will precipitate at rest. To mix the solute evenly into the solution, gently rotate the vial between the palms of your hands. Do NOT SHAKE the vial, as this causes bubbles to form and may result in dose errors. Appropriate injection sites include upper arms, abdomen, thighs, scapulae, and buttocks. Do not massage injection site, as this may increase skin irritation or increase the rate of insulin absorption. There are no oral forms of insulin. Because insulin is a protein, it is destroyed by enzymes in the gastrointestinal tract. Persons taking animal insulin products will develop antibodies over time. Antibody development can cause insulin resistance and insulin allergy. Onset of action may be delayed and duration of action extended. Human insulin produces fewer antibodies. However, when switching from animal to human insulin, doses may need to be adjusted as human insulin has a shorter duration of action. Insulins should not be mixed unless prescribed by a health care provider. When regular insulin is to be given in the same syringe with a modified insulin, always draw up the regular first (clear to cloudy).

Patient Teaching

- Because hypoglycemic reactions are most likely to occur during the insulin's peak action time (serum glucose at its lowest), learn the symptoms to watch for and the time of day or night these symptoms are more apt to occur. For example, Humulin N administered at 8 AM, hypoglycemia is possible between 4 PM and 8 PM (8–12 hours later).
- Ingestion of a rapidly absorbed form of glucose (orange juice or candy) should alleviate the symptoms of hypoglycemia. This must be followed as soon as possible by a more complex carbohydrate (e.g., skim milk, fruit, crackers) to prevent rebound hypoglycemia as cells utilize the more rapidly absorbed glucose.
- Do not skip meals, as hypoglycemia may occur.
- Learn how to safely administer insulin, including drawing up the drug and injection technique. It is important to rotate sites to prevent *lipodystrophy* (tissue atrophy or hypertrophy), which can interfere with insulin absorption.

- Family members should also learn how to give insulin injections.
- Learn serum home glucose monitoring technique.
- If hypoglycemic episodes occur regularly, notify the physician. Your diet, exercise, or insulin regimen may need to be changed.
- Contact the health care provider immediately in times of stress (e.g., surgery, dental work, acute illness, acute emotional distress), as insulin requirements may increase at this time.
- Wear a Medic-Alert tag at all times, as the behavioral changes associated with hypoglycemia or hyperglycemia can be misinterpreted, possibly delaying treatment.

ORAL HYPOGLYCEMICS

The group of drugs known as *oral hypoglycemics* may be prescribed for persons with type 2 diabetes mellitus (NIDDM) whose disease is not controlled by diet and exercise alone. They may also be used as an adjunct to insulin therapy for persons with type 1 diabetes mellitus (IDDM) to increase the number and sensitivity of insulin receptors in the cells. There are four groups of drugs in this category: sulfonylureas, biguanides, alpha-glucosidase inhibitors, and thiazolidinediones.

Sulfonylureas

The oldest and largest group of oral hypoglycemics are the sulfonylureas. They are chemically related to the sulfonamide antimicrobial drugs but lack antibacterial activity. The sulfonylureas are classified as first- and second-generation drugs, differing mainly in potency, onset and duration of action, and, to some degree, occurrence of side effects. First-generation drugs include chlorpropamide (Diabinese), tolazamide (Tolinase), tolbutamide (Orinase), and acetohexamide (Dymelor). Second-generation drugs are glipizide (Glucotrol), and glyburide (DiaBeta).

Actions and Uses

Sulfonylureas stimulate pancreatic beta cells to increase the release of endogenous insulin. They also increase tissue responsiveness to insulin, and increase the number of available insulin receptors. Second-generation agents also decrease glucose production by the liver.

Sulfonylureas are used to lower blood glucose for persons with type 2 diabetes mellitus when diet and exercise alone are not successful. However, beta cells must be functional. These drugs may also be used in combination with insulin for persons with type 1 diabetes mellitus with extreme resistance to insulin. Combinations with other oral hypoglycemics may be useful to treat severe hyperglycemia.

Side and Adverse Effects

Signs and symptoms of hypoglycemia may occur, particularly if these drugs are taken without food. Gastrointestinal effects may include nausea and heartburn. Photosensitivity and skin rash may also occur.

Interactions and Contraindications

Drugs that increase the effect of the sulfonylureas (and produce significant hypoglycemia) include insulin, alcohol, anabolic steroids, beta-adrenergic blockers, monoamine oxidase inhibitors, oral anticoagulants, sulfonamides, anticonvulsants, aspirin and other nonsteroidal anti-inflammatory drugs, chloramphenicol (Chloromycetin), and cimetidine (Tagamet). Drugs that antagonize the effect of the sulfonylureas include adrenergics, corticosteroids, thiazide diuretics, thyroid preparations, calcium channel blockers, estrogens, and phenytoin (Dilantin).

These drugs are contraindicated as the *only* antidiabetic agent for persons with type 1 diabetes mellitus (who have no functioning beta cells) and should not be taken during times of stress, surgery, or severe infection. In addition, chlorpropamide (Diabinese) should not be taken during pregnancy (**Pregnancy Category D**) or breastfeeding or by persons with renal failure. Persons who are allergic to the sulfonamide antimicrobials should avoid using sulfonylurea agents.

Biguanides

Actions and Uses

Unlike the sulfonylureas, which stimulate the release of insulin from the beta cells, metformin (Glucophage), the only drug in this category, is believed to exert its antidiabetic effect by three mechanisms: (1) decreasing glucose production by the liver, (2) decreasing intestinal absorption of glucose, and (3) improving insulin sensitivity. It has no effect on pancreatic insulin or on secretion of other hormones involved in blood glucose regulation (e.g., glucagon).

Metformin may be used for persons with type 2 diabetes mellitus as an adjunct to diet therapy when diet alone does not control hyperglycemia. It may also be used together with a sulfonylurea if necessary to manage persistent hyperglycemia.

Side and Adverse Effects

The side effects of metformin primarily affect the gastrointestinal tract. These include nausea and diarrhea, cramping, abdominal bloating, and a feeling of fullness. These side effects are temporary and can be lessened by starting with low doses with gradual increases as necessary, and taking the drug with food. Less common side effects are a metallic taste and vitamin B_{12} and folic acid deficiency. Lac-

tic acidosis may occur in persons with renal disease. Metformin does not cause hypoglycemia if given alone. If given with sulfonylureas or insulin, the potential for hypoglycemia exists.

Interactions and Contraindications

Drugs that increase the effects of metformin are furosemide (Lasix), nifedipine (Procardia), cimetidine (Tagamet), and digoxin. Acarbose (Precose) may decrease metformin levels.

Metformin is contraindicated for persons with hepatic or renal disease, alcoholism, or cardiopulmonary disease.

Alpha-Glucosidase Inhibitors

Actions and Uses

The two drugs in this category are acarbose (Precose) and miglitol (Glyset). They inhibit alpha-glucosidase enzymes (sucrase, maltase, and amylase) in the gastrointestinal tract and pancreas to delay digestion of complex carbohydrates into glucose and other simple sugars. This results in delayed glucose absorption with smaller increases of blood glucose after meals. They do not alter insulin secretion.

As with metformin, these drugs may be used alone with diet therapy, or in combination with a sulfonylurea and diet to control hyperglycemia.

Side and Adverse Effects

Most side effects involve the gastrointestinal tract: diarrhea, flatulence, and abdominal pain. High doses may elevate liver enzymes. They do not cause hypoglycemia if given alone. If administered with sulfonylureas or insulin, the potential for hypoglycemia exists.

Interactions and Contraindications

Drugs that may decrease the effect of acarbose and miglitol are intestinal adsorbents (e.g., charcoal) and digestive enzyme preparations containing carbohydrase-splitting enzymes (e.g., amylase and pancreatin). In addition, drugs that induce hyperglycemia may also decrease their effects: thiazide diuretics, corticosteroids, phenothiazines, estrogens, phenytoin (Dilantin), and isoniazid (INH).

These drugs are contraindicated for persons with diabetic ketoacidosis (DKA), cirrhosis of the liver, inflammatory bowel disease, ulcerations of the colon, partial intestinal obstruction, or chronic bowel disease.

Thiazolidinediones

The first (and only) drug in this category to be approved for use in the United States is troglitazone (Rezulin). Because this drug works by decreasing insulin resistance, it is also referred to as an *insulin-enhancing agent.*

Actions and Uses

Troglitazone decreases insulin resistance by increasing sensitivity of insulin receptors in the liver, skeletal muscles, and adipose tissue. This increases glucose uptake and utilization in skeletal muscles, increases glucose uptake and decreases fatty acid output in adipose tissue, and decreases production of glucose and triglyceride synthesis by the liver. It has no known effect on insulin secretion.

Troglitazone is used to manage type 2 diabetes mellitus for persons whose hyperglycemia is not adequately controlled despite at least 30 U of insulin per day.

Side and Adverse Effects

Side effects include headache, dizziness, peripheral edema, nausea, diarrhea, and rhinitis. It does not cause lactic acidosis in persons with renal disease. However, recent findings have shown that acute liver failure and death have occurred in a few patients receiving this drug.

Interactions and Contraindications

Concurrent use with the antilipemic drug cholestyramine (Questran) will decrease absorption of troglitazone. Troglitazone will antagonize the effects of oral contraceptives, perhaps by as much as 30%. Use of troglitazone with sulfonylureas increases the risk of hypoglycemia.

This drug is contraindicated as the *only* treatment for persons with type 1 diabetes mellitus or as treatment of DKA. It should be used cautiously in persons with congestive heart failure or hepatic disease.

Nursing Implications (for Troglitazone)

Initial and periodic monitoring of liver function tests must be undertaken. If the daily dose is missed with the usual meal, it may be taken at the next meal. Instruct patients to report promptly signs of liver impairment (e.g., anorexia, jaundice, dark urine, clay-colored stools). Women using birth control pills may need higher doses or other means of birth control.

Nursing Actions (for All Oral Hypoglycemics)

Obtain a thorough medication history prior to beginning therapy, particularly drug and food allergies (especially to sulfonamides). Assess and report blood glucose levels as ordered by health care provider. Assess the patient's knowledge of diabetes mellitus, proper diet, and appropriate exercise. Begin, or arrange for, appropriate patient and family teaching as necessary.

Patient Teaching
• Learn the signs and symptoms of hypoglycemia.
• Learn home blood glucose monitoring technique.
• Do not to take any over-the-counter drug without consulting the health care provider (because of the possibility of interactions).
• Insulin may be required during times of stress, surgery, or severe infection (because blood glucose levels will be elevated).
• Take with food to avoid gastric irritation.
• Use orange juice, sugared drinks, or hard candy for hypoglycemic reactions; follow as soon as possible with more complex carbohydrates (e.g., skim milk, crackers, cheese).
• To work optimally, acarbose (Precose) and miglitol (Glyset) should be taken with the first bite of each meal.

GLUCOSE-ELEVATING DRUGS

Drugs that act to raise blood glucose levels are also known as *insulin antagonists* or *hyperglycemics.* The two drugs in this category used to treat hypoglycemia are glucagon and diazoxide (Proglycem).

Glucagon

Actions and Uses

Glucagon is the pancreatic hormone secreted by the alpha cells in the islets of Langerhans. In the liver, glucagon stimulates glycogenolysis (breakdown of glycogen to glucose) and gluconeogenesis (conversion of fat to glucose), thereby releasing glucose into the blood. Additional actions include increased heart rate and myocardial contractility, and improved atrioventricular conduction.

Glucagon is the treatment of choice for insulin-induced hypoglycemia when the person is semiconscious or unconscious and unable to ingest oral forms of sugar. It may be administered subcutaneously, intramuscularly, and intravenously. It has now been synthesized in the laboratory and is available in tablet form for use when a quick response to hypoglycemia is indicated. Recently, intravenous glucagon has been used to treat the cardiotoxic effects of beta-adrenergic blockers, quinidine, and tricyclic antidepressants.

Interactions and Contraindications

Glucagon is incompatible with sodium chloride solution or additive (it will form a precipitate).

Use cautiously in persons with pheochromocytoma (a rare, potentially fatal adrenal medullary tumor) or those who may not have adequate liver glycogen stores.

Nursing Implications

Glucagon should be considered incompatible in a syringe with any other drug. Use only special diluent supplied by manufacturer for reconstitution; flush intravenous lines with 5% dextrose instead of sodium chloride. Patient usually begins to recover from diabetic coma within 5 to 20 minutes after subcutaneous or intramuscular injection. Give oral carbohydrates as soon as possible after patient awakens. After recovery, headache, nausea, and weakness may persist. Teach family members how to administer subcutaneous or intramuscular glucagon.

Diazoxide

Actions and Uses

Diazoxide (Proglycem) is chemically related to the thiazide diuretics. The oral form increases blood glucose by inhibiting insulin release from the beta cells and stimulating release of epinephrine from the adrenal medulla. The intravenous form of the drug has a vasodilating effect which reduces peripheral vascular resistance and lowers blood pressure.

The oral form of the drug is used to treat chronic hypoglycemia due to hyperinsulinism caused by pancreatic cancers. It is not indicated for treatment of acute hypoglycemic reactions due to diabetes mellitus. The intravenous form of the drug may be used to treat malignant hypertension (a specific form of hypertensive crisis with a sudden onset; diastolic blood pressure exceeds 140 mm Hg).

Side and Adverse Effects

Oral diazoxide may cause hyperglycemia and glycosuria in diabetic or prediabetic persons. An increase in hair growth on the back and shoulders may occur, especially in women and children, but will disappear when the drug is discontinued.

Interactions and Contraindications

Sulfonylureas will antagonize the effects of oral diazoxide. Concurrent use with thiazide diuretics and phenytoin (Dilantin) may intensify hyperglycemia, and oral diazoxide may increase phenytoin metabolism, causing loss of seizure control.

Oral diazoxide should not be used for diabetic hypoglycemia, for persons with impaired renal function, cerebral or cardiac circulation, or by patients taking corticosteroids or estrogen-progesterone combinations.

Nursing Implications

Monitor blood glucose and serum electrolytes periodically (hypokalemia potentiates hyperglycemic effect). Although oral diazoxide usually does not produce marked changes in blood pressure, periodic blood pressure checks should be done.

Instruct patients to report palpitations, dizziness, fainting, or severe headache.

REVIEW QUESTIONS: UNIT 13

1. A patient with multiple sclerosis is receiving corticotropin as part of her drug therapy. She asks the nurse why the health care provider recommended use of a salt substitute. The nurse's best response is:
   A. "Patients with multiple sclerosis cannot tolerate regular salt."
   B. "If regular salt is used with corticotropin, the risk of ulcer development is increased."
   C. "Use of salt substitutes, which contain potassium instead of sodium, helps prevent edema and low potassium levels."
   D. "Your health care provider can best explain that to you."

2. Why is it important to teach patients taking vasopressin to avoid using over-the-counter cold preparations without consulting the health care provider?

3. A child is taking somatropin as part of therapy for pituitary dwarfism. His parents tell the nurse that he has been complaining of hip pain for a week. The nurse's best response is:
   A. "This pain just means he is starting to grow."
   B. "You need to call your health care provider. The pain could indicate a problem with his hip or upper leg."
   C. "Children often complain of pain. This is nothing to worry about."
   D. "He probably just strained a muscle while playing. The pain should go away soon."

4. A patient tells the nurse that she has been taking her Synthroid every day for 7 days. She asks why she has not seen an improvement in her condition. The nurse's best response is:
   A. "It may take 1 to 2 weeks for you to notice a therapeutic effect from the drug."
   B. "Your drug dose is probably too low."
   C. "Your body must be resistant to this drug."
   D. "Your health care provider should be notified right away."

5. Teaching for patients taking iodine solutions to treat hyperthyroidism should include information that:

   A. there are no special precautions related to this drug.

   B. the drug should be diluted and taken through a straw to prevent tooth discoloration.

   C. the drug must be taken on an empty stomach to produce its effects.

   D. iodized table salt and shellfish are perfectly safe to eat.

6. Thiazide diuretics may be contraindicated for persons taking calcitriol because of the potential for:

   A. hypocalcemia.

   B. hyponatremia.

   C. hypervitaminosis D.

   D. hypercalcemia.

7. Patients taking calcitonin should contact the health care provider before taking which over-the-counter drugs?

   A. Cough syrups

   B. Cold preparations

   C. Antacids

   D. Analgesics

8. A patient taking hydrocortisone for treatment of rheumatoid arthritis tells the nurse that she is tired of having a "moon face" and "hump" on the back of her neck and she is going to stop taking the drug. The nurse's best response is:

   A. "Increase the dose of hydrocortisone to promote fat metabolism, which will decrease the excess fat deposits."

   B. "Continue taking the medication, as sudden changes in your drug therapy can cause serious adverse reactions."

   C. "Stop taking the drug, as these are symptoms of a steroid allergy."

   D. "Discontinue the drug immediately as these are symptoms of overstimulation of the adrenal glands."

9. A patient has been prescribed cortisone for asthma. He tells the nurse that he is also taking furosemide (Lasix) for hypertension. Teaching for this patient should include which of the following points?

   A. These two drugs cannot be taken together because of their antagonistic effects.

   B. There is a greater risk for sodium loss with this combination of drugs.

   C. Be sure to add potassium-rich foods to your diet or take a potassium supplement.

   D. There are no special precautions to be aware of if these two drugs are taken together.

10. Aldosterone, the primary endogenous mineralocorticoid, is a potent hormone that acts in the kidney to produce which of the following effects?

    A. Sodium and potassium retention

    B. Sodium and potassium excretion

    C. Sodium excretion and potassium retention

    D. Sodium retention and potassium excretion

11. The practice of giving the total 48-hour dose of a corticosteroid in a single dose every other day is called alternate-day therapy. Which statement contains INCORRECT information about alternate-day therapy?

    A. All corticosteroids can be scheduled using alternate-day therapy.

    B. Alternate-day therapy may decrease the incidence of Cushing's syndrome.

    C. Alternate-day therapy may delay or lessen the development of chronic endocrine suppression.

    D. Alternate-day therapy would be an appropriate initial step in a program of corticosteroid withdrawal.

12. An insulin-dependent diabetic patient asks why he received regular insulin with his usual NPH insulin following his surgery. The nurse's response should be:

    A. "Surgery increases tissue metabolism and the need for insulin."

    B. "Insulin production is decreased even further with the stress of surgery."

    C. "Physiologic stress increases serum glucose and the need for insulin."

    D. "An increased insulin dose is necessary to prevent hypokalemia."

13. A 13-year-old boy has just been diagnosed with type 1, or insulin-dependent, diabetes mellitus (IDDM). He asks why he must inject his insulin instead of taking an insulin pill. The nurse's best response is:

    A. "Insulin levels are often too high if the drug is given orally, because its metabolism and absorption are unpredictable."

    B. "Oral preparations of insulin deteriorate quickly and cannot be stored."

    C. "Injection of insulin causes the body to begin producing its own insulin, so that you won't always have to take the drug."

    D. "Insulin cannot be given orally because it is destroyed by the enzymes in the gastrointestinal tract before it can be absorbed."

14. A patient is to begin therapy with an oral hypoglycemic agent from the sulfonylurea class. As part of the assessment prior to starting the medication, it is important to obtain a drug allergy history. The patient should not take this drug if he is allergic to:

    A. insulin.

    B. sulfonamides.

    C. aminoglycosides.

    D. aspirin.

15. Oral hypoglycemic drugs are not effective as the only treatment for IDDM because:

    A. persons with IDDM have little or no endogenous insulin to be released.

    B. persons with IDDM are generally allergic to these drugs.

    C. paradoxical hyperglycemia is likely to occur.

    D. oral hypoglycemic drugs counteract the effects of other drugs that the patient may be taking.

DRUGS THAT AFFECT THE REPRODUCTIVE SYSTEM

OBJECTIVES

1. Discuss the normal hormonal feedback system that regulates the male and female reproductive systems.

2. List disorders that are treated with estrogens and progestins.

3. Identify the various estrogen and progestin drugs, their actions, uses, side effects, contraindications, and interactions used in the treatment of disorders of the male and female reproductive systems.

4. Discuss nursing actions and patient teaching associated with estrogen and progestin therapy.

5. Discuss therapeutic and adverse effects of oral contraceptives.

6. Identify the androgens and antiandrogens, their actions, uses, side effects, contraindications, and interactions that affect the male and female reproductive systems.

7. Discuss nursing actions and patient teaching related to the use of male reproductive agents.

This unit includes discussion of drugs that affect both male and female reproductive systems. Some of these drugs are classified as hormones and some are not.

The gonads, or sex glands, of the female are the ovaries and those of the male are the testes. Activity of the gonads is regulated by the gonadotropins follicle-stimulating hormone (FSH) and luteinizing hormone (LH) from the anterior pituitary gland. The same gonadotropins are produced by males and females, but they act on different organs to produce different sex hormones. Luteinizing hormone controls the female hormone progesterone and male hormone testosterone, whereas follicle-stimulating hormone controls estrogen and ovum release in females and spermatogenesis in males.

CHAPTER 45

ESTROGENS, PROGESTINS, AND ORAL CONTRACEPTIVES

*T*he female reproductive system consists of the ovaries, fallopian tubes, uterus, vagina, and, externally, the vulva. The feedback system (see Unit 13) regulates the female hormonal cycle. The hypothalamus secretes gonadotropin-stimulating hormone (GSH), which stimulates the pituitary gland, causing a rise in the production of follicle-stimulating hormone (FSH). This increase in FSH causes estrogen levels to rise and the ovum to mature. On or about day 10 of the monthly cycle, estrogen levels peak, inhibiting FSH release. Estrogen levels begin to drop by day 14, stimulating release of luteinizing hormone (LH). LH causes progesterone levels to rise in preparing the endometrium for implantation of the fertilized egg. In the absence of fertilization, about day 23, high progesterone levels inhibit LH release. The cycle starts again in 28 to 30 days (Figure 45–1).

FIGURE 45–1

Hormonal Activity During Ovulation

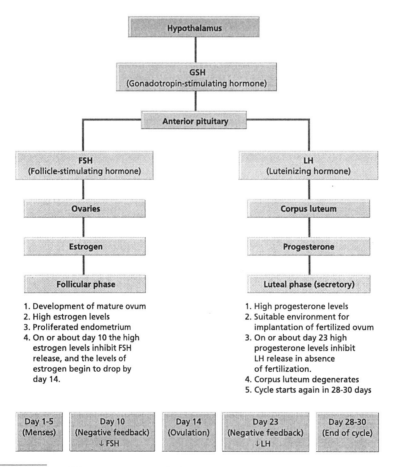

From Lilley & Aucker (1998). *Pharmacology and the Nursing Process*, 2nd ed. St. Louis: Mosby, p.432.

ESTROGENS

There are three major naturally occurring estrogens: estradiol, estrone, and estriol. They are all synthesized from cholesterol in the ovaries, have the same basic structure as steroids, and are sometimes called *steroid hormones*. Estradiol, the most potent of these, is metabolized to estrone, which is half as potent. Estrone is further metabolized to estriol, which is the least potent. The synthetic forms of estrogen are either steroidal or nonsteroidal. The nonsteroidal forms do not have the basic steroid structure but can still act on estrogenic tissues in the body. The synthetic agents are most often prescribed, as the natural estrogen extracts are generally inactive in oral form.

Some of the more commonly used synthetic steroidal estrogens include conjugated estrogens (Premarin), estradiol (Estrace), estradiol valerate (Delestrogen), ethinyl estradiol (Estinyl), estropipate (Ogen), esterified estrogens (Estratab), and estrone (Gynogen). Synthetic nonsteroidal preparations include chlorotrianisene (Tace), diethylstilbestrol (DES), diethylstilbestrol diphosphate (Stilphostrol), and dienestrol (Ortho Dienestrol Vaginal).

Routes of administration are drug-dependent and include oral, intramuscular, intravenous, topical, intravaginal, and transdermal.

Actions and Uses

The primary action of estrogen is development and maintenance of the female reproductive system. Secondary actions involve the development of secondary sex characteristics (feminization): onset of menses, breast development, higher pitched voice, broader hips, and increased subcutaneous fat. Estrogen also has several effects on other body functions: calcium and phosphorus are retained and used in bone formation; the kidneys retain more sodium and water; glucose, cholesterol, and lipids are decreased; and coagulation factors are increased.

There are a number of therapeutic uses for estrogens in both men and women. In women, in addition to use as oral contraceptives, some indications for estrogen therapy are hypogonadism, to relieve symptoms of menopause (surgical or natural), to prevent postmenopausal osteoporosis, and to treat atrophic vaginitis (shrinkage of vagina and/or urethra). Estrogens are also used to treat dysmenorrhea (painful menstruation), dysfunctional uterine bleeding, and endometriosis. They are sometimes used as palliative treatment of advanced, inoperable breast cancer (*palliative treatment* may improve quality of life, but may shorten or have no effect on length of life). Use of estrogen-containing drugs for the prevention of postpartum breast engorgement or to suppress lactation is no longer recommended because the required higher doses increase the risk of thrombophlebitis.

In men, estrogens may be used therapeutically to treat inoperable prostatic or testicular cancer, to slow tumor growth (therapeutic treatments are expected to increase both quality and length of life).

Side and Adverse Effects

Because of the possibility of hypertension and increased coagulability of the blood, the most serious adverse effects of the estrogens involve thromboembolic events. These include thrombophlebitis, cerebrovascular accident (CVA), and myocardial infarction (MI), especially in women over age 30 who smoke cigarettes. Other side and adverse effects may include amenorrhea, dysmenorrhea, breakthrough bleeding, changes in menstrual flow, enlarged uterine fibroids, and infertility. Breast changes may include tenderness, enlargement, and sometimes secretions. Gastrointestinal side effects may be nausea, abdominal cramps, bloating, and jaundice. Jaundice may be a result of altered liver function or a symptom of blockage of the biliary tree (estrogen increases concentration of cholesterol in bile, which increases the risk of the formation of gallstones). Side effects involving the skin may include *chloasma* (hyperpigmentation of face known as the "mask of pregnancy") and *linea negra* (pigmented line down center of abdomen from sternum to pubis), photosensitivity, and dermatitis. High estrogen doses may produce psychiatric depression, which can progress to psychosis, particularly if there is a history of depressive illness.

Adverse effects occur in men because estrogens antagonize androgenic hormones. This causes symptoms of feminization to occur: higher pitched voice, gynecomastia (breast enlargement), loss of facial and body hair, increased fat around hips, testicular and penile atrophy, and impotence. Decreased libido (sexual drive) and depression may occur.

Sodium and water retention, with increased levels of renin and angiotensin, may cause edema, hypertension, and weight gain in both men and women. Edema may also aggravate other conditions such as asthma, heart disease, renal disease, migraine headaches, or epilepsy.

Interactions and Contraindications

Estrogens can decrease the effect of oral anticoagulants and may inhibit the metabolism of phenytoin, resulting in phenytoin toxicity. Concurrent use with rifampin and certain antibiotics may decrease estrogenic effects. Toxic responses may occur with use with tricyclic antidepressants. Estrogens may increase the steroid effects of corticosteroids. Smoking decreases estrogenic effects and increases the risk of thrombophlebitis.

Estrogens are contraindicated in patients with breast cancer (due to stimulation of cancer cell growth), except as palliative treatment in cases of metastatic disease. It is also contraindicated in the following conditions: active or history of thrombophlebitis or thromboembolic disease (except when being used in the palliative treatment of breast or prostatic cancer), abnormal genital bleeding, and known or suspected pregnancy. Cautious use is warranted in breastfeeding women because estrogens decrease the quantity and quality of milk and may be excreted in the milk (low-dose birth control pills may be prescribed after lactation is well established). Use in prepubescent females must be carefully evaluated because of premature closure of epiphyses. Caution should be used in patients for whom fluid retention may be a problem, who have renal insufficiency or metabolic bone diseases associated with hypercalcemia.

Nursing Actions

Obtain baseline vital signs, weight, relevant symptoms, and menstrual history. Determine whether the patient has contraindications to use of estrogens or has pre-existing conditions for which cautious use is indicated. Inject intramuscular forms deep in large muscle masses and rotate injection sites. Even if symptoms of feminization and impotence occur in men who are taking estrogens as part of the treatment of reproductive malignancies, the drug will not be stopped unless the patient requests it. The symptoms will disappear when the drug is discontinued. If the patient is also taking phenytoin, be alert for signs of phenytoin toxicity (nystagmus, sedation, and lethargy). Communicate to the health care provider all medications the patient is taking. Because estrogens are often prescribed on a cyclic regimen, verify that patients are taking medications exactly as ordered. If the drug is prescribed for prepubescent girls, radiographs may be ordered periodically to monitor bone growth and for early epiphyseal plate closure.

Patient Teaching
• Menstrual changes, dysmenorrhea, amenorrhea, breakthrough bleeding, and breast changes may disappear after a few weeks or months of therapy. These symptoms should be reported to the health care provider but are not necessarily reasons to stop the drug. • Stop smoking, or decrease the number of cigarettes smoked. • Report signs and symptoms of adverse effects to the health care provider. • Take the oral drug with meals to decrease gastrointestinal upset. • Use sunblock and/or cover exposed areas of the body. • Perform monthly breast self-examinations and schedule annual pelvic and breast examinations with the health care provider. • Report suspected pregnancy immediately. Consult the health care provider if breastfeeding. • Discuss signs of depression or mood changes with the health care provider as soon as noted.

• Avoid the use of estrogen vaginal creams prior to intercourse; they can be absorbed through the skin of the penis and cause reduced potency and some degree of feminization. Use of condoms and application of cream after intercourse will prevent these effects.
• Take the medication exactly as prescribed.

ANTIESTROGENS

Actions and Uses

The primary drug in this category, tamoxifen citrate (Nolvadex), has potent antiestrogenic effects. It acts to block estrogen receptor sites in tissues high in estrogen receptors, such as breast tissue, which deprives estrogen-dependent tumors of estrogen. It may also stimulate the production of a substance known as transforming growth factor-beta, which inhibits the growth of most breast cancers. There have also been other positive consequences of tamoxifen treatment: increased bone mineral density in postmenopausal women and reduction in cholesterol levels.

Tamoxifen is a primary drug for treating advanced breast cancer in postmenopausal women. In premenopausal women with metastatic breast cancer, tamoxifen is an alternative to oophorectomy and radiation. It is also used as adjunct therapy for women with breast cancer following mastectomy, axillary node dissection, and breast irradiation. Tamoxifen is presently under investigation as a potential preventive agent for breast cancer in high-risk women. The drug is given orally.

Side and Adverse Effects

Because tamoxifen blocks the effects of estrogen, menopausal symptoms will occur: headaches, menstrual changes, vaginal bleeding, growth of facial and body hair, thinning of hair on head, hot flashes, and decreased libido. Photosensitivity, rashes, and dryness of skin may occur, as well as nausea, vomiting, anorexia, edema, blurred vision, bone pain, thrombocytopenia, and leukopenia. Some potentially fatal liver abnormalities have occurred, including fatty liver, hepatic necrosis, and hepatitis. Liver enzymes may be elevated. The adverse effect of most concern is development of endometrial cancer, which has been associated with long-term use of tamoxifen.

Interactions and Contraindications

Concurrent use of tamoxifen and oral anticoagulants increases the risk of bleeding. Hypercalcemia and elevated thyroxin levels have been reported.

Cautious use is indicated in persons with cataracts or other visual disturbances, women who are lactating, and those with leukopenia or thrombocytopenia.

Pregnancy Category D.

Nursing Actions

Review medical history and prescription and over-the-counter drug use for possible contraindication to drug therapy. Obtain baseline menstrual history and weight. Review baseline liver function tests, white blood cell and platelet counts. Report abnormal findings to the health care provider. Administer analgesics as needed for bone pain.

Patient Teaching

- Use sunblocks and protective clothing and avoid direct sunlight when possible.
- Take the medications with food to minimize gastrointestinal upset.
- Avoid the addition of salt to foods and limit ingestion of high-sodium foods to minimize edema.
- Bone pain usually indicates that tamoxifen will produce a good response. Take analgesics as necessary.
- Avoid persons with colds, flu, or other contagious diseases.
- Maintain good nutrition and hygiene.
- Bruising may occur even with mild trauma.
- Avoid pregnancy during tamoxifen therapy; use condoms, diaphragms, and/or spermicidal preparations on all occasions of intercourse.
- Report occurrence of jaundice, dark urine, anorexia, and right upper quadrant pain.

PROGESTINS

Progestational drugs consist of both natural and synthetic agents. Progesterone is the primary natural hormone. Because oral forms of progesterone are relatively inactive and parenterally administered progesterone causes local reactions and pain, synthetic derivatives were developed that are effective orally and are also more potent. These are known as *progestins*, and the more commonly used ones are medroxyprogesterone (Provera, Depo-Provera, Cycrin), hydroxyprogesterone (Gesterol L.A.), norethindrone (Norlutin), norgestrel (Ovral), megestrol (Megace), progesterone (Progestasert), and norethindrone acetate (Micronor).

Actions and Uses

The primary action of progesterone is to induce favorable conditions for fetal growth and development and to preserve the pregnancy. It is necessary for placental development, for increasing uterine muscle fibers and mammary gland maturation during pregnancy, as well as for inhibition of uterine contractions during pregnancy. Progesterone also inhibits anterior pituitary production of gonadotropic hormones, thus preventing development of other ova and ovulation.

Other changes produced by progesterone include decreasing endometrial tissue proliferation, increasing vaginal mucosa thickness, increasing basal body temperature, and producing withdrawal bleeding in the presence of estrogen. Exogenous progestins produce all the same responses as those of natural progesterone.

Progestins are useful in the treatment of primary and secondary amenorrhea; uterine bleeding caused by hormone imbalance, fibroids or uterine cancer; as palliative or adjunct treatment of certain other cancers and endometriosis; alone or in combination with estrogen to prevent contraception; and to alleviate the symptoms of premenstrual syndrome (PMS). An unlabeled use of progesterone is in the treatment of preterm labor in the late stages of pregnancy. (Unlabeled uses do not appear on a drug label or in the manufacturer's literature; they are clinical indications other than those for which the drug was primarily approved, but which now have accepted use supported by medical literature). Although progesterone has been used in the first trimester of pregnancy to prevent repeated abortion or to treat threatened abortion, there is no evidence that this effective. However, there is evidence that progesterone may be harmful to the fetus in the first 4 months, so this use is not recommended.

Progestins may also be used in certain cases of infertility. Because of the negative feedback system, exogenous administration of progesterone will cause the anterior pituitary gland to decrease production of follicle-stimulating hormone (FSH) and luteinizing hormone (LH), which prevents the ovary from developing and releasing ova. The theory is that when the progesterone is stopped, the anterior pituitary will rebound with a surge of FSH, which will stimulate the development of ova, and ovulation will follow.

Medroxyprogesterone (Cycrin, Provera) is the most commonly used progestin in the treatment of hormone imbalance, primary or secondary amenorrhea, and functional uterine bleeding. Norethindrone (Norlutin) and norgestrel (Ovral) are primarily used alone or in combination with estrogens as oral contraceptives. Megestrol (Megace) is most commonly used to treat endometrial and breast cancers, as well as weight loss in patients with acquired immunodeficiency syndrome (AIDS).

Side and Adverse Effects

The more common side effects of progestins include nausea, vomiting, menstrual changes, breakthrough bleeding, breast tenderness and secretions, acne, rashes, and photosensitivity. Sodium retention may cause edema, weight gain, hypertension, and headaches. Mental depression, insomnia, and decreased libido may occur. The most serious adverse effects of progestins include liver dysfunction, thrombophlebitis, pulmonary embolism, and sudden partial or complete loss of eyesight.

Interactions and Contraindications

Hyperglycemia may occur, requiring alterations in dosages of antidiabetic drugs. Concurrent use of medroxyprogesterone (Cycrin, Provera) or norethindrone (Norlutin) and aminoglutethimide (Cytadren) or rifampin (Rifidin) decreases the effects of the progestin.

Progestins are contraindicated in patients with history of liver disease, thrombophlebitis or thromboembolic disorders, undiagnosed vaginal bleeding, or suspected breast cancer. Progestins should not be used during pregnancy, as these drugs are known to cause heart and limb defects as well as masculinization of a female fetus and hypospadias in a male fetus. The effect of progestins on breastfeeding infants is not known. Cautious use is indicated for patients with hypertension, diabetes, congestive heart failure, depression, or a family history of breast or reproductive tract cancer. **Pregnancy Category X.**

Nursing Actions

Obtain baseline blood pressure, weight, relevant symptoms, and menstrual history. Determine use of other prescription and nonprescription drugs. Communicate this information to the health care provider. Check whether the patient has contraindications to the use of progestins or has pre-existing conditions for which cautious use is indicated. Inject intramuscular forms of the drug deep in large muscle masses and rotate injection sites minimize tissue irritation.

Patient Teaching
• Report suspected pregnancy immediately. Consult the health care provider if you are breastfeeding.
• Take oral progestins with meals to decrease gastrointestinal upset.
• Perform monthly breast self-examinations and schedule annual pelvic and breast examinations with the health care provider.
• Use sunblock and/or cover exposed areas of the body.
• Report chest pain, leg pain, blurred vision, headache, neck stiffness and pain, edema, yellow discoloration of skin or sclera, clay-colored stools, and vaginal bleeding.
• Discuss signs of depression or mood changes with the health care provider as soon as they are noted.

CONTRACEPTIVE DRUGS

Oral Contraceptives

Oral contraceptives are the most effective nonsurgical form of birth control currently available. They are closely related to estrogen and progestin because they contain varying amounts of these drugs in combination. A few oral contraceptives contain progestins only. There are three types of combination oral contraceptives:

- **Monophasic**: the dose of estrogen and progestin remains the same throughout the cycle.
- **Biphasic**: the amount of estrogen remains the same, but the amount of progestin rises in the second half of the cycle.
- **Triphasic**: estrogen amounts remain the same or may vary throughout the cycle, while the progestin varies throughout the cycle. This form more closely follows the normal hormonal levels of the monthly cycle.

Advantages of oral contraceptives are their effectiveness (98–99% if taken as directed) and convenience for those who wish to have spontaneous intercourse without having to stop to insert or apply protective devices. Primary disadvantages include placing the burden of contraception solely on the woman, the significant number of adverse effects and risks involved, and no protection against sexually transmitted diseases.

Action and Uses

Combination oral contraceptives inhibit ovulation by suppressing the gonadotropins FSH and LH. They also alter the quality of cervical and vaginal mucus (inhibits sperm penetration) and change the characteristics of the endometrium (reducing the likelihood of implantation). The mechanism of action of the progestin-only contraceptives is not clearly understood. They alter cervical mucus and exert a progestational effect on the endometrium, which apparently produces cellular changes that are hostile to implantation of a fertilized ovum. In some women, progestins also prevent ovulation.

In addition to their use in preventing pregnancy, oral contraceptives are used to regulate menses in women who have no pattern to their menstrual cycle, and to treat hypermenorrhea (excessive bleeding with menstruation) and endometriosis.

Side and Adverse Effects

Side and adverse effects of oral contraceptives are all of those associated with estrogens and progestins. Some of the less serious side effects common to combination oral contraceptive use are nausea, vomiting, edema, uterine cramping, breakthrough bleeding, breast tenderness, and rashes.

Interactions and Contraindications

Many drugs decrease the effectiveness of oral contraceptives. The more clinically relevant categories include barbiturates, certain antibiotics, griseofulvin, isoniazid, and rifampin. Drugs that may be less effective themselves when taken concurrently with oral contraceptives include anticonvulsants, beta-blockers, guanethidine, hypnotics, hypoglycemic drugs, oral anticoagulants, theophylline, tricyclic antidepressants, and vitamins.

The use of oral contraceptives is contraindicated for women with known or suspected breast cancer, pregnancy, history of or current thrombophlebitis or thromboembolic disorders, undiagnosed abnormal vaginal bleeding, cerebrovascular or heart disease, and benign or malignant estrogen-dependent liver tumors. **Pregnancy Category X.**

Nursing Actions

Review medical history and prescription and over-the-counter drug use for possible contraindications or interactions associated with oral contraceptives. Determine menstrual history for regularity of periods, duration of flow, and occurrence of pain. Assess for family and patient history of potential contraindications. Non-breastfeeding mothers may begin using oral contraceptives 4 to 6 weeks after delivery even if they have not yet resumed their menstrual periods. Breastfeeding mothers may use low-dose oral contraceptives once lactation is well established (6 to 8 weeks after delivery). However, the effect of these hormones on breastfeeding infants is not known.

Patient Teaching

- Use an additional form of birth control during the first month of therapy, until the next period.
- Because manufacturers often package oral contraceptives in cases with flowers, birds, butterflies, and so on, it is very important to keep them in a place safe from children, who may think they are candy.
- Women with diabetes need to carefully monitor fingerstick blood glucose levels and be alert for symptoms of hyperglycemia.
- Fluid retention may change the shape of the eyeball, causing contact lenses to fit improperly. Obtain annual eye examinations and notify the care provider of oral contraceptive use.
- Notify health care providers and dentists of oral contraceptive use.
- If doses of oral contraceptives are missed, the likelihood of conception is increased. If one pill is missed, two may be taken the next day. If more than two or three pills are missed, and

---

there is a chance that pregnancy could occur, use another form of birth control in addition to the remaining oral contraceptives.
- If several pills are missed in one cycle, and it is possible that a pregnancy could have occurred, stop the oral contraceptive, use another form of contraception, and notify the health care provider as soon as possible.
- Notify the health care provider of the occurrence of side effects.
- Stop smoking, or decrease number of cigarettes smoked.

Medroxyprogesterone (Depo-Provera)

The intramuscular form of the progestin medroxyprogesterone (Depo-Provera) is used as a longer acting but not permanent form of contraception. The action of this hormone provides 3 months of protection against pregnancy. Advantages include long-term reversible contraception and spontaneous sexual activity. Disadvantages are uncomfortable injections, the necessity to keep appointments for subsequent injections exactly on schedule to maintain contraception, and lack of protection against sexually transmitted diseases. If the injections are received at 3-month intervals, contraception effectiveness is 99%.

Side and adverse effects, interactions, and contraindications are the same as those of progestins.

Nursing Actions

Prior to use, assess the patient for pregnancy or history of breast cancer. Patients who have a history of diabetes mellitus, hypertension, liver or kidney disease, thrombophlebitis, or heart disease may need to be monitored more closely for complications of these diseases. Assess injection sites for redness and irritation. If the patient is breastfeeding, it is recommended that the injection be given 6 weeks after delivery; however, since there is no evidence of harm to the infant from the very small amount of progestin found in breast milk, some health care providers may order medroxyprogesterone prior to 6 weeks postpartum.

Patient Teaching

- Keep scheduled appointments for repeat injections exactly as prescribed.
- Menstrual bleeding may decrease, become irregular, or stop altogether. When the injections are discontinued, the menstrual cycle usually returns to normal within a few months.

(Continued on p. 218)

> - Weight-bearing exercises and adequate calcium will help prevent mineral loss from bone. Report bone and muscle pain to the health care provider.
> - If pregnancy is suspected despite the use of medroxyprogesterone, notify the health care provider as soon as possible.

> - The bandage may be removed after about 3 days. Observe the site for irritation.
> - Report bone or muscle pain, abdominal pain, or unusual vaginal or breast discharge.
> - Some periods may be missed. Notify the health care provider if pregnancy is possible.
> - Breastfeeding women may have Norplant inserted 6 weeks after delivery without apparent effects on the newborn.

Levonorgestrel (Norplant)

The Norplant system consists of six thin Silastic capsules containing the progestin levonorgestrel. With the use of local anesthesia, they are implanted under the skin of the inner aspect of the woman's upper arm in a fan-shaped pattern.

Action and Uses

Levonorgestrel acts by inhibiting ovulation and thickening cervical mucus, which interferes with sperm motility. The implants release their hormones very slowly, providing 5 years of protection against pregnancy. The implants can be removed at any time to reverse the contraceptive effect, and they may be replaced after 5 years if further contraception is desired. Advantages include long-term reversible contraception without the use of estrogen, and the opportunity for spontaneous sexual activity. Disadvantages are initial high cost, possible irritation or infection of insertion sites, and lack of protection against sexually transmitted diseases. Effectiveness rate is 99%.

Side and Adverse Effects

Side effects include breakthrough and heavy bleeding, increased facial and body hair, weight gain, and increased ovarian cysts. There have been reports of the capsules being visible or traveling up the arm, scarring of insertion sites, and removal difficulties in some women, requiring a minor surgical procedure.

   Interactions and contraindications are the same as those of progestins.

Patient Teaching

- The contraceptive effect begins within 24 hours if implants are inserted during the menstrual period. If inserted at any other time in the cycle, use another form of contraception until the next period.
- Avoid heavy lifting and protect insertion sites from trauma for about 3 days. Some bruising and swelling may occur.

FERTILITY DRUGS

Infertility is defined as the inability to conceive a child after 12 months of unprotected sexual intercourse. *Primary infertility* means the couple have never borne a live infant, *secondary infertility* if they have. Causes of infertility are numerous and may include female factors, male factors, or couple factors. In about 20% of cases, no specific cause can be found. Some of the female disorders are amenable to treatment with fertility drugs. These drugs include clomiphene (Clomid), gonadorelin (Lutrepulse), chorionic gonadotropin (Pregnyl), urofollitropin (Metrodin), and menotropin (Pergonal).

   If the pituitary gland and ovaries are normal, but activation of follicular (and ova) development is absent, clomiphene can stimulate the hypothalamus and pituitary to signal the ovaries to develop ovarian follicles. In cases of dysfunctional pituitary gland, there is an insufficient supply of gonadotropins to properly stimulate the ovary. Menotropins, gonadorelin, chorionic gonadotropin, and urofollitropin may be useful in treating this type of infertility because they stimulate the release of FSH and LH. When primarily LH release must be stimulated, chorionic gonadotropin and gonadorelin are used.

Actions and Uses

Clomiphene stimulates the release of FSH and LH, which results in development and maturation of the ovarian follicle, induces ovulation, and causes development and function of the corpus luteum. *Menotropins* and *urofollitrophins* are pharmacologically similar to FSH and LH, providing the necessary stimulus for ovulation. *Chorionic gonadotropin* and *gonadorelin* have pharmacologic effects that are identical to those of LH, which triggers release of the mature ovum.

   Clomiphene is used to induce ovulation in anovulatory women; it may also be used in the treatment of menstrual abnormalities, gynecomastia, and fibrocystic breast disease.

   Menotropin is used to induce ovulation in anovulatory women and stimulate spermatogenesis in men. *Gonadotropin* and *gonadorelin* are used in conjunction with menotropin to treat female infertility; they may also be used in males to treat prepubertal cryptorchidism and hypogonadotropic hypogonadism.

Side and Adverse Effects

Side effects include dizziness, headache, tachycardia, nausea, bloating, abdominal pain, constipation, blurred or double vision, photophobia, fatigue, nervousness, and breast pain. Some of the more serious effects are depression, thrombophlebitis, ovarian hyperstimulation with ovarian cyst development and possible rupture, and multiple pregnancy.

Interactions and Contraindications

There are no known significant drug interactions with these drugs.

Contraindications include pregnancy, undiagnosed vaginal bleeding, uterine fibroids, ovarian cysts, mental depression, history of or current liver dysfunction or thromboembolic disease. Clomiphene is contraindicated with pituitary or ovarian failure.

Cautious use is indicated in patients with hypertension, seizure disorders, or diabetes mellitus. **Pregnancy Category X.**

Nursing Implications

Thorough health histories, including sexual and reproductive histories, and complete physical examinations of the couple are necessary prior to treatment. Allow the couple to explore and air their feelings regarding their infertility. Placing blame on one another or their families can be devastating to their relationship. Couples frequently complain of a lack of spontaneity in their lovemaking because their activities are often dictated by the calendar or hormone test; encourage them to use imagination to keep their relationship relaxed and comfortable. Be sure couples understand all instructions regarding the treatment plan and medications (i.e., use, dose, route, timing) to ensure compliance and safe self-administration. Teach the couple to administer intramuscular forms of the drugs.

Patient Teaching

- Methods of natural family planning can be used to determine the time of ovulation to maximize chances of conception.
- Stop the drug and report severe abdominal pain to the health care provider immediately (possible rupture of ovarian cyst).
- Avoid driving or working with hazardous equipment because of potential for dizziness or visual disturbances.
- If pregnancy is suspected, stop the drug immediately and notify the health care provider.
- Report adverse effects to the health care provider.
- Take medication at the same time every day to maintain blood levels.

CHAPTER 46

ANDROGENS AND ANABOLIC STEROIDS

*T*he primary structures of the male reproductive system are the penis, scrotum, and testes. The testes are the male gonads and are a pair of glands located in the scrotum. They have both reproductive (androgenic) and endocrine activity. Channels in the testes, called *seminiferous tubules*, are the site of spermatogenesis, the process by which mature sperm cells are produced.

In the male, the same two gonadotropic hormones are produced by the anterior pituitary as are found in the female. In the male, however, follicle-stimulating hormone (FSH) stimulates the seminiferous tubules to produce sperm. Luteinizing hormone (LH, also known as *interstitial cell-stimulating hormone [ICSH]* in men), stimulates the interstitial cells in the testes to produce testosterone. Beginning at puberty, the hypothalamus begins to secrete gonadotropin-stimulating hormone (GSH), which triggers the anterior pituitary to secrete ICSH, thus causing the testes to increase production of testosterone. When serum testosterone levels are adequate, the anterior pituitary secretes FSH, which stimulates the gonads to produce sperm. This causes the hypothalamus to decrease secretion of GSH, which signals the anterior pituitary to decrease release of ICSH. As serum ICSH levels fall, interstitial cells decrease production of testosterone. When serum testosterone is inadequate, GSH levels are also low and sperm count is decreased. The hypothalamus releases GSH, the anterior pituitary increases secretion of ICSH, testosterone levels rise, and the cycle repeats. Through this negative feedback system, homeostasis of male hormones is maintained.

The male hormones, testosterone and its derivatives, are called *androgens*. For pharmaceutical use, natural forms of testosterone are obtained from bull testes. Synthetic forms of the drug are called *anabolic steroids*. *Anabolism* refers to the building up phase of metabolism, and these agents promote building of new body tissue. Anabolic steroids closely resemble the natural hormone but have much higher anabolic activity. Because of their muscle-building properties, anabolic steroids have great potential for misuse by athletes, especially those for whom larger muscles and greater strength are an advantage. There may be serious consequences to the misuse of anabolic steroids. For this reason, the U.S. Drug Enforcement Administration has classified anabolic steroids as controlled (Schedule III) substances.

This classification means that misuse of these drugs can lead to physical or psychological dependence.

The natural androgens include testosterone (Delatestryl), testosterone cypionate (Depo-Testosterone), testosterone enanthate (Andro L.A.), testosterone propionate (Testex), and testosterone transdermal (Androderm, Testoderm). These drugs must all be given subcutaneously, intramuscularly, or transdermally, as oral testosterone is metabolized and destroyed by the liver before it reaches the circulation. Synthetic androgens, which may be given orally or buccally, include danazol (Danocrine), methyltestosterone (Android, Testred), fluoxymesterone (Halotestin), nandrolone phenpropionate (Durabolin), and stanozolol (Winstrol).

ANDROGENS

Actions and Uses

The primary action of androgens is development and maintenance of the male reproductive system, including sperm production. Additional actions are development of secondary sex characteristics (masculinization): male hair distribution (facial, pubic, chest, and axillae), laryngeal enlargement and thickening of vocal cords (deepening of voice), and defining body musculature and fat distribution.

In addition to its androgenic activity, testosterone is also involved in development of muscle tissue and bone, inhibition of protein catabolism (the breaking down phase of metabolism), and retention of nitrogen, phosphorus, potassium, and sodium. Testosterone also appears to have an erythropoietic effect, which stimulates production of red blood cells.

The primary use for androgens, as with all endocrine drugs, is replacement therapy. However, there are a number of therapeutic uses for androgens in both men and women. In men, some of these uses are primary or secondary hypogonadism, postpubertal cryptorchidism, benign prostatic hypertrophy, and osteoporosis. Androgens may be useful as palliative treatment of male reproductive tumors (*palliative treatment* means that quality of life may be improved, but expected life span may be lessened). Although the tumor may grow faster in the presence of androgens, their ability to increase body mass and strength as well as promoting a feeling of well-being may contribute to better quality of life for persons with this terminal illness. For both men and women, androgens are used to reverse the catabolic effects of long-term corticosteroid therapy, and, because of their ability to stimulate production of red blood cells, they may be used to treat aplastic anemia or anemia associated with chronic renal failure. Inadequate penile development occasionally occurs in neonates. Intramuscular or topical application of low-dose testosterone for no longer than 3 months may promote penile growth. If necessary, treatment may be repeated later in childhood. The primary use of androgens in children is for boys with hypogonadism (gonadal deficiency).

In women, androgens may be indicated for endometriosis or fibrocystic breast disease. Metastatic or inoperable breast tumors may respond to androgen therapy. Androgens suppress or override the effects of estrogen in estrogen-dependent tumors, causing them to grow more slowly or even atrophy.

Side and Adverse Effects

Adverse reactions include nausea, vomiting, diarrhea, hypoglycemia, pruritus, jaundice, edema, and decreased libido (sexual drive). Serum sodium, calcium, potassium, phosphorus, and cholesterol are elevated, while clotting factors are decreased. Men may experience *priapism* (persistent, painful erections) or *gynecomastia* (breast enlargement), which should disappear when the drug dose is decreased. *Impotence* (inability to have or maintain an erection) may occur. Long-term use may increase acne and male-pattern baldness.

Long-term androgen therapy in women will produce symptoms of decreased estrogen: menstrual irregularities or amenorrhea (absence of menses), hot flashes, headache, decreased libido, vaginitis, and sleep disorders. Symptoms of masculinization (or virilism) may appear, such as increased facial and body hair (hirsutism), breast atrophy, deepening voice, clitoral enlargement, and increased muscle mass. With the exception of the voice changes, and possibly the hirsutism, these symptoms are usually reversed when the drug is stopped. Short-term therapy does not usually cause these effects.

Because androgen therapy in children accelerates bone growth, premature closure of epiphyseal plates may occur.

Although rare, very serious adverse effects involving the liver may occur. A life-threatening consequence of long-term androgen therapy may be the development of *peliosis* of the liver, formation of blood-filled cavities. Other serious hepatic effects are cholestatic hepatitis, hepatic tumors, hepatic necrosis, jaundice, and altered liver function.

The hypothalamus is unable to distinguish between endogenous hormones and those taken as medications.

Therefore, administration of these drugs initiates the negative feedback system and signals the anterior pituitary to decrease secretion of ICSH and FSH in men and LH and FSH in women. When the drug is stopped, it may take weeks to months for the male gonads to produce adequate testosterone and sperm and the female gonads to produce estrogen, progesterone, and ova. The result may be infertility and changes in secondary sex characteristics.

Interactions and Contraindications

Androgens can potentiate the effects of oral anticoagulants. Androgens antagonize calcitonin and parathyroid hormone (which may cause calcium loss from bones). Because androgens can cause hypoglycemia, doses of insulin and oral hypoglycemic drugs may need to be reduced. Concurrent use with corticosteroids increases the potential for edema. Barbiturates, phenytoin (Dilantin), and phenylbutazone (Butazolidin) decrease the effects of androgens.

Androgen therapy is contraindicated for persons with nephrosis, hepatic dysfunction, hypercalcemia, pituitary insufficiency, benign prostatic hypertrophy or prostatic cancer, and history of myocardial infarction. Men with breast cancer and women with non-estrogen-dependent breast cancer are not treated with androgens. Cautious use is indicated for persons with hypertension, hypercholesteremia, coronary artery disease, gynecomastia, renal disease, or seizure disorder. With the exception of danazol (Danocrine), which is sometimes listed as pregnancy category C, these drugs are all **Pregnancy Category X**. They are also contraindicated in lactating women.

Nursing Actions

Review medical history and prescription and over-the-counter drug use for possible contraindications to drug therapy. Record baseline height and weight, vital signs, and serum electrolytes. Assess and record urinary patterns, including any difficulty urinating or emptying the bladder. Evaluate renal, liver, and cardiac laboratory tests and report abnormal findings to the health care provider. Administer each dosage form exactly as ordered. Intramuscular forms should be injected deep into the upper outer quadrant of the gluteal muscle. Rotate injection sites to prevent tissue irritation or abscess. For replacement therapy, the transdermal forms are preferable. Testoderm is always applied to scrotal skin; Androderm to body skin and never to scrotal skin. Be sure patients clearly understand the side effects that may occur and the importance of continuing medication despite the occurrence of these effects. Report side effects to the health care provider. Testosterone and related products are Schedule III controlled substances under the Anabolic Steroids Control Act and are accounted for as are narcotic drugs.

Patient Teaching

- Report the occurrence of side effects to the health care provider.
- Do NOT stop taking the medication without consulting the health care provider.
- Do not swallow, chew, or eat the buccal tablet.
- Take fluoxymesterone or danazol with food or milk to minimize gastric irritation.
- Report weight gain of more than 2 pounds in a week and/or persistent headaches (because these are signs of possible hypernatremia).
- If edema occurs, a low sodium diet may be indicated.
- Drink 2000 to 3000 mL of fluid per day to prevent calcium kidney stones.
- Weight-bearing exercises help prevent calcium loss from bones.
- Report changes in sexual function or oligospermia.
- It may take 3 to 4 months to see the therapeutic effects of androgenic agents.
- Children will need x-rays of the wrists and hands every 6 months to evaluate bone growth and check for possible premature closure of epiphyses.
- For women taking danazol (Danocrine):
  — Perform routine breast examinations and report abnormal vaginal bleeding or discharge to the health care provider.
  — Anovulation and amenorrhea may last 2 to 3 months after the drug is discontinued.
  — Symptoms of masculinization will usually disappear after the drug is discontinued.

ANDROGEN INHIBITORS

Actions and Uses

Androgen inhibitors are drugs that block the effects of endogenous androgens. The first group is known as *5-a-reductase inhibitors* because they inhibit the enzyme 5-a-reductase, which plays a key role in the growth and maintenance of the prostate gland. When androgens are secreted in large amounts, the prostate enlarges, causing a condition known as *benign prostatic hypertrophy (BPH),* which may respond to treatment with a 5-a-reductase inhibitor. The only drug in this category is finasteride (Proscar, Propecia). Finasteride works by preventing the conversion of testosterone to 5-a-dihydrotesterone (DHT), which is the primary androgen responsible for prostatic growth.

Although finasteride exerts its effects mainly in the prostate, 5-a-reductase processes in other areas of the body may be affected, such as hair follicles. It has been found that men taking finasteride also experienced hair growth. Stud-

ies are currently underway to evaluate the effect of finasteride on both male- and female-pattern baldness. Results so far have been encouraging.

Another androgen inhibitor is the antiandrogen flutamide (Eulexin), which acts by preventing androgens from binding to their receptors. Leuprolide (Lupron) and goserelin (Zoladex) inhibit the secretion of pituitary gonadotropins, which leads to a decrease in testosterone.

All three of these drug groups may be used to treat BPH, although leuprolide and goserelin are more frequently used in the treatment of prostatic cancer. Leuprolide and goserelin may also be used to treat women with endometriosis or breast cancer. Leuprolide has had some limited use as a male contraceptive.

Side and Adverse Effects

Common side effects of all androgen inhibitors are hot flashes, loss of libido, and impotence, with possible decreased volume of ejaculate. Drug-specific effects include the following:

- *finasteride*: nausea, vomiting, diarrhea, jaundice, hepatitis, and anemia
- *flutamide*: rash, edema, gynecomastia or *galactorrhea* (excessive or spontaneous milk flow not related to lactation; may occur in men or women), depression and anxiety
- *leuprolide*: peripheral and facial edema, cardiac arrhythmias, myocardial infarction, nausea, vomiting, diarrhea, constipation, anorexia, gastrointestinal bleeding, myalgia (muscle pain), bone pain, dysuria, hematuria, fatigue, rash, hair loss, hypoglycemia
- *goserelin*: headache, gynecomastia, nausea, bone pain and bone loss; in women, vaginal dryness and spotting, breakthrough bleeding

Interactions and Contraindications

There are no established drug interactions. Contraindications specific to each drug are as follows:

- *finasteride*: obstructive intestinal and lower urinary tract disorders, ileus, gastrointestinal hemorrhage. Cautious use is indicated for persons with glaucoma. **Pregnancy Category X.**
- *flutamide*: cautious use in cases of severe liver disease. **Pregnancy Category D.**
- *leuprolide*: do not use following orchiectomy or estrogen therapy. **Pregnancy Category X.**
- *goserelin:* cautious use with urinary tract obstruction and in children. Safety and efficacy in children younger that 18 years old are not known. **Pregnancy Category X.**

Nursing Actions/Patient Teaching

The nursing actions should also be implemented in patient teaching. For all of the following drugs:

- Review medical history and use of prescription and over-the-counter drug use for possible contraindications to therapy.
- Record baseline height, weight, vital signs, serum electrolytes, and liver function tests.
- Assess and record urinary patterns, including difficulty urinating or emptying the bladder.

Finasteride (Proscar, Propecia)
- Pregnant women or women who may become pregnant should avoid skin contact with drug (because it may cause birth defects).
- Monitor urine output for decreased output or decreased flow.
- Impotence and decreased libido may occur during therapy.
- Advise the patient to avoid exposing a pregnant woman or one who may become pregnant to his semen.

Flutamide (Eulexin)
- The dose may have to be reduced if gynecomastia or galactorrhea occur.
- Liver function tests will be ordered periodically.
- Report upper abdominal pain, jaundice, dark urine, respiratory problems, sore throat, fever and chills, and facial rash.
- Decreased libido, impotence, and hot flashes may occur during therapy.

Leuprolide (Lupron)
- Teach the patient and family member to administer the intramuscular or subcutaneous form of the drug.
- Check the injection site daily: if redness and swelling occur, report to the health care provider, as this may be a reaction to the preservative, benzyl alcohol.
- Monitor urine output and report hematuria and decreased output.
- Transient bone pain and dysuria may continue for several weeks of continuous therapy.
- Decreased libido, impotence, and hot flashes may occur during therapy.

Goserelin (Zoladex)
- Teach the patient and a family member to administer subcutaneous injection in the upper abdominal wall, exactly according to manufacturer's directions.
- Transient bone pain may occur in first weeks of therapy.
- Decreased libido, impotence, and hot flashes may occur during therapy.

REVIEW QUESTIONS: UNIT 14

1. Patients taking estrogens need to be regularly assessed for:
   A. increased intraocular pressure.
   B. bradycardia.
   C. decreased urinary output.
   D. hypertension.

2. Which of the following instructions should be included in patient teaching for tamoxifen?
   A. Report bone pain to the health care provider immediately and stop taking the drug.
   B. The drug cannot be taken with food.
   C. Use sunblocks and protective clothing when out-of-doors.
   D. Sodium supplements are necessary to prevent hyponatremia.

3. Which of the following statements indicates that the client needs additional teaching about birth control pills?
   A. "I will elevate my legs and take aspirin if I experience leg pain."
   B. "I will monitor my weight and have my blood pressure checked monthly."
   C. "I may gain weight while I am taking these pills."
   D. "I know nausea is common, but it should go away in a few weeks."

4. A 76-year-old male is started on estrogen for metastatic prostate cancer. Which of the following statements leads the nurse to believe he understands the information about his medication?
   A. "I will take my pill on an empty stomach."
   B. "I may experience impotence, but it should go away when the drug is stopped."
   C. "If my breasts become enlarged I will apply ice to them."
   D. "I may have some hair loss from this drug."

5. When androgens are administered to older adult males, which of the following may occur?
   A. Rapid bone growth
   B. Loss of pubic hair
   C. Gynecomastia
   D. Prostatic enlargement

6. If a patient develops symptoms of hypercalcemia during androgen therapy, the nurse needs to instruct him to:

    A. remain in bed to avoid injury.

    B. drink 2000 to 3000 mL/day of fluid to prevent kidney stones.

    C. reduce the dose of the medication.

    D. discontinue the medication.

7. Physical changes that occur with the use of anabolic steroids in women include:

    A. increased distribution of hair on face and body.

    B. increased menstrual flow.

    C. increased endurance.

    D. thinning of skin.

8. Androgen therapy has been ordered for an 11-year-old boy who is experiencing hypogonadism. Which of the following statements made by this boy leads the nurse to believe that he has understood the teaching regarding the medication?

    A. "I may have some temporary visual changes."

    B. "If I experience acne, the drug will need to be stopped."

    C. "I will need to have x-rays every 6 months."

    D. "I can expect to lose weight as a result of taking this drug."

DRUGS THAT AFFECT THE INTEGUMENT

OBJECTIVES

1. List the classifications of drugs used to treat or prevent integumentary disorders.

2. Explain the actions, side and adverse effects, interactions, and contraindications of drugs used for integumentary disorders.

3. Describe nursing assessment data to be collected when patients are treated with specific agents for integumentary disorders.

4. Identify nursing interventions including patient teaching relevant to each major classification of drugs used to treat or prevent integumentary disorders.

CHAPTER 47

DRUGS USED TO TREAT DISORDERS OF THE SKIN AND NAILS

ANATOMY AND PHYSIOLOGY OF THE SKIN

The skin is an organ that covers the body surface. It consists of two layers: the epidermis and the dermis. The outer layer is the *epidermis*, where pigment that determines skin color is produced. The inner layer, the *dermis*, contains connective tissue, sweat glands, nerve endings, and hair roots. Hair, nails, and sebaceous glands are appendages of the skin.

The functions of the skin are protection, regulation of body temperature, secretion, sensation, and synthesis of vitamin D. The skin protects underlying tissues from trauma and pathogens, prevents excess fluid loss from those tissues, and conveys macrophages to areas invaded by infectious agents. Temperature regulation is achieved primarily by altering the diameter of blood vessels and controlling sweating. Dilated superficial blood vessels permit loss of heat from the body surface, whereas constricted vessels limit heat loss. Increased sweating promotes heat loss as water evaporates from skin surfaces. In addition to sweat, the skin secretes sebum, an oily, acidic substance that helps waterproof the skin and deter bacterial growth. Numerous nerve endings in the skin detect touch, pressure, pain, and temperature. The synthesis of vitamin D in the skin is activated by exposure to sunlight. Vitamin D is essential for the utilization of calcium and phosphorus, which are needed for bone development and play a role in neuromuscular activity.

DRUGS USE TO PREVENT OR TREAT SKIN DISORDERS

Skin disorders requiring medical intervention may be local infectious and inflammatory conditions, abnormalities in skin cell reproduction, and infestations by parasites. Classifications of drugs used for skin disorders include anti-infectives, anti-inflammatory agents, keratolytics, anti-acne drugs, antipsoriatics, pediculicides, and scabicides.

Anti-infectives

The skin is susceptible to infections caused by bacteria, viruses, and fungi. For superficial infections, topical anti-infectives are often employed, although systemic therapy is sometimes indicated. Specific anti-infectives are covered in Chapter 5. General points to remember when using topical anti-infectives are the following:

- Assess for allergies before applying; withhold the drug and notify the physician if the patient indicates history of allergy to this drug.
- Use a gloved finger or tongue blade to apply the drug.
- Monitor treated area for increasing redness, itching, or burning, which may indicate allergy or inflammation.
- Do not apply occlusive dressings without an order.

Anti-inflammatory Agents

Anti-inflammatory agents are covered in Chapter 4, but we will briefly discuss them here. The most important topical anti-inflammatory agents are glucocorticoids.

Actions and Uses

Many disorders, local and systemic, cause skin inflammation and itching. Topical glucocorticoids are often effective in suppressing this inflammatory response and providing symptomatic relief.

Side and Adverse Effects

With topical glucocorticoids, local reactions are more likely than systemic reactions. Irritation may occur at the site of application. However, glucocorticoids can be absorbed through the skin, so systemic adverse effects are possible. The risk of systemic effects is greater with prolonged therapy, application over a large area, and use of occlusive dressings. Changes in the skin associated with glucocorticoids include thinning of the skin, stretch marks, purpura (splotchy red-purple spots caused by bleeding into the skin), acne, and excessive hair growth.

Systemic effects of glucocorticoids are potentially serious and are covered in detail in Chapter 43. Among the more important adverse systemic effects are increased risk of infections, bone demineralization, muscle wasting, elevated blood glucose, hypokalemia, and retention of water and sodium.

Interactions and Contraindications

The only important drug interactions occur due to the systemic effects of glucocorticoids. Glucocorticoids decrease the effects of oral hypoglycemics, insulin, diuretics, and potassium supplements. The effects of digitalis may be increased.

Topical corticosteroids should not be applied to areas with poor circulation or infection, including acne and herpes simplex. Other contraindications are rosacea, skin atrophy, and perioral dermatitis.

Nursing Actions

Assess treated area for increased irritation, which may indicate contact dermatitis or allergy. Monitor for systemic effects: fluid retention, weight gain, increased blood pressure, and mood swings, among others. Assess for subtle signs of infection (sore throat, low-grade fever) since the body's response to infection may be suppressed.

Patient Teaching

- Apply after a bath or shower for best effects.
- Do not cover the topical agent with a dressing unless directed by the physician.
- Avoid contact with the eyes.
- Report weight gain, swelling, and sore throat.

Keratolytics

By definition, keratolytics are agents that dissolve keratin, the substance that contributes to the dry, tough characteristic of the outmost skin layer.

TABLE 47–1

Prototype Keratolytics

Prototype	Specific Considerations
salicylic acid	Low concentrations (3–6%) are used to treat dandruff, seborrheic dermatitis, acne, and psoriasis. Higher concentrations are used to treat warts and corns. People with impaired circulation should not apply keratolytics to corns because of risk for tissue injury. Salicylates are absorbed through the skin, so excess use can cause salicylate toxicity characterized by tinnitus and excessively deep respirations.
resorcinol	Used to treat acne, eczema, psoriasis, and seborrheic dermatitis.
sulfur	Used to treat acne, eczema, psoriasis, and seborrheic dermatitis. Do not apply if patient is allergic to sulfur.

Actions and Uses

Keratolytics are used to promote shedding of the outermost layer of the epidermis. Some conditions that may be treated with keratolytics are dandruff, seborrheic dermatitis, acne, and psoriasis. Agents used for their keratolytic action are salicylic acid, resorcinol, sulfur, and benzoyl peroxide. See Table 47–1.

Side and Adverse Effects

For most purposes, low concentrations of keratolytics are used, so serious adverse effects are uncommon. Excessive use may cause dryness and peeling.

Interactions and Contraindications

Applied topically, keratolytics have minimal interactions with other drugs.

People who are allergic to salicylic acid (aspirin) or sulfur should not be treated with agents that contain those substances.

Nursing Actions

Assess the affected skin before and after treatment.

Patient Teaching

- Follow directions in terms of frequency of application and areas to be treated.
- Avoid contact with the eyes or mouth.
- Wash your hands after applying the drugs.
- Notify the physician of excessive dryness, irritation, or tenderness in the treated area.

Anti-acne Drugs

A variety of drugs may be used in the treatment of acne, including isotretinoin (Accutane), tretinoin (Retin-A), benzoyl peroxide (Oxy 10), and topical and systemic antibiotics. Topical or oral forms of erythromycin and tetracycline may be used, in addition to topical clindamycin. See Table 47–2. Antibiotics are covered in Chapter 5.

TABLE 47–2

Anti-acne Agents

Type	Prototype	Specific Considerations
Vitamin A derivative	Isotretinoin (Accutane)	Side and adverse effects: inflammation of the lips and mucous membranes, itching, conjunctivitis, elevated serum triglycerides, nausea, vomiting, abdominal pain, muscle aches, photosensitivity, and bone and joint pain. More serious adverse effects: inflammatory bowel disease, benign intracranial hypertension, fetal deformity.
	tretinoin (Retin-A)	The patient should wash the affected areas with soap and water, pat dry, and wait 30 minutes before applying a thin layer of the drug.
	azelaic acid (Azelex)	Adverse effects less than tretinoin. Can decrease pigmentation in dark-skinned people. Wash and dry skin, then gently massage into affected areas twice daily.
	adapalene (Differin)	Applied at bedtime after washing. May cause excessive dryness
Comedolytic	benzoyl peroxide (Oxy 10)	May be given with antibiotics, most often erythromycin. Applied like tretinoin (above). If excessive dryness occurs, a milder strength of the drug may be recommended.

Vitamin A Derivatives

Actions and Uses

Isotretinoin and tretinoin are derivatives of vitamin A that are generally reserved for the treatment of severe acne. Isotretinoin is taken orally and works by decreasing sebum production, inhibiting inflammation, altering keratinization, and inhibiting bacterial growth. Tretinoin, which is applied topically, increases epidermal cell turnover, causing comedone plugs to be expelled. Both drugs cause a temporary worsening of acne before beneficial effects begin to become apparent.

Side and Adverse Effects

Both isotretinoin and tretinoin can cause excessive dryness and irritation of the skin. The patient may be very sensitive to sunlight, necessitating sunscreens or avoidance of bright sunshine.

Interactions and Contraindications

Risk of isotretinoin toxicity increases if given with tretinoin, etretinate, or vitamin A. Isotretinoin is very likely to cause severe fetal deformities if taken during pregnancy; therefore, patients must avoid pregnancy while taking this drug. Therapy is initiated on the second or third day of the menstrual period after a negative pregnancy test. **Pregnancy Category X.**

Antipsoriatics

Psoriasis is a skin condition characterized by bright red lesions that may be covered with silvery scales. Drugs most often used to treat this condition are tar derivatives, corticosteroids, and keratolytics. In difficult cases, etretinate (Tegison), methotrexate sodium, and calcipotriene (Dovonex) or methoxsalen (Oxsoralen) may be used.

Antipsoriatics work in a variety of ways to reduce or prevent the abnormal growth of epidermal cells. Their side and adverse effects are also quite varied. Therefore, this information will be presented in table format with specifics provided about each type of drug. Note that topical corticosteroids are covered earlier in this chapter and systemic corticosteroids are discussed in Chapter 43.

TABLE 47–3

Antipsoriatics

Type of Antipsoriatic	Prototype	Specific Considerations
anthralin	Anthra-Derm	May cause redness, irritation, and photosensitivity. Avoid contact with eyes. Gently wash and dry affected areas. Use a disposable glove to apply *only to lesions*. Rub in gently. Leave on for prescribed time, then wash off. Stains clothing, intact skin, and hair.

coal tar derivatives (keratolytic)	Estar gel	Irritates the skin; causes photosensitivity. Apply at bedtime with gloved hand and cover with loose dressing. Advise patient to wear old bedclothing since the agent stains. Apply zinc oxide or petrolatum jelly to adjacent skin to protect it.
retinoid derivative: possible anti-inflammatory and immunomodulatory actions	etretinate (Tegison)	Oral drug. For severe cases that do not respond to more conservative treatment. Serious adverse effects: peeling of skin, hair loss, dry mucous membranes, bone and joint pain, muscle cramps, fatigue, headache, eye irritation, elevated serum lipids, fetal malformations. **Pregnancy Category X.** ⚠
Antineoplastic	methotrexate (Folex)	Given PO or IV. Give PO drug 1 hour or 2 hours after meals. IV infusion should not exceed 10 mg/minute. Very toxic: diarrhea, oral ulcers, hepatotoxicity, blood dyscrasias, fetal malformations. ⚠ Used only in severe cases that do not respond to conservative treatment. **Pregnancy Category X.**
Vitamin D$_3$ analogue	calcipotriene (Dovonex)	Applied topically. May irritate skin. Hypercalcemia with excess use.
Photosensitive agent	methoxsalen (Oxsoralen)	Given orally to patients treated with photochemotherapy (PUVA). Reserved for patients with extensive lesions that have not responded to more conservative treatment. Can cause skin itching and redness, and nausea. Accelerates skin aging and increases risk of skin cancer. Advise patient to avoid sun exposure during the 24 hour period before treatment and 8 hours after taking the drug. Take with food or milk to decrease gastrointestinal irritation. Patient must wear fully protective sunglasses during UVA treatments and for the next 24 hours.

Pediculicides and Scabicides

Pediculosis is an infestation with lice, an ectoparasite, that causes intense itching. There are three types of lice infestations: head lice, pubic lice, and body lice. With head lice and pubic lice, the parasites primarily reside in the respective area of the body. Body lice, on the other hand, actually live in clothing and seek the skin only to feed. Each type of lice has a different treatment. Scabies is caused by a mite that burrows under the skin to lay eggs.

Actions and Uses

Pediculicides are agents used to treat lice infestations. *Scabicides* are agents used to eradicate mite infestations.

Side and Adverse Effects

Pediculicides and scabicides generally have few adverse effects when used as directed.

Nursing Actions and Patient Teaching

- Most infestations are treated by patients at home, although treatment is sometimes required by hospitalized patients. Key patient teaching points are noted in Table 47–4.

TABLE 47–4

Pediculicides and Scabicides

Drug	Indications	Specific Considerations
permethrin (Nix, Elimite)	Nix: drug of choice for head lice Elimite: drug of choice for scabies	First shampoo and dry the hair, then saturate the hair with permethrin. Wait 10 minutes, then rinse. Repeat in 7 days if needed. Massage cream into the skin from head to toe. Leave on 8–14 hours before washing. Permethrin may cause local burning, itching or numbness, and redness.
malathion (Ovide)	Head lice	Apply to dry hair and gently massage until scalp is moist. Allow to air dry. Do not use hair dryer because solution is flammable. Wash with shampoo 8–12 hours after application. Use fine-tooth comb to remove dead lice and nits (eggs). May be mildly irritating. Repeat in 7 days if needed.
crotamiton (Eurax)	Scabies	Massage into skin from chin to toes. Attend to skin folds and creases, but avoid eyes, mucous membranes, and inflamed areas. Repeat in 24 hours. Bathe 48 hours after second application. Repeat in 7 days if needed.

(Continued on p. 230)

Drug	Indications	Specific Considerations
pyrethrins plus piperonyl butoxide (RID, et al.)	Pubic and head lice	Apply to infested region and rinse with warm water. Avoid contact with eyes and mucous membranes. Repeat in 7 days. Use fine tooth comb to remove nits.
lindane (Kwell, et al.)	Scabies, lice	Apply to entire body from chin to toes using no more than 1 ounce of cream or lotion. Wash off after 8–12 hours. Itching may persist, but does not warrant repeat treatment. Not recommended for infants or people with seizure disorders because it is absorbed through the skin and can cause convulsions. Head lice: apply shampoo to dry hair, leave on 4 minutes, and rinse with warm water. Pubic lice: same as for head lice. Sexual partners should be treated to prevent reinfestation. Do not apply to eyebrows. Body lice: apply thin layer of ointment or cream to affected areas and leave on 8–12 hours before washing off.

REVIEW QUESTIONS: UNIT 15

Case Study

Mr. Mike Pickell has moderately severe psoriasis (see text Care Plan, textbook Chapter 47) for which anthralin cream is prescribed. He is to apply the cream once daily.

1. Patient teaching for application of anthralin cream should include:

    A. gently wash and dry affected areas.

    B. apply thin layer of cream all over the body.

    C. allow the cream to be absorbed; do not wash off.

    D. cream will not stain clothing.

2. Adverse effects of anthralin cream include:

    A. bone marrow depression.

    B. joint pain.

    C. hepatotoxicity.

    D. redness.

Mr. Pickell's condition worsens and is not responding to the anthralin. Etretinate (Tegison) is prescribed.

3. Which statement of true of etretinate?

    A. It has fewer side effects than anthralin but is more expensive.

    B. It is applied topically.

    C. It is reserved for serious cases because side effects can be severe.

    D. It is an antineoplastic agent.

4. Which antipsoriatics are clearly contraindicated during pregnancy?

    A. methotrexate (Folex)

    B. anthralin (Anthra-Derm)

    C. coal tar (Estar-Gel)

    D. methoxsalen (Oxsoralen)

DRUGS THAT AFFECT THE EYES AND EARS

OBJECTIVES

1. List the classifications of drugs used to treat disorders of the eyes and ears.

2. Explain the actions, uses, side and adverse effects, interactions, and contraindications of drugs used to treat disorders of the ear and eye.

3. Identify nursing interventions relevant to drugs used to treat eye and ear disorders.

CHAPTER 48

OPHTHALMIC AGENTS

ANATOMY AND PHYSIOLOGY OF THE EYE

Structures that comprise the visual system include the eyeball, eyelids, eyelashes, conjunctiva, and extraocular muscles. The tissue layers of the eyeball are the sclera, the choroid, and the retina. The sclera is the tough outer layer that is white except for the clear area over the iris. Important structures in the middle layer, the choroid, are the ciliary muscle and the iris. The iris is a muscle that controls the diameter of the pupil, thereby controlling the amount of light that enters the eye. In dim light, the iris contracts, which dilates the pupil. In bright light it relaxes and the pupil constricts. The lens is a clear structure behind the iris that is attached to the ciliary muscle. Contraction and relaxation of the ciliary muscle alters the shape of the lens, permitting it to focus on objects at various distances. The retina is the structure that receives images and conveys them to the brain via the optic nerve.

The interior eyeball is divided into two chambers separated by the lens. The anterior chamber, located between the iris and the cornea, is filled with aqueous humor, a clear, watery fluid. Aqueous humor is produced in the ciliary body and flows over the lens, through the pupil, and out through the trabecular meshwork into the canal of Schlemm (Figure 48–1). The production and outflow of aqueous humor must remain balanced so that the pressure within the chamber, referred to as intraocular pressure (IOP) remains within the normal range of 12 to 21 mm Hg. The posterior chamber is filled with vitreous humor, a clear gelatinous material that helps hold the retina in place.

Lacrimal glands above the eyes secrete tears to keep the eye moist and provide oxygen and some nutrients to the cornea. Fluid drains from the conjunctival sac through the lacrimal duct into the nose. This pathway is important in relation to drugs because it provides an avenue for topical drugs that have been applied to the eye to enter the body.

FIGURE 48–1

The Flow of Aqueous Humor Through the Eye

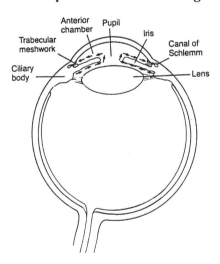

Fluid is produced by the ciliary body. It flows through the pupil into the anterior chamber and out through the trabecular meshwork and the canal of Schlemm.

From Linton, Matteson, and Maebius (2000). *Introductory Nursing Care of Adults*, 2nd ed. Philadelphia: W.B. Saunders, p. 1087.

DISORDERS OF THE EYE

The term *ophthalmic* refers to the eye; therefore, ophthalmic drugs are those intended for topical instillation in the eye. Eye disorders that may respond to pharmacologic agents include infections, inflammation, and glaucoma. Glaucoma is abnormally increased intraocular pressure that can lead to blindness. In addition to treating eye disorders, ophthalmic agents are often used to permit inspection of the interior of the eye, facilitate access for surgical procedures, prevent movement of eye structures during treatments, and block sensation in the external eye. Classifications of ophthalmic drugs include autonomic agents, diuretics, prostaglandins, anti-infectives, anti-inflammatory agents, local anesthetics, and lubricants. It should also be noted that many drugs used to treat problems unrelated to the eye may affect the eye and vision.

It may be helpful to define some terms that will be encountered in this unit:

- **Miosis**: constriction of the pupil
- **Miotic**: causing the pupil to constrict
- **Mydriasis**: dilation of the pupil
- **Mydriatic**: causing the pupil to dilate
- **Cycloplegia**: paralysis of the ciliary body so the lens is unable to accommodate
- **Cycloplegic**: causes paralysis of the ciliary body so the lens is unable to accommodate

There are also some abbreviations physicians may use in writing orders specifically for ophthalmic drugs. They are as follows:

- **OD**: right eye
- **OS**: left eye
- **OU**: both eyes

There are some general points to remember when administering or teaching the patient to administer ophthalmic agents.

- Wash your hands.
- Use only *ophthalmic* preparations in the eye.
- Roll the bottle between your hands to warm the solution.
- Be sure you have the correct drug for the correct eye. It is not unusual for patients to have different drugs for each eye.
- Be sure you have the correct drug strength. Many drugs are available in more than one strength.
- Have the patient tilt the head back and slightly toward the affected side, and look at the ceiling.
- Brace your hand on the patient's cheek so if the patient moves, you will not hit the eye with the container.
- Retract the lower lid and instill the medication in the sac.

- Do not allow the container to touch the eye or the eyelid; this would contaminate the medication.
- Apply gentle pressure to the lacrimal duct (at the inner canthus of the eye) for 1 minute to minimize the amount of medication entering body fluids.
- If more than one ophthalmic drug is to be administered, allow 5 minutes between medications.

AUTONOMIC AGENTS

Autonomic drugs are covered in detail in Unit 6. This section addresses only drugs used for ophthalmic purposes. When used properly, topical ophthalmic drugs should have minimal systemic effects. However, drugs are instilled in the conjunctival sac, which is drained by the lacrimal duct. Through this route, some drug is usually absorbed into the body. In sufficient amounts, the drugs may produce systemic side and adverse effects.

Adrenergics

Ophthalmic adrenergics include epinephrine hydrochloride 0.25–2% (Adrenalin Chloride, Glaucon), dipivefrin (Propine), and tetrahydrozoline hydrochloride 0.05% (Visine, Murine).

Actions and Uses

Ophthalmic adrenergics decrease the production of aqueous humor, dilate the pupil, and constrict blood vessels in the external eye. They are used to treat open angle glaucoma, reduce redness and itching, and dilate the pupil for examinations and surgical procedures.

Side and Adverse Effects

Topical adrenergics may cause a transient burning sensation. Because they dilate the pupil, the eye will be photosensitive (sensitive to light). Some patients complain of headache when using these preparations. Systemic effects of adrenergic ophthalmic preparations such as tachycardia, hypertension, anxiety, and cardiac dysrhythmias are rare. Chronic use of tetrahydrozoline may increase intraocular pressure.

Contraindications and Interactions

Patients with known eye disease should use ophthalmic adrenergics only on the advice of a physician. These agents are used with caution in people with cardiac disease, hyperthyroidism, diabetes mellitus, hypertension, and bronchial asthma. Patients on monoamine oxidase inhibitors and tricyclic antidepressants are at risk for hypertensive episodes if given adrenergics.

Nursing Actions

Monitor pulse and blood pressure. Anticipate pupil dilation. Assess the patient's ability to carry out activities.

Patient Teaching
• If you have any eye disease, consult your physician before using over-the-counter adrenergic drugs such as Visine.
• Because your pupils will be dilated, your eyes will be sensitive to light. You will need to protect your eyes from bright light.
• Discontinue use if you develop eye pain or headaches and notify your physician.
• Remove contact lenses before instilling tetrahydrozoline drops.

Antiadrenergics

Antiadrenergics are also called *adrenergic blockers* or *beta blockers*. Examples of antiadrenergic ophthalmic drugs are levobunolol hydrochloride 0.5% (Betagen Liquifilm), betaxolol 0.25–0.5% (Betoptic), and timolol maleate 0.25–0.5% (Timoptic).

Actions and Uses

Antiadrenergics reduce intraocular pressure in open-angle glaucoma by decreasing the production of aqueous humor.

Side and Adverse Effects

Upon instillation, antiadrenergics may cause a transient burning sensation. Other adverse effects include dry eyes, photosensitivity, and blurred vision. If sufficient drug is absorbed systemically, the patient may develop bradycardia or bronchospasm.

Interactions and Contraindications

The systemic effects of antiadrenergics enhance other cardiac depressants and antihypertensives. Antiadrenergics are contraindicated with heart failure, atrioventricular heart block, sinus bradycardia, and cardiogenic shock. Betaxolol is *least* likely to cause bronchospasm in patients with asthma.

Nursing Actions

Assess heart rate and respriations. Monitor blood glucose in people with diabetes mellitus.

Patient Teaching
• Report difficulty breathing to your physician.
• Keep appointments to monitor intraocular pressure.

Cholinergics

Cholinergic agents used for eye disorders include carbachol (Isopto Carbachol), demecarium (Humorsol), and pilocarpine (Pilocar, et al.).

Actions and Uses

Cholinergic agents are also known as *parasympathomimetics* because their effects are like those caused by stimulation of the parasympathetic nervous system. The systemic effects of cholinergics are discussed in Chapter 17. Cholinergic ophthalmic agents are classified as direct-acting (e.g., carbachol, pilocarpine) and indirect-acting (e.g., demecarium). The effects are the same, but the mechanisms of action differ. Cholinergic drugs have two important effects on the eye: (1) contraction of the iris, which constricts the pupil , and (2) contraction of the muscles of the ciliary body. Pupil constriction (miosis) improves the outflow of aqueous humor, which reduces intraocular pressure. Therefore, these drugs are useful in the treatment of some types of glaucoma.

Side and Adverse Effects

Both direct- and indirect-acting cholinergics cause slow adaptation to changes in light. Because of the pupil constriction, the patient may have difficulty seeing well enough to drive at night. Other side effects are brow ache and increased perspiration, salivation, and bronchial secretions. In addition, indirect-acting agents can cause cataracts, cysts on the iris, and corneal toxicity.

Contraindications and Interactions

Cholinergics are contraindicated with inflammation of the iris, uvea, and ciliary body as well as some types of glaucoma.

Topical anti-inflammatory agents may decrease the effects of direct-acting cholinergics. Indirect-acting cholinergics can cause respiratory and circulatory collapse if used with succinylcholine during general anesthesia.

Nursing Actions

Inspect the eye for signs of irritation or inflammation.

<table>
<tr><td colspan="1">

Patient Teaching

- Always use these medications exactly as ordered; glaucoma often has no symptoms but must be treated to avoid damage to the eye and to your vision.
- You may have difficulty seeing well enough to drive safely at night.
- Report any changes in your vision to your physician.

</td></tr>
</table>

Anticholinergics

Anticholinergic ophthalmic drugs include atropine sulfate (Isopto Atropine), homatropine hydrobromide (Isopto Homatropine), cyclopentolate hydrochloride (Cyclogyl), scopolamine hydrobromide (Isopto Hyoscine), and tropicamide (Mydriacyl Ophthalmic).

Actions and Uses

The systemic effects of anticholinergics are discussed in Chapter 18. In relation to the eye, anticholinergics relax the smooth muscles of the ciliary body and the iris. The effects are mydriasis, which is dilation of the pupil, and cycloplegia, which is loss of accommodation.

These drugs are used to dilate the pupil to permit inspection of the interior of the eye and to measure refraction. They also are used to rest the eye by limiting movement in inflammatory conditions. The drug of choice for ocular examinations is tropicamide because of its short duration of action.

Side and Adverse Effects

When anticholinergics are used on an occasional basis for eye examinations, the risk of adverse effects is small. However, mydriasis can cause blurred vision, light sensitivity, and increased intraocular pressure. With regular use, the classic systemic side effects of anticholinergics, which include dry mouth, constipation, urinary retention, fever, and tachycardia, may be manifested as well.

Interactions and Contraindications

Anticholinergics are contraindicated with glaucoma, gastrointestinal or urinary retention, asthma, and myasthenia gravis. Patients receiving other anticholinergics are at increased risk for adverse effects.

Nursing Actions

Assess for systemic effects.

<table>
<tr><td colspan="1">

Patient Teaching

- Until the effects of this drug wear off, your eyes will be more sensitive to light because your pupils are dilated; wear sunglasses when outside.
- Do not attempt to drive until your vision returns to normal.

</td></tr>
</table>

DIURETICS

The two types of diuretics used to treat eye disorders are carbonic anhydrase inhibitors and hyperosmotic drugs.

Oral Carbonic Anhydrase Inhibitors

Actions and Uses

Acetazolamide (Diamox) is the carbonic anhydrase inhibitor most often used to treat open-angle, secondary, or angle closure glaucoma when the patient does not respond to preferred drugs. It is usually given orally, but can be given intravenously in urgent situations. In the eye, acetazolamide reduces the rate of formation of aqueous humor, thereby reducing intraocular pressure. Systemically, it causes diuresis and has an anticonvulsant effect. Diuresis poses a threat of hypokalemia.

Side and Adverse Effects

Common effects of acetazolamide are fatigue, diarrhea, nausea, vomiting, anorexia, weight loss, and numbness in the limbs, lips, and mouth. Patients may note a metallic taste in the mouth. On rare occasions, confusion and severe muscle weakness have been attributed to this drug. With long-term use, adverse effects can include acidosis (because of the increased renal excretion of bicarbonate), renal and liver toxicity, and bone marrow depression.

Interactions and Contraindications

By causing potassium loss, acetazolamide increases the risk of digitalis toxicity. It enhances the effects of amphetamines and diminishes the effects of methenamine.

Acetazolamide is contraindicated in people with severe renal disease, adrenal insufficiency, hypochloremic acidosis, and allergy to sulfonamides. It is used cautiously with diabetes mellitus, gout, and obstructive pulmonary disease.

Nursing Actions

Withhold the drug and notify the physician if the patient reports allergy to sulfonamides. Monitor serum electrolytes and be alert for muscle weakness and cardiac dysrhythmias that suggest hypokalemia. Monitor blood cell counts for indications of bone marrow depression. Inspect the skin for pallor and bruising. Assess respiratory status for deep breathing typical of acidosis.

Patient Teaching

- You can expect increased urine output while on this drug.
- Notify your physician of weakness, palpitations, vomiting, or diarrhea.
- Report unexplained or prolonged bleeding, fever, sore throat, or fatigue.

Topical Carbonic Anhydrase Inhibitor

Dorzolamide (Trusopt) is a carbonic anhydrase inhibitor that is administered topically. Like acetazolamide, it lowers intraocular pressure by reducing the production of aqueous humor. However, it does not pose a risk of electrolyte imbalances or acidosis. Like most topical ophthalmic agents, it can irritate the eye. Patients commonly report a transient stinging sensation when the drug is instilled. Other adverse effects are blurred vision, tearing, eye dryness, and photosensitivity. Inflammation of the conjunctiva and the eyelids represent an allergic response and require discontinuing use of this drug.

Hyperosmotic Drugs

Actions and Uses

Hyperosmotic agents increase the osmolarity of the serum, which draws water into the blood, expanding the blood volume and resulting in increased urine output. The increased osmotic serum pressure also draws water from the intraocular fluid. These agents are most often used for rapid reduction of intraocular pressure in acute angle closure glaucoma, but may be employed in limited situations with open angle glaucoma. Agents used to reduce intraocular pressure include mannitol and urea, which are given intravenously, and glycerin and isosorbide, which are given orally.

Side and Adverse Effects

Hyperosmotic agents may cause dry mouth, headache, nausea, and vomiting.

Interactions and Contraindications

Excess loss of potassium with diuresis increases the risk of digitalis toxicity. Hyperosmotic diuretics are contraindicated with severe dehydration or electrolyte depletion and with

increasing oliguria. Because these drugs increase the blood volume initially, they should not be used if the patient has fluid volume excess, as in congestive heart failure and pulmonary edema.

Nursing Actions

Monitor fluid intake and output. Assess for fluid volume excess: bounding pulse, hypertension, edema, crackles in the lungs, anxiety. Check serum electrolyte studies and monitor for changes in mental status, neuromuscular activity, and cardiac rhythm.

Patient Teaching

- You will have increased urine output after receiving this drug
- Report shortness of breath, palpitations, or weakness

PROSTAGLANDINS

Actions and Uses

Latanoprost (Xalatan) is a prostaglandin used to treat open-angle glaucoma and ocular hypertension. This drug lowers intraocular pressure by increasing the outflow of aqueous humor. An advantage of latanoprost is that it is effective with a single daily dose.

Side and Adverse Effects

Latanoprost typically causes transient irritation, burning, and blurred vision. The conjunctiva may appear very red. People with brown iris pigmentation may have a darkening of the brown color. Less frequent effects include dry eyes, eye pain, crusting and edema of the lids, and photosensitivity. Systemic effects are uncommon but can include upper respiratory infection symptoms, chest and musculoskeletal pain, and allergic skin reactions.

Interactions and Contraindications

There are no significant interactions with latanoprost. The only contraindication is allergy.

Nursing Actions

Nursing actions are the same as patient teaching.

Patient Teaching

- Remove contact lenses prior to using these drops and wait 15 minutes before reinserting the contacts.
- Permanent darkening of eye color may occur, especially if you have green-brown, blue/gray-brown, or yellow-brown irises.
- Eye discomfort should pass quickly; if it persists, notify your physician.

LOCAL ANESTHETICS

Actions and Uses

Because of the sensitivity of the eye and the blink reflex, local anesthesia is necessary to safely and comfortably perform some diagnostic and surgical eye procedures. Examples of topical ophthalmic anesthetics are tetracaine hydrochloride (Pontocaine) and cocaine hydrochloride. Injectable agents, used for surgical procedures, include procaine hydrochloride (Novocain) and lidocaine hydrochloride (Xylocaine). Local anesthetics interfere with the initiation and conduction of nerve impulses so that the treated area lacks sensation.

Side and Adverse Effects

With topical anesthetics, the patient may have a transient stinging sensation. Long-term use, which is not recommended, can cause keratitis.

Interactions and Contraindications

There are no significant drug interactions with topical ophthalmic anesthetics.

They are contraindicated with known allergy.

Nursing Actions

Because it lacks sensation, the eye is susceptible to injury. If ordered, apply a patch or shield. Monitor children or confused adults until the anesthetic effects wear off. Most topical agents have a duration of action less than 20 minutes. Injected agents may last as long as 12 hours.

Patient Teaching

- Until sensation returns, your eyes are susceptible to injury. Avoid rubbing the anesthetized eye.

ANTI-INFECTIVES

Anti-infective agents are discussed in Chapter 5. Depending on the site of an eye infection, anti-infectives may be given topically, orally, or by injection into the subconjunctival space or aqueous humor. Table 48–1 provides information about specific topical drugs used to treat bacterial, fungal, and viral infections of the external eye.

TABLE 48–1

Ophthalmic Anti-infectives

Type of Anti-infective	Prototypes	Comments
Antibacterial	Bacitracin ointment (AK-Tracin, Polysporin)	Use: superficial *Staphylococcus* infection. Penetrates cornea and conjunctiva. Apply $1/2$ inch ointment in lower conjunctival sac.
	Chloramphenicol (AK-Chlor solution, Chlorofair solution and ointment, Chloromycetin solution and ointment, Chloroptic solution and ointment)	Use: Gram-positive and gram-negative infections of anterior eye
	Erythromycin Ointment (Ocu-Mycin, Ilotycin)	Use: Gram-positive infections. Trachoma. Prevention of ophthalmia neonatorum.
	Gentamicin solution and ointment (Gentak, Genoptic, Gentaciden, Gentrasul, Garamycin)	Use: Gram-negative external eye infections. Bacterial corneal ulcers. Infected burns.
	Tobramycin (Tobrex 0.3% solution and ointment; TobraDex 0.3% solution and ointment)	Use: Gram-negative and gram-positive aerobes. Superficial external eye infections. Sometimes used in combination with corticosteroids.
	Tetracycline suspension and ointment (Achromycin 1%)	Broad-spectrum. Effective against many bacteria, *Rickettsia, Chlamydia, Mycoplasma,* and spirochetes. Prevents gonococcal ophthalmia neonatorum.

(Continued on p. 238)

Type of Anti-Infective	Prototypes	Comments
	Sulfonamides (Sulfacetamide sodium ophthalmic solution and ointment) Sulfisoxazole solution and ointment (Gantrisin)	Broad-spectrum. Effective against many bacteria, *Actinomyces, Chlamydia, Toxoplasma,* and plasmodia.
Antiviral Drugs	Idoxuridine solution (Herplex 0.1% solution)	Use: Herpes simplex keratitis (herpes simples virus infection of the cornea); infection may recur.
	Vidarabine Ointment (Vira-A 3%)	Use: Herpes simplex keratitis (herpes simplex virus infection of the cornea). Effective against cytomegalovirus and varicella-zoster virus.
	Trifluridine solution (Viroptic 1%)	Use: Drug of choice for herpes keratitis (herpes simplex virus infection of the cornea)
Antifungal Drugs	Natamycin (Natacyn 5% solution)	Broad-spectrum. Use: Drug of choice for initial treatment of fungal keratitis. Also used to treat conjunctivitis and blepharitis. Only commercially prepared topical antifungal for the eye.
	Amphotericin B (Fungizone)	Used to treat corneal ulcers caused by *Fusarium, Candida, Aspergillus, and Alternaria.* Prepared in the pharmacy from preparations intended for systemic use.
	Miconazole (Monistat)	Broad-spectrum. Used to treat corneal fungal infections. Prepared in the pharmacy from preparations intended for systemic use.

ANTI-INFLAMMATORY AGENTS

Exposure to allergens can evoke an inflammatory response in the eye. Treatment is important because inflammation can result in scar formation that could impair vision. The two categories of drugs used to reduce ocular inflammation are topical corticosteroids and nonsteroidal anti-inflammatory drugs (NSAIDs).

Corticosteroids

Corticosteroids, including dexamethasone, prednisolone acetate, prednisolone sodium phosphate, fluorometholone, and medrysone are available under numerous trade names. See Table 48–2.

TABLE 48–2

Ophthalmic Corticosteroid Preparations

Generic Name	Trade Names
dexamethasone	Maxidex, Decadron Phosphate MSD, Decadron Phosphate
prednisolone acetate	Econopred, Econopred Plus
prednisolone sodium phosphate	Inflamase, AK-Pred, Metreton, Inflamase Forte
fluorometholone	FML Forte, FML
medrysone	HMS

Action and Uses

Corticosteroids inhibit the antigens that stimulate the inflammatory response. They reduce capillary permeability and suppress the influx of white blood cells. When inflam-

mation is associated with infection, anti-infective agents must be used along with corticosteroids. If used alone, the corticosteroids mask signs of infection, possibly permitting progression of the infection with serious consequences.

Side and Adverse Effects

Side and adverse effects of topical corticosteroids include blurred vision, tearing, eye pain, nausea, vomiting, and a burning sensation in the eyes. In people with a predisposition to glaucoma, intraocular pressure may rise when corticosteroids are used. Long-term use can cause ocular hypertension and cataracts. Systemic effects of corticosteroids are described in Chapter 43.

Interactions and Contraindications

There are no significant drug interactions with the ophthalmic corticosteroids. They are contraindicated in the presence of infection unless anti-infectives are used at the same time.

Nursing Actions

Assess and document redness and discomfort. Report lack of improvement.

Patient Teaching
• Do not stop using oral corticosteroids suddenly; taper the dose as prescribed.   • Notify the physician if the condition does not improve or if vision deteriorates.

Nonsteroidal Anti-inflammatory Drugs

Topical NSAIDs used to treat eye conditions include flurbiprofen sodium (Ocufen), suprofen solution 1% (Syntex), diclofenac solution (Voltaren, Cataflam), and ketorolac (Toradol, Acular).

Actions and Uses

Topical NSAIDs suppress inflammation associated with surgical procedures and allergies and may be given preoperatively to prevent pupil constriction during certain surgical procedures.

Side and Adverse Effects

These drugs may cause irritation manifested by burning or stinging sensations, or itching. Tearing and swelling of the eyelids are associated with an allergic response.

Interactions and Contraindications

Ophthalmic NSAIDs are contraindicated in patients who are allergic to any NSAIDs. In the treatment of recurrent anterior uveitis, NSAIDs may be given with topical corticosteroids. Some sources recommend administering ophthalmic NSAIDs at least 10 minutes apart from other ophthalmic drugs. Check specific drug information before using.

MISCELLANEOUS OPHTHALMIC AGENTS

Lubricants

Dry eyes can be caused by a variety of problems and can result in damage to the cornea. Eye lubricants (artificial tears) are used to restore the normal moisture to the external eye. Preparations include drops, ointments, and inserts. Inserts are small rods placed in the conjunctival sac that release a lubricant over a 24-hour period. Lubricants have no adverse effects.

Dyes

Dyes, including fluorescein and rose bengal, are used to reveal foreign bodies and superficial injuries to the cornea. The only common adverse effect of the topical dyes is occasional transient stinging, which is more common with rose bengal than with fluorescein. Both dyes also can stain the skin. To decrease irritation with rose bengal, a topical anesthetic may be applied first. Irrigation of the eye following the procedure reduces staining of the eyelids.

Fluorescein can be given intravenously prior to retinal angiography for study of retinal blood vessels. Tell the patient the skin may have a yellowish cast for as long as 12 hours, and the urine will be bright yellow-orange for 24 hours.

People can have serious allergic reactions to these dyes, so it is vital to assess allergies before administering dyes in any form.

OTIC AGENTS

ANATOMY AND PHYSIOLOGY OF THE EAR

The major sections of the ear are the external ear, the middle ear, and the inner ear. The auricle, or pinna, is the visible external part of the ear. The external auditory canal is a passageway that extends from the external opening to the tympanic membrane. The tympanic membrane, commonly referred to as the *eardrum*, vibrates in response to sound waves that enter the external canal.

The middle ear extends from the tympanic membrane to the oval window. It is an air-filled space that contains three small bones (ossicles): the malleus, the incus, and the stapes. Sound waves received by the tympanic membrane are relayed by vibrations of these bones to the oval window, which lies between the middle and inner ears. The eustachian tube, which extends from the middle ear to the nasopharynx, creates an air passage so that air pressure remains the same on both sides of the tympanic membrane. The mastoid process is a bony structure made of air cells that are directly connected to the middle ear.

The inner ear consists of the membranous labyrinth and the bony labyrinth. The membranous labyrinth contains endolymph, a fluid that moves with changes in body position. The parts of the bony labyrinth are the vestibule, semicircular canals, and cochlea. The vestibule and semicircular canals maintain posture and balance. Part of the cochlea, the organ of Corti, transmits stimuli from the oval window to the acoustic nerve. It is the end organ of hearing.

DISORDERS AFFECTING THE EAR AND HEARING

Hearing requires a patent canal, an intact tympanic membrane that can vibrate, intact and moveable ossicles, and functional sensory receptors. Balance requires normal function of the vestibule and semicircular canals.

The external ear is vulnerable to infections, inflammation, and trauma. In addition, the external canal can become obstructed by foreign bodies or by excessively dry *cerumen* (earwax). Anything that impairs the passage of sound waves from the external ear to the organ of Corti can affect hearing. For example, fluid in the middle ear, fixed ossicles, and

nerve damage could all result in temporary or permanent hearing loss. Balance is affected by conditions in the inner ear, including infections and Ménière's disease.

Drugs used to treat disorders affecting the ear and hearing include anti-infectives, anti-inflammatory agents, antiemetics, cerumenolytics, local anesthetics, and drying agents. Anti-infectives are covered in Chapter 5, anti-inflammatory agents in Chapter 4, antiemetics in Chapter 35, and local anesthetics in Chapter 10. Therefore, they will be discussed here only in relation to the ear.

It should also be noted that many drugs used for various conditions are *ototoxic*, meaning they can temporarily or permanently harm the acoustic nerve. When giving an drug that is ototoxic, be sure to tell the patient to report any *tinnitus* (ringing in the ears) or changes in hearing or balance. Often, the toxic effects resolve if the drug is discontinued promptly.

Drugs used to treat disorders of the ear may be administered systemically or topically. When administering topical drugs into the ear, remember the following:

- Only *otic* drugs are intended for the external ear.
- Warm the solution by rolling the container between your hands.
- Tilt the patient's head away from you and brace your hand on the patient's cheek.
- Do not contaminate the container by touching it to the patient's skin.
- Instruct the patient to keep the ear up for several minutes so the drug will flow into the ear.

You will need to know some common abbreviations used in orders for otic drugs. These include the following:

- **AD**: right ear
- **AS**: left ear
- **AU**: both ears

ANTI-INFECTIVES

Actions and Uses

For infections of the external ear, topical solutions are often ordered. Chloramphenicol (Chloromycetin Otic) is an example of an antibacterial agent used for ear infections. It is effective against both gram-positive and gram-negative organisms. Neomycin sulfate, colistin sulfate, and polymyxin B sulfate are other anti-infectives that are sometimes used in various combinations with corticosteroids to treat infection and inflammation of the ear.

Side and Adverse Effects

Topical chloramphenicol may be irritating to the tissues lining the ear canal. Local irritation is manifested as itching, tenderness, redness, and swelling. Patients can have serious allergic reactions ranging from urticaria (hives) to anaphylaxis. Bone marrow depression is possible, especially with prolonged or frequent use. If the patient has a perforated tympanic membrane, the drug can enter the middle ear and exert ototoxic effects.

Interactions and Contraindications

Chloramphenicol can enhance the effects of oral hypoglycemics, phenytoin, warfarin, and other bone marrow depressants, and can antagonize the effects of clindamycin and erythromycin. These interactions are less likely with topical than with systemic administration.

Chloramphenicol otic is contraindicated with known allergy and in patients with a perforated tympanic membrane.

Nursing Actions

Assess for allergy before administering these drugs. Inspect the external canal and tympanic membrane. Do not administer otic drugs in the presence of a ruptured tympanic membrane. Assess for possible signs of bone marrow depression: easy bruising or bleeding, fatigue and pallor, and signs of new or worsening infection.

Patient Teaching
• Notify your physician if you have burning, pain, or redness in the affected ear.
• Use exactly as prescribed; do not exceed recommended dosage or period of use.

ANTI-INFLAMMATORY AGENTS

Corticosteroids are used for their anti-inflammatory properties. Preparations intended for otic use include desonide-acetic acid (Otic Tridesilon) and hydrocortisone-acetic acid-propylene glycol (VoSol-HC Otic, Acetasol HC).

Actions and Uses

Topical corticosteroids are the most often used anti-inflammatory agents for external ear conditions. These drugs sup-

press the symptoms of inflammation (redness, swelling, itching) that occur in response to local tissue irritation, infection, or trauma. They are often used in combination with anti-infectives.

Side and Adverse Effects

Indications of local irritation include itching, burning, tenderness, swelling, and redness. Other possible adverse effects are delayed healing, excessive dryness, excessive hair growth, acneiform eruptions, loss of pigmentation, and secondary infection. With short-term therapy, systemic effects are unlikely but can occur, especially in young children and with occlusive dressings. Systemic effects of corticosteroids are covered in Chapter 43.

Interactions and Contraindications

Interactions of otic corticosteroids are most significant in relation to systemic effects as addressed in Chapter 43. Otic corticosteroids are contraindicated with a perforated tympanic membrane, herpes simplex in the external auditory canal, vaccinia, and varicella.

Nursing Actions

Assess for improvement or worsening of symptoms. Be alert for signs of systemic effects such as weight gain.

Patient Teaching
• Use only as prescribed.
• Notify your physician if symptoms do not improve.

ANTIEMETICS

Antiemetics are drugs used to prevent or treat nausea and vomiting. Ménière's disease and other conditions affecting the inner ear result in dizziness with nausea and vomiting. Meclizine (Antivert) is an antiemetic often used to manage these symptoms.

CERUMENOLYTICS

Cerumen, commonly called *ear wax*, can accumulate and harden in the external auditory canal. Agents used to soften cerumen so it can be removed are called *cerumenolytics*. Examples are triethanolamine polypeptide oleate-condensate (Cerumenex Drops) and carbamide peroxide (Auro Ear Drops, Debrox, E-R-O, Murine Ear Drops).

Actions and Uses

Cerumenolytics contain glycerin that softens cerumen and effervescent oxygen that loosens the impacted material. Fifteen to 30 minutes following instillation of the agent, gentle irrigation with warm water is done to flush the debris from the canal. The process can be repeated daily for up to 10 days until the canal is clear.

Side and Adverse Effects

Cerumenolytics are irritating and may cause burning, itching, tenderness, redness, swelling, and hives.

Interactions and Contraindications

These drugs should not be instilled if the patient has a perforated tympanic membrane.

Nursing Actions

Inspect the external canal for impacted cerumen following treatment. Note the effectiveness of the irrigation.

Patient Teaching
• These drugs are for occasional use only. • If the agent gets on the skin around the ear, wash it off promptly.

ANESTHETICS

Local anesthetics may be used to relieve pain and itching related to inflammation or to facilitate removal of impacted cerumen. Examples are benzocaine (Americaine-Otic), benzocaine-antipyrine (Auralgan, et al.), and benzocaine-antipyrine phenylephrine (Tympagesic). Remember that anesthetics only treat the symptoms, and other drugs may be needed to treat the underlying problem. Otic local anesthetics are contraindicated during pregnancy and lactation and in children under age 1. Assess for allergy to local anesthetics before administering these drugs.

DRYING AGENTS

Drying agents such as acetic acid or boric acid are often added to anti-infective agents. In this case, drying agents reduce the risk of recurrent irritation of the external ear canal. Drying agents are also used alone to inhibit bacterial growth. They may be recommended after swimming for people who are prone to ear infections. Like other otic preparations, drying agents may be locally irritating, causing tenderness, itching, and swelling.

REVIEW QUESTIONS: UNIT 16

Case Study

Mr. Don Dickson is recovering from cataract surgery this morning in the outpatient surgery center. His physician prescribes anti-infective ophthalmic drops and corticosteroid drops for him to use at home.

1. What would be most critical to ask before teaching Mr. Dickson about the anti-infective ophthalmic drops?
   A. Do you have any allergies?
   B. Are you taking any over-the-counter drugs?
   C. What kind of work do you do?
   D. Do you have any pain in your eye?

2. Patient teaching should include which of the following?
   A. Press the outer canthus of the eye after instilling the drops.
   B. Instill the drops in the upper conjunctival sac.
   C. Touch the tip of the dropper to the conjunctival sac to stabilize it.
   D. Wait 5 minutes between instilling the anti-infectives and the corticosteroids.

3. Which statement is correct about topical drugs for the eye?
   A. There is no risk of systemic effects.
   B. They are used for diagnostic and treatment purposes.
   C. Only topical drugs applied to the eye can affect the pupil.
   D. Ophthalmic drugs have no serious side or adverse effects.

Match the term on the left with the definition on the right.

4. _____ mydriatic	A.	right eye
5. _____ cycloplegia	B.	causing the pupil to constrict
6. _____ miotic	C.	causing the pupil to dilate
7. _____ miosis		
8. _____ mydriasis	D.	paralysis of ciliary body
9. _____ cycloplegic	E.	left eye
10. _____ OD	F.	dilation of the pupil
11. _____ OS	G.	constriction of the pupil
12. _____ OU	H.	both eyes
	I.	causing paralysis of ciliary body

Case Study

Mr. Javier Riojas has been hospitalized with an acute episode of Ménière's disease. He will be discharged with meclizine (Antivert).

13. Meclizine is classified as a/an:

   A. anti-infective.

   B. ceruminolytic.

   C. antiemetic.

   D. anesthetic.

14. A positive response to meclizine would be:

   A. patient sleeping soundly.

   B. patient states nausea is relieved.

   C. patient's blood pressure decreases.

   D. patient states pain in ear is diminished.

Match the term on the left with the definition on the right.

15. _____ tinnitus	A. left ear
16. _____ cerumen	B. right ear
17. _____ AD	C. both ears
18. _____ otic	D. ringing in the ears
19. _____ ototoxic	E. earwax
20. _____ AS	F. related to the ear
21. _____ AU	G. toxic to the ear

DRUGS THAT AFFECT MENTAL AND EMOTIONAL STATUS

OBJECTIVES

1. Describe the anatomy and physiology of the nervous system as it relates to mental health concepts.

2. List the drug classifications used to treat individuals with mental illness.

3. Explain the actions, side effects, adverse events, interactions, and contraindications of drugs used to treat anxiety, psychosis, and depression.

4. Describe nursing assessment data to be collected when patients are on specific drugs that affect the central and peripheral nervous system related to the treatment of mental illness.

5. Identify nursing interventions, including patient and family teaching, relevant to each major classification of drugs used to treat patients with mental illness.

Anatomy and Physiology of the Central Nervous System

The brain, brain stem, and spinal cord make up the central nervous system. The peripheral nervous system is made up of sensory and motor nerves as well as the ganglia outside the central nervous system. Most mental illnesses are directly related to the brain (central nervous system); occasionally, however, the peripheral nervous system is involved as well.

The brain functions by transmitting information in the form of electrical and chemical messaging units that allow the billions of nerve cells (neurons) to talk with one another. Impulses travel across the neurons by way of electrical conduction until they get to the end of the neuron. Nerve cells do not touch one another. Instead, there is a tiny space between each neuron called the *neurosynaptic junction*. When the electrical nerve impulse reaches this junction, the electrical charge ends and the neuron produces chemical messengers that are quickly released at the distal end of the neuron into the neurosynaptic junction. These chemical messengers, known as *neurotransmitters*, quickly enter the space between the two neurons and are picked up by the next neuron, which is then "turned on" and continues the nerve impulse on through the next neuron. Medications used to treat mental illness generally act on these messenger systems, especially the neurotransmitters.

The brain is the seat of all mental processes. These processes include cognition (thinking), perception and interpretation of outside stimuli (information in the environment), executive thinking and decision making (assessing a situation, making sense of it, planning, and taking action), memory (short- and long-term), feelings and emotions, and coordination of motor function (body movements) to name a few.

The physiology of the central nervous system has primarily to do with electrical and biochemical messenger unit systems and how they work. Neurons within the brain "talk" to one another in a process known as *neurotransmission*. Neurotransmission is made possible by way of electrical and chemical messengers, as discussed previously. As an impulse (nerve signal) travels along a neuron itself, it moves along by changing its electrical charge from one end of the neuron. Because this electrical charge cannot pass directly to the next neuron, the neurons use neurotransmitters to pass along a signal through the neurosynaptic junction (the space between the neurons). Nurses are particularly concerned with the neurotransmitters serotonin, epinephrine, norepinephrine, dopamine, and gamma-aminobutyric acid (GABA). Almost all of the drugs used to treat mental illnesses involve one or more of these neurotransmitters.

Drugs Used to Treat Mental Illness

Drugs used to treat mental illnesses generally act to create some balance or adjustment of neurotransmitter levels in the brain. Certain mental illnesses are believed to be related to either too much of one or more neurotransmitters (such as dopamine in psychotic disorders) or too little of one or more neurotransmitters (such as serotonin and norepinephrine in depression). Medications used to treat persons with certain mental illnesses are specific to the neurotransmitter imbalance believed to be related to that illness.

Classifications of drugs discussed in this unit include anxiolytics (drugs used in the treatment of anxiety), neuroleptics/antipsychotics (used in the treatment of psychoses), and antidepressants (used in the treatment of depression and certain other disorders).

CHAPTER 50

ANXIOLYTICS

nxiolytics, also known as *anti-anxiety drugs*, are designed to bring relief to the patient suffering from anxiety. Although anxiety can be viewed as a symptom, the patient may actually have a diagnosed anxiety disorder. There are many disorders that are classified as anxiety disorders. *The Diagnostic and Statistical Manual of Mental Disorders, 4th Edition* classifies anxiety disorders in the following manner:

1. Panic disorder without agoraphobia

2. Panic disorder with agoraphobia

3. Agoraphobia without history of panic disorder

4. Specific phobia

5. Social phobia (social anxiety disorder)

6. Obsessive-compulsive disorder

7. Posttraumatic stress disorder

8. Acute stress disorder

9. Generalized anxiety disorder (includes overanxious disorder of childhood)

10. Anxiety disorder due to a general medical condition

11. Substance-induced anxiety disorder

12. Anxiety disorder not otherwise specified

ANXIOLYTICS

There are six major categories of anxiolytics: benzodiazepines, barbiturates, antidepressants, antihistamines, and newer agents (non-benzodiazepines, non-barbiturates). Each category of anxiolytic has its own special considerations and nursing implications. This chapter will review each category and the associated nursing implications.

Benzodiazepines

Actions and Uses

Benzodiazepines are the most commonly used category of anti-anxiety drugs in the world. Benzodiazepines are also among the safest of the anxiolytic drugs. These drugs work by enhancing the level of gamma-aminobutyric acid (GABA) in the brain. GABA is the neurotransmitter that is involved in down-regulating (slowing down) certain parts of the central nervous system (CNS). When GABA is enhanced, anxiety usually decreases.

Some of the drugs listed in this category are also helpful in the treatment of insomnia and stress-related conditions. Anxiolytics have other effects as well. Some are also used as muscle relaxants, some as antiseizure medications, and some are used to induce partial anesthesia. This chapter will focus primarily on the use of these medications in treating persons with anxiety.

Dosages are specific for each medication in this category. Also of importance are the different "half-lives" of these medications. *Half-life* refers to how long it takes for the body to rid itself of at least half the drug. The longer the half-life, the longer a portion of that drug stays in the person in an active state. In some cases, a longer half-life is desirable. In others, it is not. Benzodiazepines with a very short half-life may be helpful in panic and sleep disorders, but they may also result in rebound anxiety. Benzodiazepines with a long half-life provide more of a blanket type of protection from anxiety. However, benzodiazepines with very long half-lives may result in residual effects the next day as well as cumulative increases over time. The benzodiazepines, their usual total daily doses, and half-lives are given in Table 50–1.

TABLE 50-1

Benzodiazepines

Drug Name (Generic/Trade)	Half-Life (Hours)	Usual Adult Total Daily Dose Range (mg/day)
Alprazolam (Xanax)	12–20	0.5–4
Chlordiazepoxide (Librium)	12–100	15–100
Clonazepam (Klonopin)	18–50	0.5–10
Clorazepate (Tranxene)	30–100	7.5–60
Diazepam (Valium)	20–90	2–40
Halazepam (Paxipam)	20–100	80–160
Lorazepam (Ativan)	10–20	2–4
Oxazepam (Serax)	5–15	15–90
Prazepam (Centrax)	30–200	10–60

Adapted from Stuart, G., & Laraia, M. (1998) *Principles and Practice of Psychiatric Nursing*, 6th ed. St. Louis: Mosby, p. 578.

Side and Adverse Effects

Common side effects of the benzodiazepines are drowsiness, sedation, ataxia, vertigo, feelings of detachment, increased irritability or hostility, anterograde amnesia, tolerance, dependency, and rebound anxiety. Rare side effects include nausea, headache, confusion, gross psychomotor impairment, depression, and paradoxical rage reaction (which is extremely rare [Laraia, 1998]).

Interactions and Contraindications

Benzodiazepines are considered CNS depressants. As such they have the potential to depress certain vital functions such as respiratory rate, cognition (thinking, attention, concentration, and memory) and motor coordination. All of these medications have the potential to cause drowsiness and decrease mental alertness. When taking one of these medications, the use of alcohol is contraindicated because alcohol intensifies the effects of the benzodiazepine. Other CNS depressants (narcotics, other benzodiazepines, and barbiturates) should be administered with great caution, as their actions can potentiate the effects of the benzodiazepines, resulting in a greater chance for, and severity of, CNS depression. If the patient has had an allergic reaction to one benzodiazepine, the use of another from the same family may be contraindicated.

The elderly may be more sensitive to the effects of these medications and often the dose may need to be adjusted to a smaller amount. Watch for confusion, disorientation, decreased attention and concentration, and impaired memory in the elderly. Also monitor for psychomotor changes.

All sedative-hypnotics cross the placental barrier during pregnancy. If given in the predelivery period, the drug may contribute to depression of neonatal vital functions. Benzodiazepines also pass through the nursing mother's milk and therefore breastfeeding while on these medications is usually contraindicated.

Nursing Actions

The nurse must assess the patient receiving these medications for therapeutic response. Ask patients to rate their anxiety on a scale of 1 to 10 before administering the dose and then again some time after the dose has been given. Document the patient's response as well as any side effects to the medication. The nurse must also assess the patient for any side effects following administration of the dose (as listed above) and intermittently if given on an outpatient basis. Ongoing assessment as to adequate respiratory effort, alertness, level of consciousness, and gross motor movement are important considerations. It has been suggested that an effective sedative (anxiolytic) agent should reduce anxiety and exert a calming effect with little or no effect on motor or mental functions. The extent of central nervous system depression caused by an anxiolytic should be the minimal and consistent with desired therapeutic effect (Trevor & Way, 1998). The nurse must also monitor for signs of abuse, since benzodiazepines may be habit-forming and physically addicting.

Patient Teaching

- Take the medication exactly as prescribed.
- Never increase the dose of these medications on your own. This medication may be habit-forming; both psychological and physical dependency can develop.
- Do not suddenly discontinue this medication without supervision, as sudden discontinuation may result in withdrawal symptoms including seizures.
- The medication must not be transferred to anyone else for any reason.
- Driving and operating dangerous machinery should be avoided until the exact effects of the medication are known and there is no interference with attention, concentration, judgment and motor coordination.

Barbiturates

Actions and Uses

Barbiturates are another category of anti-anxiety medication with a significant sedative quality. Barbiturates also act on the neurotransmitter GABA. It is felt that barbiturates act by prolonging the flow of GABA at the receptor site. Barbiturates are used less often now than they once were, since the benzodiazepines just discussed are generally considered safer and just as effective. Nevertheless, barbiturates are still used in some settings. Table 50–2 lists the common barbiturates.

TABLE 50–2

Barbiturates

Drug Name (Generic/Trade)	Half-Life (Hours)	Usual Adult Total Daily Dose Range (mg/day)
Secobarbital (Seconal)	19–34	100–200
Pentobarbital (Nembutal)	15–48	100–200
Amobarbital (Amytal)	8–42	100–200
Butabarbital (Butisol)	34–42	100–200
Phenobarbital	24–140	100–200

Adapted from Stuart, G., & Laraia, M. (1998) *Principles and Practice of Psychiatric Nursing*, 6th ed. St. Louis: Mosby, p. 580.

Side and Adverse Effects

Common side effects of the barbiturates are similar to those of the benzodiazepines, except that barbiturates have a more linear effect toward anesthesia and coma. They are considered less safe that benzodiazepines for this reason. In large doses, barbiturates may actually induce anesthesia. Drowsiness, sedation, ataxia, vertigo, feelings of detachment, increased irritability or hostility, anterograde amnesia, tolerance, dependency, and rebound anxiety may occur. Rare side effects include nausea, headache, confusion, gross psychomotor impairment, depression, and paradoxical rage reaction and depressed respirations (Laraia, 1998). There is a lesser margin of safety in this category of anxiolytic/sedative.

Interactions and Contraindications

Barbiturates are also central nervous system depressants. They have more of a potential to depress vital functions such as respiratory rate, cognition (thinking, attention, concentration, and memory), and motor coordination than benzodiazepines. They cause drowsiness, sedation, and decreased mental alertness. The use of alcohol is contraindicated when taking these medicines because alcohol significantly intensifies the effects of the barbiturates. Other CNS depressants (narcotics, other barbiturates, and benzodiazepines) should be administered with great caution as their actions can potentiate the effects of barbiturates, resulting in a greater potential severity of CNS depression. If the patient has had an allergic reaction to one barbiturate, the use of another from the same family may be contraindicated.

Once again, the elderly are more sensitive to the effects of these medications and often the dose needs to be adjusted to a smaller amount. The nurse must watch for confusion, disorientation, decreased attention and concentration, and impaired memory in the elderly as well as psychomotor changes.

All barbiturates cross the placental barrier during pregnancy. If given in the predelivery period, the drug may contribute to depression of neonatal vital functions. Barbiturates also pass through the nursing mother's milk, and therefore breastfeeding while on these medications is contraindicated.

Nursing Actions

Again, the nurse must assess the patient receiving these medications for therapeutic response. Ask patients to rate their anxiety on a scale of 1 to 10 before administering the dose and then again some time after the dose has been given. Document the patient's response as well as any side effects to the medication. The nurse must also assess the patient for any side effects following administration of the dose (as listed above) and intermittently if given on an outpatient basis. Ongoing assessment as to adequate respiratory effort, alertness, level of consciousness, and gross motor movement are important considerations. Observe for daytime sedation after administration the previous day. A "hangover" effect may occur (sluggishness, fatigue, drowsiness, decreased motor coordination).

Patient Teaching

- It is very important to take the medication exactly as prescribed.
- Never increase the dose of these medications on their own. This medication may be habit-forming, and both psychological and physical dependency may develop.
- Do not suddenly discontinue this medication without supervision, as sudden discontinuation may result in withdrawal symptoms, including seizures.
- Do not drink alcohol while taking this medication. The interaction of alcohol with barbiturates may be even more dangerous than with benzodiazepines.
- The medication must not be transferred to anyone else for any reason.
- Driving and operating dangerous machinery should be avoided.

ANTIDEPRESSANTS IN THE TREATMENT OF ANXIETY

Antidepressants are usually used to treat depression; however, persons with panic disorder and persons with obsessive-compulsive disorder (types of anxiety disorders) often respond well to certain antidepressants. Most antidepressants work by enhancing levels of the neurotransmitters se-

rotonin, norepinephrine, or both. These two neurotransmitters tend to increase neurotransmission. This will be discussed in further detail in Chapter 52.

As mentioned earlier, the benzodiazepines and the barbiturates work by enhancing levels of GABA. The antidepressants, however, do not directly affect the neurotransmitter GABA. Nevertheless, some antidepressants have been found to be effective in the selective treatment of certain anxiety states and disorders, as listed earlier.

Actions and Uses

In panic disorder, the antidepressant paroxetine (Paxil) seems to be very helpful. Paroxetine is known as a selective serotonin reuptake inhibitor (SSRI); thus, it blocks the reuptake of serotonin at the distal end of the neuron, thereby allowing more serotonin to remain in the neurosynapse between the two neurons. This increases the amount of serotonin in the neurosynaptic space, allowing for more transmission to take place. The result in this case is better management of panic. The usual daily dose of paroxetine is 10 to 40 mg. It is not uncommon, however, for someone treated with paroxetine to also be on a benzodiazepine as well. Often, patients treated with paroxetine will experience relief of panic or anxiety gradually over time. It takes 3 to 4 weeks or more for this effect to reach its peak. This is in contrast to the benzodiazepines, which work quickly; that is, shortly after they are administered.

Two antidepressants that work well in the treatment of the anxiety disorder obsessive-compulsive disorder are clomipramine (Anafranil) and fluvoxamine (Luvox). Clomipramine is a type of antidepressant known as a *tricyclic*. The usual daily adult dose of clomipramine is 100 to 200 mg; however, the dose is started lower and titrated up as tolerated. Clomipramine results in an increase in both serotonin and norepinephrine. When increased, these neurotransmitters increase neurosynaptic transmission across the neurons as well. Fluvoxamine (Luvox) is another SSRI. The usual daily adult dose of fluvoxamine is 100 to 300 mg, starting with a lower dose and gradually titrated up as tolerated. Again, its action is to support more transmission across the neurosynaptic junction. These medications also take a few weeks to reach their maximum usefulness.

Side and Adverse Effects

Anticholinergic side effects including dry mouth, blurred vision, constipation, tachycardia, urinary retention, and cognitive dysfunction may occur, as well as weight gain and orthostatic hypotension, especially with clomipramine. Drowsiness may also occur. With fluvoxamine, nervousness, headache, sexual dysfunction, and insomnia may occur as well as nausea and diarrhea.

Interactions and Contraindications

All antidepressants may lower the seizure threshold. Therefore, antidepressants must be used with great caution in patients with a history of head injury or seizure disorder. Antidepressants may be contraindicated in the presence of a seizure disorder. Paroxetine and clomipramine are contraindicated in a patient currently using monoamine oxidase inhibitors (MAOIs). There must be a 14-day washout period after an MAOI is discontinued before starting a patient on either of these two drugs. Fluvoxamine is contraindicated in patients using astemizole or cisapride. Clomipramine is contraindicated in patients with myocardial infarction.

Nursing Actions

Assess the patient for a therapeutic response to the medication and well as for any adverse or side effects. Document and report findings. Provide sugar-free hard candy or gum for patients who experience dry mouth. Monitor for changes in sleep pattern or other changes based on side effect profile. Assess urinary output and report any suspicion of urinary retention at once. Provide for plenty of fluids and a diet with sufficient fiber to avoid constipation. If constipation occurs, report and treat as directed. Monitor for signs of serotonin syndrome and report at once.

Patient Teaching
• It is very important to take the medication exactly as described.
• Do not discontinue the drug without supervision, as this may lead to withdrawal symptoms.
• Get out of bed slowly to avoid dizziness and fainting.
• Avoid hazardous activities until the effects of the medication are known and you are free from adverse side effects related to cognition and motor function.
• Do not drink alcohol while taking this medication.
• Drink plenty of fluids and use hard candy or gum for dry mouth.
• If insomnia persists, report to the health care provider managing the medication.
• If sexual side effects persist, contact the health care provider to discuss.

ANTIHISTAMINES

Two antihistamines have been helpful in the treatment of anxiety. These are diphenhydramine (Benadryl) and hydroxyzine (Atarax, Vistaril). Generally, these medications are not as effective as the benzodiazepines, but they may provide some relief. Antihistamines cause sedation, which may provide temporary relief from anxiety. They are not habit-forming, nor can one become physically dependent on them. They do, however, lower the seizure threshold and therefore may be contraindicated in patients with a history of seizure disorders. The usual dose of diphenhydramine is 25 to 50 mg qid. The usual dose of hydroxyzine is 50 to 100 mg qid.

Non-Benzodiazepine Anxiolytics

A single non-benzodiazepine medication available for the treatment of anxiety is Buspirone (BuSpar). Buspirone is a potent anti-anxiety agent without addictive potential. Buspirone is an effective anxiolytic that does not have muscle relaxant or anticonvulsant activity. It is considered safe because it does not interact with other CNS acting drugs, has no sedative-hypnotic properties, and is not a significant CNS depressant. Usual daily adult dose is 20 to 30 mg in divided doses.

Actions and Uses

Buspirone is effective in the treatment of anxiety, but not of panic. Its onset of action is very gradual, usually taking several weeks to reach its maximal potential. It is appealing because of its nonaddictive potential; however, it does take time to work and requires that the patient can tolerate waiting some time for relief.

Side and Adverse Effects

Dizziness, drowsiness, and nausea have been reported by patients taking buspirone. No physical dependence has been reported.

Interactions and Contraindications

These drugs are contraindicated in the concomitant administration of MAOIs.

Nursing Actions

Assess baseline anxiety and assess for changes in level of anxiety. Observe for any side effects, report, and document. Monitor for vertigo. Have the patient monitor dizziness and avoid operating hazardous machinery and driving until vertigo subsides.

Patient Teaching

- This medication does not relive anxiety immediately and does not work in the same way as other anti-anxiety medications. The full effect is not expected until 4 weeks or more of therapy.
- Use relaxation techniques, deep breathing exercises, and other coping strategies to manage stress and anxiety.

REFERENCES

American Psychiatric Association (1994). *Diagnostic and Statistical Manual of Mental Disorders* (4th ed.). Washington, D.C.: Author.

Laraia, M.T. (1998). "Psychopharmacology." In Stuart, G.W., & Laraia, M.T. (Eds.) *Principles and Practices of Psychiatric Nursing* (6th ed.). St. Louis: Mosby, pp. 571–603.

Laraia, M.T., and Stuart, G.W. (1995). *Quick Psychopharmacology Reference*. St. Louis: Mosby.

Trevor, A.J., and Way, W.L. (1998). "Sedative and Hypnotic Drugs." In Katzung, B.G. (Ed.). *Basic and Clinical Pharmacology*. Stamford, CT: Appleton & Lange, pp. 354–371.

CHAPTER 51

NEUROLEPTICS/ANTIPSYCHOTICS

*N*euroleptics, also known as *antipsychotics*, are a class of drugs designed to treat patients suffering from psychotic symptoms such as auditory and visual hallucinations, delusions, bizarre behaviors (called *positive symptoms*) and other significant alterations in thought process, as well as the so-called *negative symptoms* such as a decrease or loss of normal function, limited range and intensity of emotional expression (flat affect), restricted thought and speech (alogia), lack of initiation of goal-directed behavior (avolition/apathy), inability to experience pleasure or to maintain social contacts (anhedonia/asociality) and attentional impairment (Moller & Murphy, 1998).

In recent years, newer neuroleptics (called *atypicals*) have been developed that are especially good at treating the negative symptoms of schizophrenia as well as the positive symptoms. Older neuroleptics were primarily effective in treating only positive symptoms.

Neuroleptic medications are used in the treatment of psychiatric disorders in which psychosis is present. Patients with a psychotic illness have significantly altered thought processes; however, patients with a severe mood disorder may also have psychotic features. The following psychotic disorders are usually associated with psychotic (altered) thought process:

1. Schizophrenia
2. Schizophreniform disorder
3. Schizoaffective disorder
4. Delusional disorder
5. Brief psychotic disorder
6. Shared psychotic disorder
7. Psychotic disorder due to a general medical condition
8. Substance-induced psychotic disorder
9. Psychotic disorder not otherwise specified

As mentioned, some patients with severe mood disorders may also have psychotic features, in which case a neuroleptic might be ordered. These disorders are as follows:

1. Major depressive disorders, severe, with psychotic features
2. Bipolar I disorders with psychotic features
3. Bipolar II disorders with psychotic features

NEUROLEPTICS

As with other psychotropic drugs, neuroleptics have their effects on neurotransmitters. With neuroleptics, the primary neurotransmitter involved is dopamine. It is felt that the primary effect of neuroleptics results from the blockade of dopamine in two systems of the brain, the mesolimbic and the mesofrontal systems. (Potter & Hollister, 1998). Thus we think about neuroleptics as decreasing the effects of dopamine in the central nervous system. Neuroleptics do, however, have an effect on other neurotransmitters. Because of this, many side effects may result. Side effects and adverse reactions will be discussed later in this chapter.

Actions and Uses

There are four major categories of neuroleptics: phenothiazine derivatives, thioxanthene derivatives, butyrophenone derivatives, and the miscellaneous structures (atypicals). The main differences in these four categories involve potency, dose, likelihood of side effects, effects on positive symptoms, and effects on negative symptoms. The newer neuroleptics (atypicals) are particularly useful in treating patients with both negative and positive symptoms and tend to have less dangerous side effects. As mentioned, neuroleptics are used to decrease psychotic symptoms.

Some neuroleptics are "high potency–low dose" and some are "low potency–high dose." High-potency drugs are usually effective at much lower doses than the low-potency drugs. Therefore it may be helpful to remember which drugs are high potency and which drugs are low potency. Note that high potency–low dose drugs are more likely to cause cardiovascular side effects than high dose–low potency drugs. Orthostatic hypotension (a decrease in blood pressure when one changes from a lying position to an upright position) is one such effect. Although orthostatic hypotension can occur with any neuroleptic, it may occur more frequently, or more severely with high potency–low dose neuroleptic drugs.

See Table 51–1 for a list of neuroleptic categories, drug names, usual adult dosage, and preparations.

TABLE 51-1

Neuroleptic Drugs

Generic Name (Trade Name)	Drug Dosage: Equivalence (mg)	Usual Adult Dosage Range (mg/day)	Preparations
Phenothiazines			
Chlorpromazine (Thorazine)	100	100–1000	PO, IM, L
Thioridazine (Mellaril)	100	100–800*	PO, L
Mesoridazine (Serentil)	50	50–400	PO, IM, L
Perphenazine (Trilafon)	10	8–64	PO, IM, L
Trifluoperazine (Stelazine)	5	5–60	PO, IM, L
Fluphenazine (Prolixin)	4	2–60	PO, IM, L L-A
Thioxanthene			
Thiothixene (Navane)	5	2–120	PO, IM, L
Butyrophenone			
Haloperidol (Haldol)	4	2–100	PO, IM, L, L-A
Dibenzoxazepine			
Loxapine (Loxitane)	10	20–160	PO, IM, L
Dihydroindolone			
Molindone (Moban)	10	10–225	PO, L
Atypical Antipsychotics			
Clozapine (Clozaril)	50	10–600	PO
Risperidone (Risperdal)	1	1–6	PO
Olanzapine (Zyprexa)	2	5–20	PO

*Upper limit to avoid retinopathy

IM, Intramuscular; L, oral liquid, concentrate, suspension, or elixir; LA, Long-acting injectable preparations; PO, oral tablet or capsule.

Adapted from Stuart, G., & Laraia, M. (1998). *Principles and Practice of Psychiatric Nursing*, 6th ed. St. Louis: Mosby.

OTHER USES OF NEUROLEPTICS

In addition to the use of neuroleptics to treat psychotic symptoms, certain neuroleptics may be used for other purposes. Some of the older neuroleptics are effective in the treatment of nausea and vomiting. One neuroleptic commonly used for the treatment of nausea and vomiting is prochlorperazine (Compazine). It is mentioned here because this drug may cause the same side effects or adverse reactions as other neuroleptics. Patients receiving this drug should be monitored closely for extrapyramidal side effects, which will be discussed later. Prochlorperazine (Compazine) should not be administered to children. Another use of neuroleptics is in the treatment of intractable hiccoughs after less aggressive treatment has failed.

Persons with Tourette's disorder have also been treated with some success with the neuroleptic haloperidol. This medication is used to treat some symptoms of Tourette's in both adults and children.

Side and Adverse Effects

Side effects of neuroleptics are grouped into several categories. Owing to the complex nature of these side effects, each category will be presented separately. Side effects from neuroleptic medications represent one of the most common

reasons that patients with psychotic thought problems stop taking their medications. The patient's discontinuing these medications without close supervision may result in an acute episode of psychosis. This will be important when teaching patients about their medications.

Extrapyramidal Symptoms

Extrapyramidal side effects (EPS) include Parkinson's syndrome–like movements (involuntary fine motor tremors, cogwheel rigidity), akathisia (uncontrollable restlessness, inability to sit still), and acute dystonic reactions (uncontrollable spastic movements and/or muscle rigidity affecting the head, neck, eyes, and facial area as well as the limbs). Oculogyric crisis may also occur, in which case the eyes will roll upward and to the side (upward lateral gaze).

Patients on neuroleptics must be monitored carefully for these signs and symptoms. Dystonic reactions involving the head and neck may result in a compromise in the patient's airway, making breathing difficult. Be prepared to support respiratory function if this occurs.

Parkinson-like symptoms (dystonia included) can be treated with anticholinergic drugs such as benztropine (Cogentin), trihexyphenidyl (Artane), biperiden (Akineton), and procyclidine (Kemadrin). The antihistamine diphenhydramine (Benadryl) is also helpful in treating EPS. Select benzodiazepines such as diazepam (Valium), lorazepam (Ativan) and clonazepam (Klonopin) are commonly used in the treatment of extrapyramidal symptoms as well. In rare cases amantadine (Symmetrel) may be used. Some Parkinson-like symptoms may gradually subside in some patients over time; however, this is less likely to be the case in elderly patients. Dystonic reactions must be treated at once.

See Table 51–2 for a list of drugs used to treat extrapyramidal side effects of neuroleptics.

TABLE 51–2

Drugs Used to Treat Extrapyramidal Side Effects

Generic Name (Trade Name)	Adult Dosage Range (mg/day)	Preparations
Anticholinergics		
Benztropine (Cogentin)	1–6	PO, IM, IV
Trihexyphenidyl (Artane)	1–10	PO
Biperiden (Akineton)	2–6	PO
Procyclidine (Kemadrin)	6–20	PO
Antihistamines		
Diphenhydramine	25–300	PO, IM, IV
Benzodiazepines		
Diazepam (Valium)	2–6	PO, IV
Lorazepam (Ativan)	0.5–2	PO, IM
Clonazepam (Klonopin)	1–4	PO
Dopamine Agonist		
Amantadine	100–300	PO

Data from: Laraia, M.T. (1998). "Psychopharmacology." In Stuart, G.W., & Laraia, M.T. (Eds.) *Principles & Practice of Psychiatric Nursing (6th ed.).* St. Louis: Mosby.

Neuroleptic Malignant Syndrome

Neuroleptic malignant syndrome (NMS) is the most severe and life-threatening condition that can occur as an adverse reaction the neuroleptic medications. Early detection, discontinuation of the drug, and rapid treatment can prevent death. Neuroleptic malignant syndrome is characterized by fever, tachycardia, diaphoresis (sweating), muscle rigidity, involuntary muscle contractions, "pseudoseizures," elevated white blood cell count, elevated creatinine phosphokinase (CPK) enzymes, and eventually kidney failure. It is absolutely critical for the nurse to assess for and report immediately any of the signs and symptoms described here. Special procedures and medications are used to treat this condition.

Tardive Dyskinesia

Tardive dyskinesia is an extremely serious adverse reaction to a neuroleptic drug that can occur after a patient has been on the drug over an extended period of time. With tardive dyskinesia, the patient exhibits involuntary, bizarre, and repetitive motor movements of the head (face and tongue), extremities, and trunk. Although these bizarre movements usually subside when the patient is asleep, it should be remembered that they are not voluntary and are often very embarrassing to the patient and frightening to others. These effects usually do not present until the patient has been on a neuroleptic drug for more than 6 months. Unfortunately, tardive dyskinesia does not usually resolve, even after the medication has been stopped. See Table 51–3 for a listing of side effects and adverse reactions of neuroleptics.

TABLE 51–3

Side and Adverse Effects of Neuroleptics

Body System/Side Effect	Description/Assessment Priorities
Agranulocytosis	A medical emergency developing quickly with a sudden onset of sore throat, fever, fatigue, and significant decrease in circulating white blood cells—associated with the administration of clozapine
Autonomic nervous system general	Dry mouth, blurred vision, difficulty urinating, constipation, sedation
Cardiovascular	Orthostatic hypotension, elevated resting pulse rates, and ECG changes
Endocrine and sexual function	Amenorrhea, false-positive pregnancy tests, galactorrhea, gynecomastia in males, inability to ejaculate, increased libido in women, decreased libido in men, infertility, impotence, weight gain
Central nervous system:	
Parkinson's syndrome	Fine motor tremors, muscle rigidity, and loss of facial expression
Akathisia	Motor restlessness, inability to sit still, may be accompanied by anxiety
Akinesia	Loss or poverty of movements or temporary paralysis of a muscle
Dystonias	Involuntary muscle spasms/contractions of the head, jaw, face, tongue, neck, and extremities. May occur suddenly, painful and frightening, may result in airway compromise
Oculogyric crisis	Involuntary rolling of the eyes, usually in an upward, lateral movement
Neuroleptic malignant syndrome	A severe, life-threatening adverse reaction involving muscle rigidity, dystonia, akinesia, mutism, obtundation, agitation, seizure-like involuntary movements, fever, sweating, increased pulse and blood pressure; white blood count elevation and kidney failure may occur
Seizures	Generalized seizures may occur in a minority of patients; however, the incidence is slightly higher with clozapine
Skin/eyes	Photosensitivity, allergic dermatitis
Tardive dyskinesia	Delayed adverse effect involving abnormal, involuntary, repetitive, irregular movements, involving the head (tongue & facial muscles), extremities, and trunk; usually irreversible

Seizures

As noted earlier, these drugs may lower the seizure threshold. There is a risk of seizure in patients taking neuroleptics, although it is only about 1%. The risk is slightly increased (5%) in patients taking clozapine (Laraia, 1999).

Agranulocytosis

Agranulocytosis represents a medical emergency. In this side effect, the patient's white blood cell (WBC) count is seriously decreased. Most often, the patient will rapidly develop a fever, sore throat, and fatigue or other signs of infection. These symptoms must be reported and treated at once. This side effect is associated with the neuroleptic clozapine. Persons taking clozapine must have regular blood counts to carefully monitor their WBC count. If there is a significant drop in WBCs, the clozapine must be discontinued.

Photosensitivity

The patient taking neuroleptic drugs may be especially sensitive to the sun. As such, a hat should be worn when the patient is to spend more than brief periods of time out in the sun. The nurse must watch for sunburn, and sunscreen must be used to protect the skin. Further, many patients taking neuroleptics find that their eyes are more sensitive to light. In this case, sunglasses should be worn when out of doors or in very bright light.

Anticholinergic Effects

Anticholinergic effects include dry mouth, blurred vision, constipation, rapid pulse (even when resting), orthostatic hypotension (blood pressure drops when changing from a lying to a sitting or standing position).

Metabolic and Endocrine Effects

Weight gain often occurs in patients taking neuroleptic drugs. Careful nutritional planning and an exercise program tailored to the individual can help with this side effect. Women may experience amenorrhea, galactorrhea, and infertility. Men may experience a loss of libido, impotence, ejaculatory difficulties, and infertility.

Interactions and Contraindications

Neuroleptics have a central nervous system depressant effect. They should be used with caution in patients receiving other central nervous system (CNS) depressants. Use of other CNS depressants may intensify the side effects of neuroleptics. Alcohol should be avoided when patients are taking neuroleptics.

Antacids and systemic agents used to reduce the acidity of stomach contents (e.g., cimetidine) given within 2 hours of neuroleptic administration may interfere with the absorption of the drug. Therefore, these drugs should not be given within 2 hours of the neuroleptic.

As with many other psychotropic drugs (e.g., antidepressants), neuroleptics may lower the seizure threshold in patients. As such, they must be used with extreme caution in patients with a history of seizure disorders or head injury. Lowering the seizure threshold of an individual makes him or her more vulnerable to seizures.

It is not uncommon for neuroleptics to be used in combination with antiparkinsonism agents. Antiparkinsonism agents are used to treat some of the side effects of neuroleptics and will be discussed in further detail below. Patients with allergic reactions to previous treatment with neuroleptics in a particular category may be more vulnerable to an allergic reaction when given another neuroleptic from the same category.

Care should be taken when using neuroleptics in the elderly. The elderly are generally more sensitive to this class of drugs and thus may be more susceptible to potential side effects and adverse reactions. Extreme caution should be used in the administration of neuroleptics in pregnant women.

Nursing Actions

Nursing actions are based on careful baseline and ongoing assessment, monitoring for effective response to medications, patient education, and vigilant monitoring for side effects. A baseline assessment of the patient's history and mental status with particular attention to behavior and thought content, experience of hallucinations, delusions, and other psychotic signs and symptoms must be conducted to have something to compare the patient's progress to after initiation or continuation of neuroleptic medications.

Following the baseline, the nurse should assess the patient at regular intervals for both a therapeutic response to the medication and the appearance of any side effects. Therapeutic responses should be expected as the outcome of treatment, including a decrease in both the positive and negative signs of psychosis. Ongoing assessment for hallucinations, delusions, and other alterations in thought disorder must be noted and documented.

Monitor closely for side effects. Of critical importance are changes in vital signs, fever, sore throat, pain, and muscle tone and abnormal movement. Gross and fine motor movements must be assessed frequently. Fine motor tremors may be a sign of the onset of extrapyramidal signs. Severe motor movement changes such as rigidity, facial grimacing, spasms of muscle groups, restlessness and anxiety, repetitive movements, pacing, and the inability to sit still should be reported and addressed swiftly. The use of PRN (as necessary) medication should follow careful assessment to determine what

side effect the patient is demonstrating. Remember that acute dystonic reactions, neuroleptic malignant syndrome, and agranulocytosis require immediate nursing and medical intervention.

With proper nursing care, neuroleptics can be used safely and effectively in the treatment of persons with psychotic illnesses. Attention must be paid to even minor changes to recognize and take action at the early onset of any side effects. Effective patient teaching will promote better outcomes with less incidence of recurrence of disabling symptoms and rehospitalizations.

Patient Teaching

- Dry mouth, blurred vision and weight gain are common with this type of drug.
- Be sure to maintain adequate hydration.
- Use sugarless gum or hard candy for dry mouth and maintain proper oral hygiene.
- Blurred vision may improve over time.
- Avoid participating in potentially dangerous activities such as driving until the sedation has subsided and vision is adequate.
- Get up slowly out of bed or from a sitting position to a standing position, as orthostatic hypotension may occur.
- It is important to continue the medication(s) under the provider's directions and keep all outpatient appointments.
- Be sure you understand the potential side effects, and report any onset of side effects immediately to your health care provider or another health care provider if yours is not available.

REFERENCES

American Psychiatric Association. (1994). *Diagnostic and Statistical Manual of Mental Disorders* (4th ed.). Author: Washington, DC.

Laraia, M.T. (1998). "Psychopharmacology." In Stuart, G.W., & Laraia, M.T. (Eds.), *Stuart & Sundeen's Principles and Practice of Psychiatric Nursing* (6th ed.). St. Louis: Mosby.

Moller, M.D., & Murphy, M.F. (1998). "Neurobiological Responses and Schizophrenia and Psychotic Disorders." In Stuart, G.W., & Laraia, M.T. (Eds.) *Stuart & Sundeen's Principles and Practice of Psychiatric Nursing* (6th ed.). St. Louis: Mosby.

Potter, W.Z., & Hollister, L.E. (1998). "Antipsychotic Agents and Lithium." In Katzung, B.G. (Ed.). *Basic and Clinical Pharmacology* (7th ed.). Stamford, CT: Appleton & Lange.

ANTIDEPRESSANTS

*T*he antidepressants are a class of drugs used in the treatment of depression as well as certain other conditions. *Depression* is defined as "an abnormal extension or overelaboration of sadness and grief. The word *depression* can denote a variety of phenomena, a sign, symptom, syndrome, emotional state, reaction, disease, or clinical entity" (Stuart & Laraia, 1998, p. 858). Although many people feel sad and blue or "depressed" from time to time, clinical depression involves a significant level of symptoms that can interfere with a person's ability to experience full health and function in their life roles. Antidepressant medication, especially when used in combination with psychotherapy, can be very helpful in managing the signs and symptoms of depression.

The Diagnostic and Statistical Manual of Mental Disorders, 4th ed., lists depressive disorders as disorders of mood. A partial list is offered here.

1. Major depressive disorder(s)

    A.) Single episode

        1.) Mild, moderate, or severe

        2.) If severe, with or without psychotic features

    B.) Recurrent episode

        1.) Mild, moderate, or severe

        2.) If severe, with or without psychotic features

2. Dysthymic disorder

    A.) Lasts at least 2 years

    B.) Lasts at least 1 year in adolescents

3. Depressive disorder not otherwise specified

Persons with these depressive disorders commonly require antidepressant medication to recover. Antidepressants are one of the most commonly prescribed classes of drugs in the United States today.

ANTIDEPRESSANT ACTIONS

Antidepressants work to treat depression by enhancing certain neurotransmitters. You will remember from the introduction to this unit that neurotransmitters are the biochemical transporters that get released from the end of one neuron into the space between the neurons and picked up by the next neuron to facilitate neurotransmission. It is felt that in depression there are insufficient amounts of neurotransmitters available to facilitate adequate signal transmission. Thus, the antidepressants are designed to increase the availability of neurotransmitters at the neurosynaptic junction to allow for proper signal transmission. Each category of antidepressant works in a somewhat different way, but most are involved with the neurotransmitter serotonin. Some antidepressants also affect other neurotransmitters such as norepinephrine. Antidepressant categories and the drugs belonging to those categories are now discussed and are listed in Table 52–1.

SELECTIVE SEROTONIN REUPTAKE INHIBITORS

One of the most recent groups of antidepressants is the selective serotonin reuptake inhibitor group (SSRIs). The SSRIs are a group of antidepressants whose action is to block the reuptake of serotonin. Once a neuron has released its stores of serotonin into the junction between the two neurons, the next neuron captures some of the serotonin at its receptor sites. Next, the first neuron sweeps up the leftover serotonin by way of a mechanism called a *reuptake pump*. Some believe this reuptake pump acts as an off switch, halting neurotransmission and conserving leftover serotonin. In depression, however, there is not enough serotonin in the junction. The SSRI antidepressants block the reuptake pump from sweeping up the remaining serotonin, thus allowing more serotonin to stay in the junctions. Since these drugs selectively target serotonin, they are called *selective serotonin reuptake inhibitors*. These drugs tend to have less serious side effects than older antidepressants and they tend not to be lethal in an overdose.

TRICYCLIC ANTIDEPRESSANTS

Tricyclic antidepressants have been available for almost 40 years, preceding the SSRIs. Drugs in this class block the reuptake of serotonin and the reuptake of norepinephrine. Drugs in this category have been used successfully for many years. However, because they affect norepinephrine, they can cause a number of troublesome and sometimes serious side effects and adverse reactions. An overdose of one of the drugs in this category may result in cardiac electrical conduction problems (dysrhythmias) that can result in death. For this reason, these drugs are not prescribed as often as they once were. Further, while the SSRIs are commonly tolerated in single daily doses, some tricyclics must be given in divided doses.

TETRACYCLICS/OTHER AGENTS

Tetracyclics and other agents are similar in action and effect to the drugs previously listed. Some of these drugs affect specific subtypes of serotonin whereas others affect both serotonin and norepinephrine. Maprotiline (Ludiomil), for example, has the same risk in overdose as do the tricyclics. Some of the drugs in this category tend to be more sedating than others. Refer to Table 52–1 for further information.

MONOAMINE OXIDASE INHIBITORS

Monoamine oxidase inhibitors (MAOIs) are drugs that block the metabolism of norepinephrine, serotonin, and tyramine. By blocking the natural metabolism of these substances, more neurotransmitters become available for signal transmission, as noted earlier in this chapter. These drugs are very powerful, however, and must be used with extreme caution. Because the ability to metabolize tyramine (an amino acid necessary in the production of neurotransmitters) is decreased, if foods high in tyramine are ingested, or if certain other drugs (other antidepressants, cold medications and several others) are ingested while the patient is taking an MAOI, a hypertensive crisis may occur. This is a medical emergency. Special patient and family teaching is necessary regarding the foods and medicines that the patient must avoid. The patient must be counseled not to take any other medications without consulting with the person prescribing the MAOI. For these reasons, and because there are many alternatives to this category of drugs, the MAOIs are seldom used.

TABLE 52–1

Antidepressant Drugs

Drug (Trade Name)	Daily Dose Range (mg)	Considerations
SSRIs		
Citalopram (Celexa)	20–60	SSRIs can be taken once a day, making adherence to a prescribed treatment easier for the patient. SSRIs are not considered cardiotoxic; thus, an overdose is unlikely to cause life-threatening arrhythmias. Besides depression, SSRIs may be useful in panic disorder and obsessive-compulsive disorder. Some patients tolerate the medications in the AM, others in the PM.
Fluoxetine (Prozac)	10–80	
Fluvoxamine (Luvox)	50–300	
Paroxetine (Paxil)	10–60	
Sertraline (Zoloft)	50–200	
Tricyclics		
Amitriptyline (Elavil)	75–150	Tricyclics affect not only serotonin, but also epinephrine/norepinephrine and as such may cause cardiac complications. Severe and life-threatening dysrhythmias may result from an overdose. Side effects may be more problematic in this group of medications than with SSRIs.
Clomipramine (Anafranil)	25–250	
Desipramine (Norpramin)	100–300	
Doxepin (Sinequan)	75–300	
Imipramine (Tofranil)	75–200	Many of these medicines cannot be taken once a day; bid or tid dosing must be used to reach the total daily dose.
Nortriptyline (Pamelor)	75–150	
Trimipramine (Surmontil)	75–200	
Tetracyclics		
Maprotiline (Ludiomil)	75–225	At least as potentially dangerous as tricyclics, significant sedation may occur. May be given in single or divided doses.
Mirtazapine (Remeron)	15–45	
Other Agents		
Bupropion (Wellbutrin)	300–450	Divided doses (increase risk of seizures)
Nefazodone (Serzone)	200–600	Divided doses (sedating)
Trazodone (Desyrel)	50–400	Divided doses > 100 mg (sedative)
Venlafaxine (Effexor)	75–375	Divided doses
MAOIs		Not first-line (first choice) drugs.
Phenelzine (Nardil)	45–90	Strict diet restrictions. Interactions with foods containing tyramine, other antidepressants, and many other drugs can lead to life-threatening hypertensive crisis. Must be given in divided doses.
Tranylcypromine (Parnate)	30–60	

SIDE AND ADVERSE EFFECTS

Not every patient experiences side effects from antidepressants, but all patients should be taught what the common side effects of their medications are in order to recognize and report them should they occur. Some side effects may be troublesome at first (such as a headache and drowsiness or insomnia), but often most side effects lessen as the patient continues on the medication. Other side effects are more worrisome and should be reported so that they can be managed or appropriate changes can be made. When not addressed, side effects that are troublesome and persistent may lead the patient to stop taking the medication. Adherence to medication can become a serious problem.

Specific Category Side and Adverse Effects

Selective serotonin reuptake inhibitors may cause headache, anxiety, insomnia, fine motor tremors, nausea, gastrointestinal upset, diarrhea, rashes, decreased libido, and sexual dysfunction, including anorgasmia and ejaculatory disturbances.

Tricyclic antidepressants are known to cause sleepiness (which may be increased when they are taken with other sedating substances), fine motor tremor, insomnia, dry mouth, blurred vision, constipation, urinary hesitancy, confusion, orthostatic hypotension, cardiac conduction defects, arrhythmias, increased risk of seizures, weight gain, sexual disturbances, and exacerbation of psychotic symptoms.

Monoamine oxidase inhibitors may cause headache, drowsiness, dry mouth, weight gain, postural hypotension, and sexual disturbances. Again, note that if the patient takes a stimulant, or ingests foods with significant levels of tyramine, hypertension may result.

Maprotiline (Ludiomil) may cause all of the side effects of the tricyclics as well as increased risk of seizures that is dose related (the higher the dose, the higher the likelihood of seizures).

Trazodone, nefazodone, and venlafaxine may cause drowsiness, vertigo, confusion, insomnia, asthenia, dry mouth, blurred or altered vision, cardiac conduction changes, constipation, nausea, and agitation. Trazodone can cause priapism, a medical emergency in men in which there is a persistent abnormal erection of the penis, usually without sexual desire. If this condition occurs, medical attention must be provided at once.

Bupropion may cause dry mouth, vertigo, sweating, fine motor tremor, aggravation of psychosis, and a higher potential for seizures than other antidepressants. It should be noted that many of the side effects of one antidepressant may also be a side effect of others in its class. As newer drugs become available, the side effect profiles tend to improve; that is, many newer drugs have fewer side effects than their predecessors do.

INTERACTIONS AND CONTRAINDICATIONS

Occasionally a patient may be placed on more than one antidepressant at a time; however, this approach must be used very cautiously. One risk this presents is that of serotonin syndrome. Serotonin syndrome is characterized by hyperthermia, muscle rigidity, myoclonus, and rapid changes in vital signs. This syndrome constitutes a medical emergency and treatment must be instituted at once. This is especially likely to occur if a patient taking an MAOI is given an SSRI. Patients taking MAOIs should not be started on any other antidepressant until at least a 14-day washout period has been completed. If a patient taking an MAOI has the drug discontinued, generally a 7-day washout period must be completed before starting on another antidepressant.

With the exception of the SSRIs, the antidepressants must be used with extreme caution in patients with concurrent heart problems, especially dysrhythmias. Often an electrocardiogram is desired as a baseline to rule out conduction defects before starting a patient on antidepressants other than SSRIs.

Bupropion is generally contraindicated in patients with a history of head injury, seizure disorder, and eating disorders due to its significant potential to lower the seizure threshold and activate seizures in these patients. It should be noted, however, that all antidepressants might lower the seizure threshold of any individual.

All patients on antidepressants must be cautioned against using alcohol or other drugs (unless prescribed by a physician, advanced practice nurse, or physician's assistant who is aware of which antidepressant the patient is taking), as central nervous system depression may occur. Patients should consult the health care provider who ordered the medication before taking over-the-counter cold and flu medicines.

NURSING ACTIONS

The nurse must assess the patient receiving these medications for therapeutic response. Assess the patient's mood, affect, sleep pattern, anxiety, eating, weight changes, and ability to function at baseline and then regularly throughout the course of treatment. Sometimes it is helpful to ask the patient to keep a log of his or her mood and feelings. This information can then be referred to when assessing the effectiveness of the medication over time.

The nurse should assess the patient for the emergence of any side effects or adverse reactions and report them to the person prescribing the drug. In certain cases, as listed above, adverse reactions must be reported at once. Less threatening side effects can be reported as soon as it is reasonable to do so. Document the patient's response as well as any side effects to the medication.

Dry mouth can be managed by offering fluids and having the patient use sugarless gum or hard candy. Attention to oral hygiene is important. The patient should be warned about getting out of bed (or up from a chair) slowly to avoid dizziness and a potential fall if orthostatic hypotension is experienced. If the drug given is sedating, it may be ordered at bedtime. Assess for daytime sedation and sleepiness. Providing reassurance can be very helpful.

Since some patients being treated with antidepressants have suicidal ideation, the amount of medication dispensed at any one prescription fill or refill should be controlled, to limit the amount that might be ingested in an intentional overdose.

Patient Teaching

- It is very important to take the medication exactly as prescribed.
- Never increase the dose of these medications on your own.
- Do not suddenly discontinue this medication without supervision, as sudden discontinuation may result in very uncomfortable symptoms.
- Learn the potential side effects of the medication you are prescribed and report the emergence of side effects or adverse reactions to the person prescribing the medication.
- Some drugs of this type cause orthostatic hypotension, so use care when moving from a lying to a standing or sitting position.
- Urinary retention is a possibility with some medications. Notify your health care provider if you have difficulty urinating.
- If you are taking an MAOI, then foods containing significant amounts of tyramine must be avoided. These foods include Chianti and vermouth wines, draft beers, banana, aged or mature cheeses, fermented or aged proteins (meats and fish), pickled and smoked fish, yeast and protein extracts, fava beans and broad bean pods, overripe or spoiled fruits, liver, sausage, processed aged meats (pepperoni, salami, canned ham), and sauerkraut.
- Medications that must be avoided include almost any other antidepressant, decongestants or cold medicines containing decongestants, some antihistamines, meperidine (Demerol), many asthma medications, local anesthetics with epinephrine, stimulants of any kind, cocaine, and amphetamines.
- Antidepressants must not be transferred to anyone else for any reason.

- Driving and operating dangerous machinery should be avoided until the exact effects of the medication are known and there is no interference with attention, concentration, judgment, and motor coordination. It is very important that antidepressants be kept in a safe place and out of the reach of children. An overdose of antidepressants can have serious and even fatal consequences.

SUMMARY

Antidepressants can have significant beneficial effects for patients suffering from depression, anxiety, panic disorder, and obsessive-compulsive disorders as well as chronic pain and certain other conditions. These medications can be dangerous if not used exactly as prescribed. Careful ongoing assessment of the patient to monitor for therapeutic response as well as any side effects or adverse reactions is critical. Early intervention is required to manage some side effects as soon as they appear. Less severe side effects can be managed by the nurse and the patient. Patient and family teaching is essential and will facilitate patient adherence to the prescribed regime.

REFERENCES

American Psychiatric Association. (1994). *Diagnostic and Statistical Manual of Mental Disorders* (4th ed.). Author: Washington, DC.

Laraia, M.T. (1998). "Psychopharmacology." In Stuart, G.W., & Laraia, M.T. (Eds.), *Stuart & Sundeen's Principles and Practice of Psychiatric Nursing* (6th ed.). St. Louis: Mosby.

Potter, W.Z., & Hollister, L.E. (1998). "Antidepressant Agents." In Katzung, B.G. (Ed.). *Basic and Clinical Pharmacology* (7th ed.). Stamford, CT : Appleton & Lange.

REVIEW QUESTIONS: UNIT 17

1. Serotonin, epinephrine, norepinephrine, dopamine, and GABA are:

   A. neurotransmitters.

   B. anticholinergics.

   C. depressants.

   D. antipsychotics.

2. The most commonly used anti-anxiety drugs are the:

    A. antihistamines.

    B. barbiturates.

    C. benzodiazepines.

    D. antidepressants.

3. You expect CNS depressants to:

    A. increase respiratory rate.

    B. stimulate mental processes.

    C. impair motor coordination.

    D. cause tachycardia.

4. An advantage of buspirone (BuSpar) over other anti-anxiety agents is that buspirone:

    A. is not a CNS depressant.

    B. is inexpensive.

    C. is a muscle relaxant.

    D. can be taken orally.

5. Cardiovascular side effects are more common with which type of neuroleptic?

    A. High potency–low dose

    B. High dose–low potency

    C. Low potency–high dose

    D. Low potency–low dose

6. Which of the following may be an extrapyramidal drug side effect?

    A. Sedation

    B. Involuntary fine motor tremors

    C. Seizures

    D. Paralysis

7. SSRIs, tricyclics, tetracyclics, and MAOIs are all examples of:

    A. neurotransmitters.

    B. antidepressants.

    C. antibiotics.

    D. anti-anxiety agents.

8. Which of the following should be avoided by a patient who is taking an MAOI?

    A. Fresh vegetables

    B. Apples

    C. Grilled steak

    D. Smoked fish

CALCULATION AND PREPARATION OF DRUG DOSAGES

OBJECTIVES

1. State common household and metric equivalents.

2. Calculate equivalents among different systems of measurement.

3. Identify and interpret the components of a complete drug order.

4. Define common abbreviations used in medication orders.

5. Calculate drug dosages using the same and different systems of measurement.

6. Explain reconstitution and displacement.

7. Describe the measurement of insulin.

8. Calculate drop rates for intravenous infusions.

DOSAGE CALCULATIONS

I. QUICK REVIEW OF MATH SKILLS

FRACTIONS

Definitions: A *fraction* is a way of representing an amount as part of a whole. For example, $\frac{1}{2}$ represents one of two parts of something. If we use a pie to illustrate: the pie would be cut into 2 pieces. One piece of that pie would be $\frac{1}{2}$ of the whole pie.

In a fraction, the top number (in this case = 1) is called the *numerator*. The bottom number in this case = 2) is the *denominator*.

Addition with Like Denominators

1. Add the numerators

2. Put the total of the numerators over the denominator

3. Reduce to lowest terms

    a. If the numerator is larger than the denominator

    b. If both the numerator and the denominator can be evenly divided by a common number

Example: $\frac{1}{3} + \frac{1}{3} = \frac{1+1}{3} = \frac{2}{3}$

Example: $\frac{2}{3} + \frac{1}{3} = \frac{2+1}{3} = \frac{3}{3} = 1$

Example: $\frac{2}{3} + \frac{2}{3} = \frac{2+2}{3} = \frac{4}{3} = 1\frac{1}{3}$

Addition with Different Denominators

1. Find the lowest common denominator (LCD). This is the smallest number that both denominators will go into evenly.

Example: $\frac{2}{3} + \frac{3}{6}$ LCD = 6   (Both 3 and 6 go into 6 evenly)

Example: $\frac{1}{5} + \frac{4}{3}$ LCD = 15   (Both 5 and 3 go into 15 evenly)

2. Convert each denominator to the LCD by dividing the LCD by the denominator and multiplying the result by the numerator.

Example: $\frac{1}{5} + \frac{4}{3}$ LCD = 15

To convert $\frac{1}{5}$ to $\frac{x}{15}$

    a. Divide the LCD (15) by the denominator (5) = 3

    b. Multiply 3 by the numerator (1) = 3

    c. Answer: $\frac{1}{5} = \frac{3}{15}$

To convert $\frac{4}{3}$ to $\frac{x}{15}$

    a. Divide the LCD (15) by the denominator (3) = 5

    b. Multiply 5 times the numerator (4) = 20

    c. Answer: $\frac{4}{3} = \frac{20}{15}$

3. Use the LCD for the denominator and add the numerators

$\frac{3}{15} + \frac{20}{15} = \frac{23}{15}$

4. Reduce to lowest terms

$\frac{23}{15} = 1\frac{8}{15}$

Subtraction with Like Denominators

1. Subtract the numerators

2. Put the difference in the numerators over the denominator

3. Reduce to lowest terms

    a. If numerator is larger than denominator

    b. If both the numerator and the denominator can be evenly divided by a common number

Example: $\dfrac{2}{3} - \dfrac{1}{3} = \dfrac{2-1}{3} = \dfrac{1}{3}$

Subtraction with Different Denominators

1. Find the lowest common denominator (LCD).

2. Convert each denominator to the LCD by dividing the LCD by the denominator, and multiplying the result times the numerator.

Example: $\dfrac{4}{3} - \dfrac{1}{5}$ LCD = 15

To convert $\dfrac{4}{3}$ to $\dfrac{x}{15}$

   a. Divide the LCD (15) by the denominator (3) = 5

   b. Multiply 5 by the numerator (4) = 20

   c. Answer: $\dfrac{4}{3} = \dfrac{20}{15}$

To convert $\dfrac{1}{5}$ to $\dfrac{x}{15}$

   a. Divide the LCD (15) by the denominator (5) = 3

   b. Multiply 3 by the numerator (1) = 3

   c. Answer: $\dfrac{1}{5} = \dfrac{3}{15}$

3. Use the LCD for the denominator and subtract the numerators

$\dfrac{20}{15} - \dfrac{3}{15} = \dfrac{17}{15}$

4. Reduce to lowest terms

$\dfrac{17}{15} = 1\frac{2}{15}$

Multiplication of Fractions

1. Multiply the numerators

2. Multiply the denominators

3. Reduce to lowest terms

Example: $\dfrac{4}{3} \times \dfrac{1}{5} = \dfrac{4 \times 1}{3 \times 5} = \dfrac{4}{15}$

Division of Fractions

Terms used in division are dividend and divisor. The *dividend* is divided by the *divisor*. For example, 12 ÷ 2 = 6. 12 is the dividend and 2 is the divisor.

1. Invert the numerator and the denominator in the divisor

2. Multiply the numerators

3. Multiply the denominators

4. Reduce to lowest terms

Example: $\dfrac{4}{5} \div \dfrac{2}{3} = \dfrac{4}{5} \times \dfrac{3}{2} = \dfrac{4 \times 3}{5 \times 2} = \dfrac{12}{10} = 1\frac{2}{10} = 1\frac{1}{5}$

DECIMALS

A decimal is a way of writing a fraction that has a denominator which is a multiple of 10. Instead of actually writing a denominator as in a fraction, the denominator is indicated by the number of places from the left of the number to the decimal point.

For example, .9 has only one number (one place) right of the decimal. Therefore, we know that .9 represents $\frac{9}{10}$.

With .09, there are two places right of the decimal point. This represents $\frac{9}{100}$.

With .009, there are three places right of the decimal point. This represents $\frac{9}{1000}$.

You can convert fractions to decimals by dividing the numerator by the denominator.

Example: $\dfrac{1}{2} = 1.00 \div 2 = .50$

Adding Decimals

1. List the numbers to be added so that the decimal points are in line

2. Add the numbers to find the sum of the numbers

3. Place the decimal in the sum (total) in the same position as in the line of numbers being added

Example:
```
   1.50
   2.63
   3.02
   6.00
 ------
  13.15
```

Subtracting Decimals

1. Line up the numbers so the decimals are aligned

2. Subtract

3. Place the decimal in the number in the answer in the same position as in the numbers in the problem

Example:
```
   2.63
 - 1.50
 ------
   1.13
```

Multiplying Decimals

1. Multiply the numbers in the usual way

2. Count the number of places to the right of the decimals in the multiplier AND the multiplicand

3. Counting from the right end of the product, use the total number of places to locate the decimal in the product

Example: 2.63 (2 decimal places) **Multiplicand**
$\times$ 1.51 (2 decimal places) **Multiplier**
263
1315
263
3.9713 (4 decimal places) **Product**

Dividing Decimals

1. The divisor must be converted to a whole number by moving the decimal point to the right end of the number

2. Move the decimal point the same number of places to the right in the dividend

3. Divide in the usual way

4. Place the decimal in the answer directly above the decimal in the dividend

Example: 1.50 divided by .60 =
.60 = 60   (decimal moved 2 places to the right to make whole number)
1.50 = 150 (decimal moved 2 places to the right)

$$\begin{array}{r} 2.5 \text{ \textbf{quotient}} \\ \textbf{divisor} \quad 60/150.0 \text{ \textbf{dividend}} \\ \underline{120} \\ 300 \\ \underline{300} \\ 0 \end{array}$$

RATIO AND PROPORTION

A *ratio* represents the relationship between two numbers. The two numbers in a ratio are separated by a colon. To illustrate, a class has 7 students with 5 women and 2 men. The ratio of women to men is 5 to 2. This ratio would be written 5:2. If the class had 14 students with 10 women and 4 men, the ratio would be 10:4. This can be reduced to 5:2.

A *proportion* is two ratios that are equal in value. For example, 1:2 has the same value as 2:4. The two ratios in a proportion are separated by two colons. So, a proportion using the ratios just given would be written as 1:2::2:4.

Ratio and proportion are used to solve problems when one number in a proportion is unknown. It is useful when you need to convert between different systems of measurement and to determine the amounts of drugs to prepare in order to administer the prescribed dosage.

The unknown number in a proportion is represented by "X." For example: 1:X::2:4.

Because we know the other three numbers in the proportion, we can find the value of "X."

The problem can be set up two ways, but the basic mathematical operation is the same.

1. You multiply the means by the extremes. The *means* are the two numbers in the center of the proportion; the *extremes* are on either end of the proportion.

   So, in 1:X::2:4, the means are X and 2. The extremes are 1 and 4.

   a. Multiply the means

   b. Multiply the extremes

   c. Write: the product of the means equals the product of the extremes

   d. Find the value of one X

Example: You can set the problem up in a linear format like this:

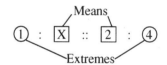

   a. X times 2 = 2X

   b. 1 times 4 = 4

   c. 2X = 4

   d. To find the value of one X, divide each side of the equation by 2.

$$\frac{2X}{2} = \frac{4}{2} \quad X = \frac{4}{2} \quad X = 2$$

2. Another way to set up the problem is:

   a. Convert the ratios to fractions by placing the first number in each ratio over the second number in that ratio

   b. Cross-multiply

   c. Solve for one X

Example:

   a. $\dfrac{1}{X} = \dfrac{2}{4}$

   b. X $\times$ 2 = 2X;   1 $\times$ 4 = 4
      2X = 4

   c. $\dfrac{2X}{2} = \dfrac{4}{2}$ $X = \dfrac{4}{2}$ $X = 2$

This chapter will use the second format for solving ratio and proportion problems. However, use whichever format you like.

II. SYSTEMS OF MEASUREMENT

METRIC SYSTEM

The metric system defines standardized units of measurement based on multiples or divisions of 10. Drug dosages and physician's drug orders commonly use the metric system.

Liquid Measurement

The basic unit of measure of liquids is the *liter*. A liter can be divided into 1000 equal portions called *milliliters* (mL). A cubic centimeter (cc) is the same as a milliliter.

Weight Measurement

The basic unit of measure of solids is the *gram* (g). One thousand grams is a *kilogram* (kg). A gram can be divided into 1000 equal portions called *milligrams* (mg). A milligram can be divided into 1000 equal portions called *micrograms* (µg).

The equivalents below are commonly used. You should memorize them:

1 L = 1000 mL
1000 g = 1 kg
1 g = 1000 mg
1000 µg = 1 mg

When using the metric system, remember the following:

1. Use Arabic numbers (1, 2, 3, etc.) rather than Roman numerals (I, IV, etc.)

2. Write the number first, then the unit of measure

3. Use decimals to express values less than a whole number

Converting Within the Metric System

When converting grams to milligrams, or liters to milliliters, just multiply the grams or liters by 1000 or move the decimal 3 places to the right.

Example: 3 g × 1000 = 3000 mg
4 L × 1000 = 4000 mL

When converting milligrams to grams or milliliters to liters, divide by 1000, or just move the decimal 3 places to the left.

Example: 1500 mg ÷ 1000 = 1.5 g
2000 mL ÷ 1000 = 2 L

It is also easy to convert numbers from one unit of measure to another in the metric system using ratio and proportion. For example, if you wish to convert 300 mg to grams:

1. Start with the known equivalent. In this case, 1 g = 1000 mg

2. State your unknown equivalent. 300 mg = X g

3. Write the proportion: $\dfrac{1000 \text{ mg}}{1 \text{ g}} = \dfrac{300 \text{ mg}}{X \text{ g}}$

4. Cross multiply: 1000X = 300

5. Find the value of one X: $\dfrac{1000X}{1000} = \dfrac{300}{1000}$

    X = .3

    Answer: 300 mg = .3 g

APOTHECARIES SYSTEM OF MEASUREMENT

The apothecaries system of measurement was used more in the past in relation to drugs than it is now. However, since it is still used by some physicians in drug orders, you must be familiar with the most common units of this system. Most often, you will convert apothecary measurements into the metric system in order to calculate dosages.

Volume

Apothecary measurements for liquids are called measures of volume. The units used to measure volume are minims, fluid drams, ounces, pints, quarts, and gallons. Volume equivalents include:

60 minims = 1 fluid dram
8 fluid drams = 1 ounce
16 ounces = 1 pint
32 ounces = 1 quart
4 quarts = 1 gallon

Weight

Apothecary measurements for solids are called measures of weight. The units used to measure weight are grains, drams, ounces, and pounds. Weight equivalents include:

60 grains = 1 dram
12 ounces = 1 pound (note this is different from the 16 ounces to a pound that we most often use)

HOUSEHOLD SYSTEM OF MEASUREMENT

Household measurements are not precise enough to use when measuring drugs because there is no standardization in the measuring devices. Nevertheless, you need to be

TABLE 53-1

Equivalents Among Systems of Measurement

Household	Apothecary	Metric
teaspoon	1 dram	4–5 mL
tablespoon	$\frac{1}{2}$ ounce	15 mL
glass/cup	8 ounces	240 mL
	1 ounce	30 mL
	1 grain	60 or 65 mg
	2.2 lbs	1 kg
	16 minims	1 mL
	15 grains	1 g

able to convert household measures into the metric measures. Household measurement equivalents are noted in Table 53–1.

EQUIVALENTS AMONG SYSTEMS OF MEASUREMENT

Sometimes the drug order and the available drug dose are in different systems of measurement. For example, the physician might order $\frac{1}{4}$ grain of codeine, but the drug label notes each tablet contains 15 mg of codeine. In this case you will need to convert the grains to milligrams in order to select the correct number of tablets. Unfortunately, equivalents among the systems of measurement are not exact. However, the most commonly used equivalent that you will need to remember is:

60 mg = 1 grain

To convert among systems of measurement, use the ratio and proportion approach. To illustrate, if you need to give $\frac{1}{4}$ grain of codeine and you have codeine tablets labeled 15 mg, covert the grains to milligrams.

Known equivalent: 1 grain = 60 mg
Unknown equivalent: $\frac{1}{4}$ grain = X mg
Proportion: $1:60::\frac{1}{4}:X$

$$\frac{1}{60} = \frac{\frac{1}{4}}{X} \quad 1(X) = 60(\tfrac{1}{4}) \quad X = 15$$

$\frac{1}{4}$ grain = 15 mg

III. INTERPRETING DRUG ORDERS

Nurses administer drugs based on legal orders written by physicians and others, including some nurse practitioners who meet state requirements for prescribing drugs.

The components of a complete drug order are:

• Name of the drug
• Dosage (amount) of the drug
• Route of administration

• Frequency of administration
• Special instructions

Examples: Amoxicillin 250 mg PO q 6 h.
Maalox 30 mL PO q 4 h while awake.
Pipracil 1.5 g IM stat.

Drug orders are typically written in a shorthand fashion using a variety of abbreviations. It is your responsibility to understand common abbreviations. If you encounter one you do not know, look it up before proceeding (Table 53–2).

Table 53-2

Common Abbreviations

Units of Measure	Routes of Administration
cc = cubic centimeter	AD = right ear
dr = dram	AS = left ear
Gm, gm, g, G = gram	AU = both ears
gr = grain	ID = intradermal
gtt, gtts = drop(s)	IM = intramuscular
kg = kilogram	IV = intravenous
L = liter	IV push, IVP = intravenous push/bolus
lb = pound	IVPB = intravenous piggyback
mEq = milliequivalent	OD = right eye
mg = milligram	OS = left eye
mL = milliliter	OU = both eyes
m, min = minim	PO, per os = by mouth
mg, mcg = microgram	R = rectal
oz = ounce	SQ, subq, subc = subcutaneous
T, tbsp = tablespoon	SL, subl = sublingual
tsp, t = teaspoon	vag = vaginal
U, u = unit	

Drug Forms

caps, cap = capsule(s)
elix = elixir
fl, fld = fluid
supp = suppository
syr = syrup
tab, tabs = tablet(s)
tinct = tincture
ung = ointment

Schedules

ac = before meals
ad lib = as desired
AM, am = morning
bid = twice daily
d = day
h, hr = hour
HS, hs = at bedtime (hour of sleep)
n, noc, noct = night
pc = after meals
PRN = as needed
q = every
qd = every day
qod = every other day
qh = every hour
q2h = every 2 hours
q6h = every 6 hours
qid = four times daily
stat = immediately
tid = three times daily

Other

$\overline{aa}$ = each
$\overline{c}$ = with
DC, disc = discontinue
KVO, TKO = keep vein open
NPO = nothing by mouth
OTC = over the counter
per = by means of
Rx = take
$\overline{s}$ = without
$\overline{ss}$ = one half

IV. CALCULATING DOSAGES

SAME SYSTEM OF MEASUREMENT

When a drug order and the available form of the drug are in the same system of measurement, you simply use ratio and proportion to determine the number or volume of the drug to administer.

Example:
Order: Isordil 20 mg PO q 6 h
Available: Isordil 10 mg tabs
How many tablets should you give?
Solution: The order and the available drug are both in milligrams (mg), so no conversion is necessary.

1. Identify the known and the unknown ratios
    a. Known ratio: 1 Isordil tablet = 10 mg
    b. Unknown ratio: X Isordil tablet(s) = 20 mg

2. Set up the proportion
    10 mg:1 tab::20 mg:X tabs
    OR

    $$\frac{10 \text{ mg}}{1 \text{ tab}} = \frac{20 \text{ mg}}{\text{X tabs}}$$

3. Cross-multiply
    a. $10 \times X = 10X$
    b. $1 \times 20 = 20$
    c. The two products are equal: $10X = 20$
4. Solve for X: $\dfrac{10X}{10} = \dfrac{20}{10}$ $X = \dfrac{20}{10}$

    X = 2 tablets

Example:
Order: Amoxicillin oral suspension 250 mg PO q 6 h
Available: Amoxicillin oral suspension 125 mg/5 mL
How many mL should you give?
1. Known and unknown ratios
    a. Known ratio: 125 mg = 5 mL
    b. Unknown ratio: 250 mg = X mL
2. Proportion: $\dfrac{125 \text{ mg}}{5 \text{ mL}} = \dfrac{250 \text{ mg}}{\text{X mL}}$

3. Cross-multiply: $125(X) = 250(5)$
    $$125X = 1250$$

4. Solve for X: $\dfrac{125X}{125} = \dfrac{1250}{125}$

    X = 10 mL

DIFFERENT SYSTEMS OF MEASUREMENT

If the drug order is written using a system of measurement that is different from the available form of the drug, you must convert them to the same system of measurement before you can calculate the dosage. It is suggested that you convert apothecary and household measurements into metric measurements.

Example:
Order: Codeine gr $\frac{1}{2}$ PO prn q 3 h for pain
Available: Codeine phosphate tablets 15 mg
How many tablet(s) should you give?

Solution:
1. Convert grains to milligrams
    a. Set up a ratio using the known equivalent of grains and milligrams
        60 mg = gr 1
    b. Set up a ratio to represent the unknown equivalent
        X mg = gr $\frac{1}{2}$
    c. Set up a proportion with the two ratios
        $$\frac{60 \text{ mg}}{\text{gr } 1} = \frac{\text{X mg}}{\text{gr } \frac{1}{2}}$$
    d. Cross-multiply
        $1 \times X = 1X$
        $60 \times \frac{1}{2} = 30$
    e. The two products are equal: $X = 30$
    f. You have determined that 30 mg is equal to $\frac{1}{2}$ grain.

2. Determine how many tablets to give
    a. Identify the known and the unknown ratios
        i. Known ratio: 1 codeine tablet = 15 mg
        ii. Unknown ratio: X codeine tablet(s) = 30 mg
3. Set up the proportion
    15 mg:1 tab::30 mg:X tabs
    $$\frac{15 \text{ mg}}{1 \text{ tab}} = \frac{30 \text{ mg}}{X \text{ tabs}}$$
4. Cross-multiply
    $15 \times X = 15X$
    $1 \times 30 = 30$
5. The two products are equal: $15X = 30$
6. Find the value of one X
    $$\frac{15X}{15} = \frac{30}{15} \quad X = \frac{30}{15} \quad X = 2 \text{ tablets}$$

V. RECONSTITUTION

Some drugs are supplied in a vial in powdered or crystalline form that must be *reconstituted* (dissolved in liquid) for administration. The manufacturer provides information about the appropriate reconstitution of each drug that includes the following:

- Type of diluent (solvent): sterile water for injection, bacteriostatic water for injection, 0.9% sodium chloride injection, or other specified solution.
- Volume of diluent: directions vary depending on the route of administration and the dose.
- Shelf life: how long the medication can be used after reconstitution.
- Storage; whether the drug should be refrigerated or stored at room temperature.

DISPLACEMENT

Let's say you have added 5 mL of diluent to a vial of penicillin. If you were to use your syringe to withdraw all the contents of the vial, it would measure more than 5 mL. The increased volume that is contributed by the dissolved powder is called *displacement.* Directions for use usually provide all the information you need to calculate your dosage. Typical directions for reconstituting a vial of an antibiotic that contains 1,000,000 units might be: Add 3.5 mL Bacteriostatic Water for Injection to yield a solution of 250,000 units per mL.

In the example just given, see if you can calculate the displacement. If each mL contains 250,000 units, there would be 4 mL of reconstituted solution (1,000,000 divided by 250,000 = 4). You only put 3.5 mL of water in the vial, so how much volume was added by the powder? 4 mL − 3.5 mL = 0.5 mL. The displacement was 0.5 mL.

What if the manufacturer just told you how much diluent to add, but did not tell you the final dilution? Suppose you were directed only to add 3.5 mL to a vial containing 1,000,000 units. The order was to give 500,000 units. To give an accurate dose, you could:

1. Add the 3.5 mL of diluent to the vial
2. Withdraw the total amount of the solution from the vial with a syringe to measure the total volume. In our example, it would be 4 mL.
3. Knowing that 4 mL = 1,000,000 units, calculate the volume needed to give 500,000 units.

$$\frac{4 \text{ mL}}{1,000,000 \text{ U}} = \frac{X \text{ mL}}{500,000 \text{ U}}$$

$1,000,000(X) = 4(500,000)$
$1,000,000X = 2,000,000$
$$\frac{1,000,000X}{1,000,000} = \frac{2,000,000}{1,000,000}$$
$X = 2 \text{ mL}$

VI. INSULIN ADMINISTRATION

People with diabetes mellitus produce insufficient insulin or are unable to use insulin normally for glucose metabolism. They may require insulin injections for normal metabolism. Insulin may be given at a fixed dosage several times a day, or the dosage may be adjusted on the basis of the patient's blood glucose reading.

When giving insulin, it is critical to select the correct insulin, syringe, and route of administration.

INSULIN

Insulin is classified by source, type, and strength in units. Insulin is classified as human, pork, or beef depending on the source. There are various brand names, but all are classified by type as rapid-acting (regular), intermediate action (NPH, Lente), and long acting (Ultralente).

It is common for patients to receive combinations of types of insulin mixed in a single injection. Commercially prepared mixtures of regular and NPH are available in limited proportions, typically 30% regular and 70% NPH or 50% regular and 50% NPH. If the patient's order calls for a different proportion of insulin types, you will have to mix them yourself.

Insulin is measured in units. It comes in 10 mL vials. The most common dosage is 100 units per mL (called U-100). Though not commonly used, a concentration of 500 units per mL is available. It is called Regular (Concentrated) Iletin.

INSULIN SYRINGES

Special syringes should be used to administer insulin. Insulin syringes include ones that hold 100 units, 50 units, 30 units, and 25 units. For most accurate measurement, the smallest available insulin syringe that will hold the

prescribed dose should be used. You must be very careful to read the markings on the syringe correctly. In some, each mark represents one unit. In others, each mark represents two units.

FIGURE 53–1

Insulin Syringes

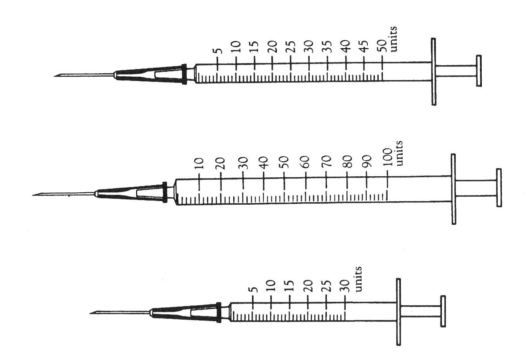

ROUTES OF ADMINISTRATION

Insulin is most commonly given subcutaneously. Some patients have programmable insulin pumps that deliver doses of insulin based on preset times and doses. In some situations, it is given intravenously. Only REGULAR insulin is given intravenously.

SLIDING SCALE

When each insulin dose is based on blood glucose, the patient is said to be on a *sliding scale*. Sliding scales are individualized for each patient. Blood glucose levels are measured and the patient's insulin dose is based on the blood glucose level. An example of a sliding scale follows:

Blood Glucose (mg/dL)	Regular Insulin
< 151	0
151–200	5 units
201–240	8 units
241–280	11 units
281–330	14 units
> 330	Notify M.D.

In this example, if the patient's blood glucose were 210, the insulin dose would be 8 units of regular insulin.

MIXING INSULIN

When you need to give two types of insulin at the same time, you can combine them in one syringe to avoid subjecting the patient to two needlesticks. Mixtures are typically combinations of regular and NPH insulins. Remember that regular insulin is clear, and NPH insulin is cloudy. The rule of thumb is "clear to cloudy," meaning you draw up the regular (clear) first, then the NPH (cloudy) as described below.

Suppose you had an order for 15 units of regular and 10 units of NPH insulin:

1. Select vials of regular and NPH as ordered.
2. Cleanse the tops of both vials with alcohol swabs.
3. Draw up 10 units of air in your syringe and inject the air into the NPH vial.
4. Draw up 15 units of air in your syringe and inject the air into the regular vial.
5. Withdraw 15 units of regular insulin.
6. Invert the NPH insulin vial and insert the needle of the syringe that already contains the regular insulin.
7. Be careful not to inject the regular insulin into the NPH vial.
8. Pressure in the NPH vial should allow you to easily withdraw 10 units of NPH.
9. Do not overfill the syringe; you cannot return excess NPH back into the vial because it is mixed with regular.
10. Check to be sure the total is (in this case) 25 units.
11. Administer the insulin.

VII. INTRAVENOUS DRUG THERAPY

The intravenous route is commonly used to administer drugs, especially antimicrobials and emergency drugs. Intravenous drugs may be given IV push or IV piggyback.

- *IV push* means the drug is injected directly into a venous access device—either through an intermittent infusion device or through a port on an established intravenous line. Drugs given IV push are usually small in volume.
- *IV piggyback* means the drug is administered at a set infusion rate through a port on an established intravenous line. IV piggyback is usually used when drugs are diluted in larger volumes of fluid, commonly 50 to 100 mL.

Your Nurse Practice Act and agency policies define what you are permitted to do in relation to intravenous therapy. It is critical that you know your limitations in terms of administering or monitoring the administration of intravenous drugs. You must be especially careful when administering intravenous drugs because the effects may occur immediately. Guidelines for intravenous drugs are as follows:

1. **Dose.** Be absolutely certain you have prepared the correct dose.
2. **Preparation.** Be sure to select a preparation intended for intravenous administration.
3. **Dilution.** Be sure the drug is properly diluted before administration.
4. **Rate.** Consult drug literature to determine how slowly the drug must be given. Rapid infusion of some drugs can have fatal consequences.

MANUAL REGULATION OF INFUSION RATES

Intravenous infusion sets have a drip chamber and a clamp on the tubing that allow control of the flow rate. You must calculate the number of drops per minute that will deliver the fluid at the desired rate. To do this, you must know the *drop factor:* how many drops equal one milliliter. *Macro* droppers deliver 10, 15, or 20 drops per milliliter. Check the box in which the tubing comes to see the drop factor for the brand you are using. *Micro* droppers deliver 60 drops per milliliter.

To calculate drop rate for a specific drug, follow these steps:

1. Calculate how many milliliters should be given in 1 hour. Divide the total amount of fluid ordered by the number of hours specified. If the order is stated in mL/hour, this is unnecessary.
2. Calculate how many drops should be given in 1 hour. Multiply the number of milliliters to be given each hour by the drop factor in the delivery set you are using.
3. Calculate how many drops should be given in 1 minute. Divide the number of drops per hour by 60 to find out how many drops should be given in 1 minute.

If you prefer to use a formula, you can calculate the flow rate this way:

$$\frac{\text{Fluid volume to be infused} \times \text{Number of drops per mL with selected infusion set}}{\text{Time in minutes}} = \text{Drops per minute}$$

Example:
Order: cephalothin sodium (Keflin) 500 mg in 100 mL 5% dextrose in water per IV piggyback q 8 h. Infuse over 1 hour. Equipment drop factor is 10.

1. Number of mL per hour: 100 mL as ordered
2. Number of drops in 1 hour: 100 mL x 10 = 1000 drops per hour
3. Number of drops per minute: 1000 divided by 60 = 16.6 = 17 drops per minute

PRACTICE PROBLEMS

Basic Math Review

1. $\dfrac{2}{7} + \dfrac{3}{7} =$

2. $\dfrac{3}{5} + \dfrac{1}{5} + \dfrac{2}{5} =$

3. $\dfrac{2}{5} + \dfrac{3}{10} =$

4. $\dfrac{1}{3} + \dfrac{4}{6} + \dfrac{7}{12} =$

5. $\dfrac{5}{9} - \dfrac{2}{9} =$

6. $\dfrac{5}{6} - \dfrac{3}{8} =$

7. $\dfrac{1}{9} \times \dfrac{2}{3} =$

8. $\dfrac{3}{5} \times \dfrac{1}{2} =$

9. $\dfrac{7}{10} \div \dfrac{3}{4} =$

10. $\dfrac{5}{6} \div \dfrac{2}{9} =$

11. $2.3 + 1.6 =$

12. $12.13 + 56 + 0.12 =$

13. $13.6 - 5.3 =$

14. $2.54 - 1.2 =$

15. $16.78 \times 3.2 =$

16. $3.04 \times .004 =$

17. $157.8 \div 52.6 =$

18. $.125 \div .06 =$

Ratio and Proportion

1. Write as ratios:

    a. $\dfrac{1}{2}$

    b. $\dfrac{2}{3}$

    c. $\dfrac{6}{10}$

2. Write these sets of fractions as a proportion:

    a. $\dfrac{1}{2}, \dfrac{2}{4}$

    b. $\dfrac{9}{10}, \dfrac{90}{100}$

    c. $\dfrac{5}{25}, \dfrac{20}{100}$

3. Solve for X

    a. 10:X::6:12

    b. 100:X::250:50

Systems of Measurement

1. State the following metric equivalents:

    a. 1000 mL = _____ L

    b. 1 kg = _____ g

    c. 1000 mg = _____ g

    d. 1 mg = _____ μg

2. Convert the following:

    a. 2 g = _____ mg

    b. 6 g = _____ kg

    c. 3 mg = _____ μg

    d. 2 L = _____ mL

    e. 500 μg _____ mg

    f. 11 kg = _____ g

    g. 500 mg = _____ g

    h. 60 mg = _____ gr

    i. 10 gr = _____ mg

    j. $\dfrac{1}{2}$ gr = _____ mg

    k. .4 mg = _____ gr

    l. $\dfrac{1}{120}$ gr = _____ mg

Determine the correct amount of the drug to give in each dose:

1. Order: cefixime (Suprax) oral suspension 400 mg PO q AM.

    Available: cefixime (Suprax) oral suspension 100 mg/5 mL.

2. Order: furosemide (Lasix) 20 mg IV push now.

    Available: furosemide (Lasix) 10 mg/mL.

3. Order: diazepam (Valium) 4 mg PO bid.

   Available: diazepam (Valium) 2 mg, 5 mg, and 10 mg tablets.

4. Order: phenytoin (Dilantin) 300 mg PO qd.

   Available: phenytoin (Dilantin) oral suspension 125 mg/5 mL.

5. Order: atenolol (Tenormin) 50 mg PO q am.

   Available: atenolol (Tenormin) 25 mg tablets.

6. Order: vancomycin (Vancocin) 125 mg PO q 6 h.

   Available: vancomycin (Vancocin) oral solution 250 mg/5 mL.

7. Order: cefuroxime (Zinacef) 1.5 g IV piggyback q 8 h.

   Available: cefuroxime (Zinacef) 750 mg/50 mL.

8. Order: meperidine (Demerol) 75 mg and promethazine HCl (Phenergan) 25 mg IM now.

   Available: meperidine (Demerol) 50 mg/mL

   promethazine HCl (Phenergan) injection 50 mg/mL

9. Order: meperidine (Demerol) 50 mg and atropine 1/150 gr IM now.

   Available: meperidine (Demerol) 100 mg/mL

   atropine sulfate 0.4 mg/mL

10. Order: acetaminophen 5 grains PO for temp > 101°F.

    Available: acetaminophen 325 mg tablets

    (Hint: remember that one grain can be 60 or 65 mg)

11. Order: Milk of Magnesia 1 ounce tonight at bedtime.

    Available: Milk of Magnesia 240 mL bottle.

12. Order: phenytoin (Dilantin) 4 mg/kg/day in three divided doses. (Patient weighs 22 lbs)

    Available: phenytoin (Dilantin) oral suspension 30 mg/5 mL

Mark the correct amount of insulin on the syringe.

1. 15 U Humulin R sc q am

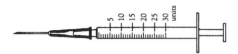

2. 35 U NPH insulin sc now

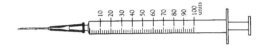

3. 10 U regular insulin and 20 U NPH sc q am

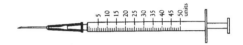

Determine the correct flow rate for each ordered intravenous drug

1. Aminophylline 300 mg IV in 50 mL 0.9% NaCl. Administer over 30 minutes.

   Drop factor: 20

2. Abelcet (amphotericin B) 250 mg in 100 mL IV piggyback over 2 hours.

   Drop factor: 60

ANSWERS TO REVIEW QUESTIONS

Unit 1

1. D
2. F
3. B
4. L
5. E
6. H
7. J
8. I
9. C
10. K
11. A
12. G
13. B
14. A
15. C
16. II
17. I
18. V
19. IV
20. III
21. Physical and chemical characteristics
22. Circulation to intended site
23. Plasma protein binding
24. Affinity for fatty tissue
25. Barriers (brain, placenta)
26. Right: drug, dose, time, route, patient
27. B
28. D
29. A
30. B

Unit 2

1. Careful intake and output, monitor blood pressure and pulse, daily weights, assess for peripheral edema, check for distended neck veins, assess lung sounds, measure abdominal girth
2. A
3. B
4. Dairy products, dark green leafy vegetables, cereals, meats, fish
5. Lethargy, tachycardia, hypotension, stomach cramps, vomiting, diarrhea, convulsions
6. Steroidal and nonsteroidal
7. A
8. D
9. C
10. A
11. C
12. C
13. D
14. B
15. A

16. A
17. D
18. A
19. B
20. B
21. D
22. A
23. C
24. B
25. D
26. A
27. D
28. C
29. B
30. A
31. B
32. B
33. A
34. C
35. A
36. D
37. C
38. B
39. A
40. A
41. B
42. A
43. C
44. B
45. D
46. C
47. A
48. B

Unit 3

1. A
2. D
3. B
4. C
5. A
6. B
7. D
8. A
9. B
10. C
11. C
12. D
13. A

Unit 4

1. C
2. A
3. B
4. C
5. A

6. D
7. A
8. A
9. B
10. D
11. C
12. B
13. Urinary incontinence is associated with atrophic vaginitis. Estrogen restores the elasticity of the vaginal tissues, which, in turn, improves control of voiding.
14. False
15. Alpha-adrenergic agonist
Refs: Saunders Nursing Drug Handbook 1999
Duthrie and Katz, chaps 5, 18, 19, 26, 27
Lehne
16. A
17. C
18. D
19. A
20. D
21. D

Unit 5

1. C
2. A
3. D
4. C
5. A
6. B
7. C
8. A

Unit 6

1. Heart, increased heart rate, increased force of heart muscle contraction
2. B
3. D
4. A
5. D
6. A
7. C
8. B
9. C
10. A
11. D
12. D
13. A
14. B

Unit 7

1. Dilate the bronchi

2. False
3. She should rinse her mouth after using the inhaler.
4. She has hypertension and cardiac disease. A sympathomimetic can raise the blood pressure and stimulate the heart, causing tachycardia and dysrhythmias.
5. A selective ß₂ agonist produces bronchodilation with less cardiac stimulation.
6. Many bronchodilators stimulate the central nervous system and the heart. Also, anxiety and tachycardia occur when a person is not getting enough oxygen.
7. Leukotriene inhibitor
8. This drug prevents acute attacks and should be taken regularly as ordered. It will not stop an acute attack.
9. The bronchodilator is used first to open the airways so that the corticosteroid can be more deeply dispersed in the lungs.
10. False. Unless used excessively for a long period of time, inhaled corticosteroids do not generally cause adverse systemic effects.

Unit 8

1. B
2. C
3. A
4. B
5. C
6. D
7. A
8. B
9. A
10. C
11. D
12. A
13. B

Unit 9

1. Improves cardiac contractility
2. Cardiac, GI, CNS
3. Give the digoxin as ordered.
4. Hypokalemia
5. Loss of excess fluid
6. B
7. Automaticity
8. New dysrhythmias, hypotension
9. Cinchonism
10. Quinidine can decrease production of prothrombin and platelets.
11. Quinidine enhances the effects of digitalis.
12. Calcium channel blocker/antagonist
13. Decreases blood pressure and heart rate
14. Verapamil causes orthostatic hypotension: the blood pressure falls with position changes.
15. Avoid sudden position changes. Exercise the legs before standing. Avoid hot baths or showers. Avoid prolonged standing in one place.
16. Hypertension usually has no symptoms, so it is not safe to stop drugs on the basis of symptoms.

17. Abruptly stopping the drug can cause blood pressure to rise dangerously.
18. Elevate legs when sitting; avoid prolonged standing in one place.

Unit 10

1. Bismuth tablets, metronidazone, tetracycline
2. To discourage emergence of drug-resistant *Helicobacter pylori*
3. Metronidizole
4. Inhibit gastric acid secretion
5. Antiandrogenic effects, central nervous system effects, inhibition of drug-metabolizing enyzmes
6. No significant interaction between famotidine and warfarin (note: cimetidine prolongs action of warfarin so that warfarin dose would need to be reduced if cimetidine prescribed)

Unit 11

1. C
2. A
3. B
4. D
5. B
6. D

Unit 12

1. Increases bone mineral density by impairing bone resorption
2. D
3. A
4. Calcitonin (Miacalcin) and raloxifene (Evista)
5. Whether she has a uterus, because estrogen replacement therapy alone increases the risk of endometrial cancer.

Unit 13

1. C
2. These preparations frequently contain epinephrine or ephedrine, which can increase blood pressure.
3. B
4. A
5. B
6. D
7. C
8. B
9. C
10. D
11. A
12. C
13. D
14. B
15. A

Unit 14

1. D
2. C
3. A
4. B
5. D
6. B

7. A
8. C

Unit 15

1. A
2. D
3. C
4. A

Unit 16

1. A
2. D
3. B
4. C
5. D
6. B
7. G
8. F
9. I
10. A
11. E
12. H
13. C
14. B
15. D
16. E
17. B
18. F
19. G
20. A
21. C

Unit 17

1. A
2. C
3. C
4. A
5. A
6. B
7. B
8. D

UNIT 18

Determine the correct flow rate

1. Aminophylline 300 mg IV in 50 mL 0.9% NaCl

    Administer over 30 minutes

    Drop factor = 20

    500 mL × 20 gtts = 1000 gtts

    1000 gtts ÷ 30 minutes = 33 gtts/min
2. Abelcel 250 mg in 100 mL over 2 hrs

    Drop factor = 60

    100 mL ÷ 2 hrs = 50 mL/hr

    50 mL × 60 gtts = 3000 gtts

    2 hrs = 60 min

    3000 gtts ÷ 60 minutes = 50 gtts/min

KEY: PRACTICE PROBLEMS

Basic Math Review

1. $\dfrac{2}{7} + \dfrac{3}{7} = \dfrac{5}{7}$

2. $\frac{3}{5} + \frac{1}{5} + \frac{2}{5} = \frac{6}{5} = 1\frac{1}{5}$

3. $\frac{2}{5} = \frac{4}{10} + \frac{3}{10} = \frac{7}{10}$

4. $1/3 = 4/12$
    $4/6 = 8/12$
   $+ 7/12 = 7/12$
   $\qquad 19/12 = 1\ 7/12$

5. $\frac{5}{9} - \frac{2}{9} = \frac{3}{9}$

6. $\frac{5}{6} = \frac{20}{24}$
   $- \frac{3}{8} = \frac{9}{24}$
   $\qquad \frac{11}{24}$

7. $\frac{1}{9} \times \frac{2}{3} = \frac{2}{27}$

8. $\frac{3}{5} \times \frac{1}{2} = \frac{3}{10}$

9. $\frac{7}{10} \div \frac{3}{4} = \frac{7}{10} \times \frac{4}{3} = \frac{28}{30} = \frac{14}{15}$

10. $\frac{5}{6} \div \frac{2}{9} = \frac{5}{6} \times \frac{9}{2} = \frac{45}{12} = 3\frac{9}{12}$

11. 2.3
     $+ 1.6$
     $\overline{3.9}$

12. 12.13
      56.00
     $+ 0.12$
     $\overline{68.25}$

13. 13.6
      $- 5.3$
      $\overline{8.3}$

14. 2.54
      $- 1.20$
      $\overline{1.34}$

15. 16.78
     $\times \quad 3.2$
     $\overline{3356}$
     $\underline{5034}$
     53.696

16. 3.04
     $\times \quad .004$
     $\overline{.01216}$

17. $526. \overline{)1578.}$
    $\qquad \underline{1578}$
    $\qquad \quad 0$

       2.08
18. $6\overline{)12.50}$
    $\quad \underline{12}$
    $\quad \ \ 50$
    $\quad \ \ \underline{48}$
    $\quad \ \ 20$

Ratio and Proportion

1. Write as ratios
   a. $\frac{1}{2} = 1{:}2$
   b. $\frac{2}{3} = 2{:}3$
   c. $\frac{6}{10} = 6{:}10$

2. Write as proportions
   a. $1{:}2{::}2{:}4$
   b. $9{:}10{::}90{:}100$
   c. $5{:}25{::}20{:}100$

3. Solve for X
   a. $10{:}X{::}6{:}12 \quad 6X = 120 \quad X = 20$
   b. $100{:}X{::}250{:}50 \quad 250X = 5000$
   $\qquad X = 20$

Systems of Measurement

1. State the following metric equivalents
   a. $1000 \text{ mL} = 1 \text{ L}$
   b. $1 \text{ kg} = 1000 \text{ g}$
   c. $1000 \text{ mg} = 1 \text{ g}$
   d. $1 \text{ mg} = 1000 \text{ µg}$

2. Convert the following
   a. $2 \text{ g} = 2000 \text{ mg}$
   $\frac{1 \text{ g}}{1000 \text{ mg}} = \frac{2 \text{ g}}{X \text{ mg}} \quad X = 2(1000)$
   $X = 2000 \text{ mg}$

   b. $6 \text{ g} = .006 \text{ kg}$
   $\frac{1 \text{ kg}}{1000 \text{ g}} = \frac{X \text{ kg}}{6\text{g}}$
   $1000X = 6$
   $X = \frac{6}{1000} \quad X = .006 \text{ kg}$

   c. $3 \text{ mg} = 3000 \text{ µg}$
   $\frac{1 \text{ mg}}{1000 \text{ µg}} = \frac{3 \text{ mg}}{X \text{ µg}} \quad X = 3(1000)$
   $X = 3000 \text{ µg}$

   d. $2 \text{ L} = 2000 \text{ mL}$
   $\frac{1 \text{ L}}{1000 \text{ mL}} = \frac{2 \text{ L}}{X \text{ mL}} \quad X = 2(1000)$
   $X = 2000 \text{ mL}$

   e. $500 \text{ µg} = 0.5 \text{ mg}$
   $\frac{1 \text{ mg}}{1000 \text{ µg}} = \frac{X \text{ mg}}{500 \text{ µg}}$
   $\frac{1000\ X}{1000} = \frac{500}{1000} \quad X = .5 \text{ mg}$

   f. $11 \text{ kg} = 11,000 \text{ g}$
   $\frac{1 \text{ kg}}{1000\text{g}} = \frac{11 \text{ kg}}{X \text{ g}} \quad X = 11(1000)$
   $X = 11,000 \text{ g}$

   g. $500 \text{ mg} = 0.5 \text{ g}$
   $\frac{1 \text{ g}}{1000 \text{ mg}} = \frac{X \text{ g}}{500 \text{ mg}}$
   $1000X = 500 \quad \frac{1000X}{1000} = \frac{500}{1000}$
   $X = 0.5 \text{ g}$

   h. $60 \text{ mg} = 1 \text{ gr}$
   i. $10 \text{ gr} = 600 \text{ mg}$
   $\frac{60 \text{ mg}}{1 \text{ gr}} = \frac{X \text{ mg}}{10 \text{ gr}} \quad X = 60(10)$
   $X = 600 \text{ mg}$

   j. $\frac{1}{2} \text{ gr} = 30 \text{ mg} \quad \frac{1}{2} = .5$
   $\frac{60 \text{ mg}}{1 \text{ gr}} = \frac{X \text{ mg}}{.5 \text{ gr}} \quad X = 60(.5)$
   $X = 30 \text{ mg}$

   k. $.4 \text{ mg} = \frac{1}{150} \text{ gr}$
   $\frac{60 \text{ mg}}{1 \text{ gr}} = \frac{.4 \text{ mg}}{X \text{ gr}} \quad 60X = .4$
   $X = \frac{.4}{60} \quad X = \frac{4}{600} \quad X = \frac{1}{150}$

   l. $\frac{1}{120} \text{ gr} = 0.5 \text{ mg}$
   $\frac{60 \text{ mg}}{1 \text{ gr}} = \frac{X \text{ mg}}{\frac{1}{120} \text{ gr}}$
   $X = 60\left(\frac{1}{120}\right) \quad X = \frac{60}{120} = .5$

Determine the correct amount

1. $\frac{100 \text{ mg}}{5 \text{ mL}} = \frac{400 \text{ mg}}{X \text{ mL}} \quad \frac{100X}{100} = \frac{2000}{100}$
   $X = 20 \text{ mL}$

2. $\frac{10 \text{ mg}}{1 \text{ mL}} = \frac{20 \text{ mg}}{X \text{ mL}} \quad \frac{10X}{10} = \frac{20}{10}$
   $X = 2\text{mL}$

3. $\frac{2 \text{ mg}}{1 \text{ tab}} = \frac{4 \text{ mg}}{X \text{ tabs}} \quad \frac{2X}{2} = \frac{4}{2}$
   $X = 2 \text{ tabs, 2 mg each}$

4. $\frac{125 \text{ mg}}{5 \text{ mL}} = \frac{300 \text{ mg}}{X \text{ mL}} \quad \frac{125X}{125} = \frac{1500}{125}$
   $X = 12 \text{ mL}$

5. $\frac{25 \text{ mg}}{1 \text{ tab}} = \frac{50 \text{ mg}}{X \text{ tabs}} \quad \frac{25X}{25} = \frac{50}{25}$
   $X = 2 \text{ tabs}$

6. $\frac{250 \text{ mg}}{5 \text{ mL}} = \frac{125 \text{ mg}}{X \text{ mL}} \quad 250X = 5(125)$
   $\frac{250X}{250} = \frac{625}{250} \quad X = 2.5 \text{ mL}$

7. a. $\dfrac{1\ g}{1000\ mg} = \dfrac{1.5\ g}{X\ mg}$ X = 1.5(1000)

   X = 1500 mg   1.5 g = 1500 mg

   b. $\dfrac{750\ mg}{50\ mL} = \dfrac{1500\ mg}{X\ mL}$

   $\dfrac{750X}{750} = \dfrac{75{,}000}{750} = 100\ mL$

8. a. $\dfrac{50\ mg}{1\ mL} = \dfrac{75\ mg}{X\ mL}$ $\dfrac{50X}{50} = \dfrac{75}{50}$

   X = 1.5 mL meperidine

   b. $\dfrac{50\ mg}{1\ mL} = \dfrac{25\ mg}{X\ mL}$ $\dfrac{50X}{50} = \dfrac{25}{50}$

   $X = \dfrac{1}{2} = 0.5$ mL promethazine

9. a. $\dfrac{100\ mg}{1\ mL} = \dfrac{50\ mg}{X\ mL}$ $\dfrac{100X}{100} = \dfrac{50}{100}$

   $X = \dfrac{1}{2} = 0.5$ mL meperidine

b. $\dfrac{60\ mg}{1\ gr} = \dfrac{X\ mg}{\frac{1}{150}\ gr}$

   $X = 60\left(\dfrac{1}{150}\right)$

   $X = \dfrac{60}{150} = 0.4$ mg

   $\dfrac{1}{150}$ gr = 0.4 mg atropine

   0.4 mg = 1 mL atropine

10. $\dfrac{65\ mg}{1\ gr} = \dfrac{X\ mg}{5\ gr}$ X = 325 mg

    1 tab = 325 mg

11. 30 mL
    No calculation necessary

12. 1. $\dfrac{2.2\ lbs}{1\ kg} = \dfrac{22\ lbs}{X\ kg}$ $\dfrac{2.2X}{2.2} = \dfrac{22}{2.2}$

    X = 10 kg

    patient wt = 10 kg

2. $\dfrac{4\ mg}{1\ kg} = \dfrac{X\ mg}{10\ kg}$ X = 40 mg

   total daily dose = 40 mg

   one dose = 40 ÷ 3 = 13.3 mg

3. $\dfrac{30\ mg}{5\ mL} = \dfrac{13\ mg}{X\ mL}$ $\dfrac{30X}{30} = \dfrac{65}{30}$

   = 2.16 mL = 2.2 mL

Intravenous Drug Flow Rates

1. a. 50 mL × 20 (drop factor) = 1000 gtts to administer

   b. 1000 gtts ÷ 30 minutes = 33 gtts/min

2. a. 100 mL × 60 (drop factor) = 6000 gtts to administer

   b. 6000 gtts ÷ 120 minutes (2 hrs) = 50 gtts/min

REFERENCE LIST

Abrams, A. C. (1998). *Clinical Drug Therapy*, 5th ed. Philadelphia: Lippincott.

American Psychiatric Association (1994). *Diagnostic and Statistical Manual of Mental Disorders*, 4th ed. Washington, D. C.: American Psychiatric Association.

Applegate, E. J. (1995). *The Anatomy and Physiology Learning System: Textbook*. Philadelphia: W. B. Saunders.

Bennett, J. C., & Plum, F. (Eds.) (1996). *Cecil Textbook of Medicine*, 20th ed. Philadelphia: W. B. Saunders.

Black, J. M., & Matassarin-Jacobs, E. (1997). *Medical-Surgical Nursing: Clinical Management for Continuity of Care*, 5th ed. Philadelphia: W. B. Saunders.

Cleveland, L., Aschenbrenner, D.S., Venable, S. J., & Yensen, J. A. P. (1999). *Nursing Management in Drug Therapy*. Philadephia: Lippincott.

Duthrie, E. H., & Katz, P. R. (1998). *Practice of Geriatrics*, 3rd ed. Philadelphia: W. B. Saunders.

Eckler, J. A., & Fair, J. M. S. (1996). *Pharmacology Essentials*. Philadelphia: W. B. Saunders.

Fahs, P. S., & Kinney, M. (1991). "The Abdomen, Thigh, and Arm Sites for Subcutaneous Sodium Heparin Injections." *Nursing Research (40)* pp. 204-207.

Ferrell, B. R., Grant, M., Virani, R., & Marugg, C. (1998). "Guidelines: Critical Areas of End of Life Care." Report of project entitled *Strengthening Nursing Education to Improve Pain Management and End of Life Care.* Supported by a grant from the Robert Wood Johnson Foundation.

Hodgson, B. B., & Kizior, R. J. (1999). *Saunders Nursing Drug Handbook 1999*. Philadelphia: W. B. Saunders.

Ignatavicius, D. D., Workman, M. L., & Mishler, M. A. (1999). *Medical-Surgical Nursing Across the Health Care Continuum*, 3rd ed. Philadelphia: W. B. Saunders.

Jaffe, M. S., & McVan, B. F. *Davis's Laboratory and Diagnostic Test Handbook.* Philadelphia: F. A. Davis.

Katzung, B. G. (1998). *Basic and Clinical Pharmacology*, 7th ed. Stamford, CT: Appleton & Lange.

Kee, J. L., & Hayes, E. R. (2000). *Pharmacology: a Nursing Process Approach*, 3rd ed. Philadelphia: W. B. Saunders.

Lehne, R. A. (1998). *Pharmacology for Nursing Care*, 3rd ed. Philadelphia: W. B. Saunders.

Lilley, L. L. & Aucker, R. S. (1999). *Pharmacology and the Nursing Process*, 2nd ed. St. Louis: Mosby.

Linton, A. D., Matteson, M. A., & Maebius, N. K. (1995). *Introductory Nursing Care of Adults*. Philadelphia: W. B. Saunders.

Matteson, M. A., McConnell, E. S., & Linton, A. D. (1997). *Gerontological Nursing*, 2nd ed. Philadelphia: W. B. Saunders.

McCorkle, R., Grant, M., Frank-Stromborg, M., & Baird, S. (1998). *Cancer Nursing: A Comprehensive Textbook*, 2nd ed. Philadelphia: W. B. Saunders.

Monahan, F. D., & Neighbors, M. (1998). *Medical-Surgical Nursing: Foundations of Practice*, 2nd ed. Philadelphia: W. B. Saunders.

Pinnell, N. L. (1996). *Nursing Pharmacology*. Philadelphia: W. B. Saunders.

Stuart, G. W., & Laraia, M. T. (1998). *Stuart & Sundeen's Principles and Practice of Psychiatric Nursing*, 6th ed. St. Louis: Mosby.

Turkoski, B. B., Lance, B. R., & Bonfiglio, M. F. (1999). *Drug Information Handbook for Nursing*, 2nd ed. Cleveland: Lexi-Comp, Inc.

Wilson, B. A., Shannon, M. T., & Stang, C. L. (1999). *Nurse's Drug Guide*. Stamford, CT: Appleton and Lange.

INDEX

Antipurines, 87
Antipyrimidines, 87
Antishock drugs, 151–152
Antitubercular drugs
    primary, 32–34
    second-line, 34
Antitumor antibiotics, 84–85
Antitussives, 118
Antiviral drugs
    for human immunodeficiency virus (HIV),
        36–39
    for non-human immunodeficiency virus
        (Non-HIV), 34–36
Anxiety, 79
Anxiolytics, 58, 246–251
Aralen (chloroquine), 41
Arava (leflunomide), 184–185
Arrhythmias, 143
Arthritis, 183
    drugs for treating, 183–186
Aspirin (acetylsalicylic acid), 18
Assessments
    health history, 11
    nursing diagnoses and, 12
    physical examination, 11
Asthma, 125
Atarax (hydroxyzine), 249
Atrial dysrhythmias, 1443
Attention deficit hyperactivity disorder
    (ADHD), 112
Atypicals, 252
Aura, 103
Autonomic drugs, for ophthalmic purposes,
    233–235
Autonomic nervous system, 91
Azathioprine (Imuran), 185–186
Azulfidine (sulfasalazine), 184

B

Balanced anesthesia, 62
Barbiturates, 58–60, 248–249
    as antiepileptic drug, 105–106
    as intravenous anesthetic agents, 63
Benadryl (diphenhydramine), 249
Benemid (probenecid), 186–187
Benzodiazepines, 60–61, 106–107, 246–247
    as intravenous anesthetic agents, 63
Beta-adrenergic drugs, 94–95
Beta-adrenergic receptors, 93
Beta-blockers, 96–98, 234
Beta-lactams, 26–27
Biguanides, 205, 206
Biologic response modifiers (BRMs), 135
Birth control drugs
    levonorgestrel (Norplant), 218
    medroxyprogesterone (Depo-Provera),
        217–218
    oral, 216–217
Bisphosphonates, 188
Bleeding, 128–129
Blocking agents, 91. *see also* Adrenergic
    blockers
Bone-forming therapy, 189
Bowel lavage agents, 168
Bowman's capsule, 172
BRMs. *See* Biologic response modifiers
    (BRMs)

Bronchodilators, 122–124
Bronchospasm, 122
Buccal routes, 5
Bulk-forming laxatives, 166–167
BuSpar (Buspirone), 249
Buspirone (BuSpar), 249

C

Caffeine, 114
Calcimar (calcitonin-salmon), 188–189
Calcitonin, 195
Calcitonin-salmon (Calcimar, Miacalcin),
    188–189
Calcium, 47–48
Cancer, antineoplastic agents for, 83–84
Cannabinoids, 164
Capsules, 2
Carbamazepine (Tegretol), 107–108
Carbonic anhydrase inhibitors
    oral, 235–236
    topical, 236
Carboxylic acids, 17–19
Cardiotonic, 140
Cardiovascular system
    anatomy and physiology of, 139
    drugs for disorders of, 139
Catecholamines, 93
Cathartics, 166
Central nervous system (CNS), 91, 244
    stimulants, 112–114
Cephalosporins, 26–27
Cerumen, 241–242
Ceruminolytic, 241–242
Chemical drug actions, 6
Chemical names, 2
Chemotaxis, 17
Chemotherapy, 83
Chloramphenicol (Chloromycetin Otic),
    240–241
Chloromycetin Otic (chloramphenicol), 240–241
Chloroquine (Aralen), 41
Cholesterol, 153
Cholinergic drugs, 99–100, 234–235
Cholinesterase inhibitors, 75
Chorionic gonadotropin (Pregnyl), 218
Clomid (clomiphene), 218
Clomiphene (Clomid), 218
Clomipramine (Anafranil), 249
Clots
    anticoagulants for, 129–130
    thrombolytics, 131
CNS. *See* Central nervous system (CNS)
Colchicine, 187
Cold remedies
    antihistamines, 119
    antitussives, 118
    intranasal glucocorticoids, 120
    nasal decongestants, 117–118
Comfort, promoting, 78–80
Compazine (prochlorperazine), 253
Confusion, 74
Constipation, 79
Contraceptive drugs
    levonorgestrel (Norplant), 218
    medroxyprogesterone (Depo-Provera),
        217–218
    oral, 216–217

Controlled substances, 3
Convulsions, 103
Corticosteroids, 238. *see also* Glucocorticoids;
    Mineralocorticoids
    for ears, 241
    inhaled, 126
Corticotropin (Acthar), 192–193
Cough, 79
Coumadin (warfarin), 130
Cross-sensitivity, 22
Cross-tolerance, 8
Cumulation, 8
Cycloplegic, 233
Cycloplegia, 233
Cyclosporine, 136
Cystitis, 179
Cytadren (aminoglutethimide), 202
Cytotec (misoprostol), 159–160
Cytotoxic drugs, 136–137
Cytovene (ganciclovir), 35–36

D

Dantrium (dantrolene), 69
Dantrolene (Dantrium), 69
DDAVP (desmopressin), 193–194
Decimals, 263–264
Delirium, 74, 79
Dementia, 74
    vascular, 76
Denominator, 262
Depakene (valproic acid), 108–109
Depakote (valproic acid), 108–109
Depolarizing drugs, 67
Depo-Provera (medroxyprogesterone), 217–218
Depression, 79, 247
Desmopressin (DDAVP), 193–194
Diabetes mellitus, 203
    type 1, 203–205
    type 2, 205–207
Diabetic ketoacidosis, 203
Diamox (acetazolamide), 235–236
Diapid (lypressin), 193–194
Diarrhea, 169
    absorbents for, 170
    antibiotic therapy for, 170
    drugs for, 169–170
Diazoxide (Proglycem), 208
Digestive system
    anatomy and physiology of, 156
    drugs for disorders of, 156
Digitalis glycosides, 140–141
Diphenhydramine (Benadryl), 249
Displacement, 269
Distribution, drug, 6
Diuretics, 174, 178, 235–236
    carbonic anhydrase inhibitors, 176
    loop, 175–176
    osmotic, 176–177
    potassium-sparing, 177
    thiazide, 175
Donepezil, 75
Dopamine, 93
Dopaminergic drugs, 110–111
Dopram (doxapram), 113–114
Dorzolamide (Trusopt), 236

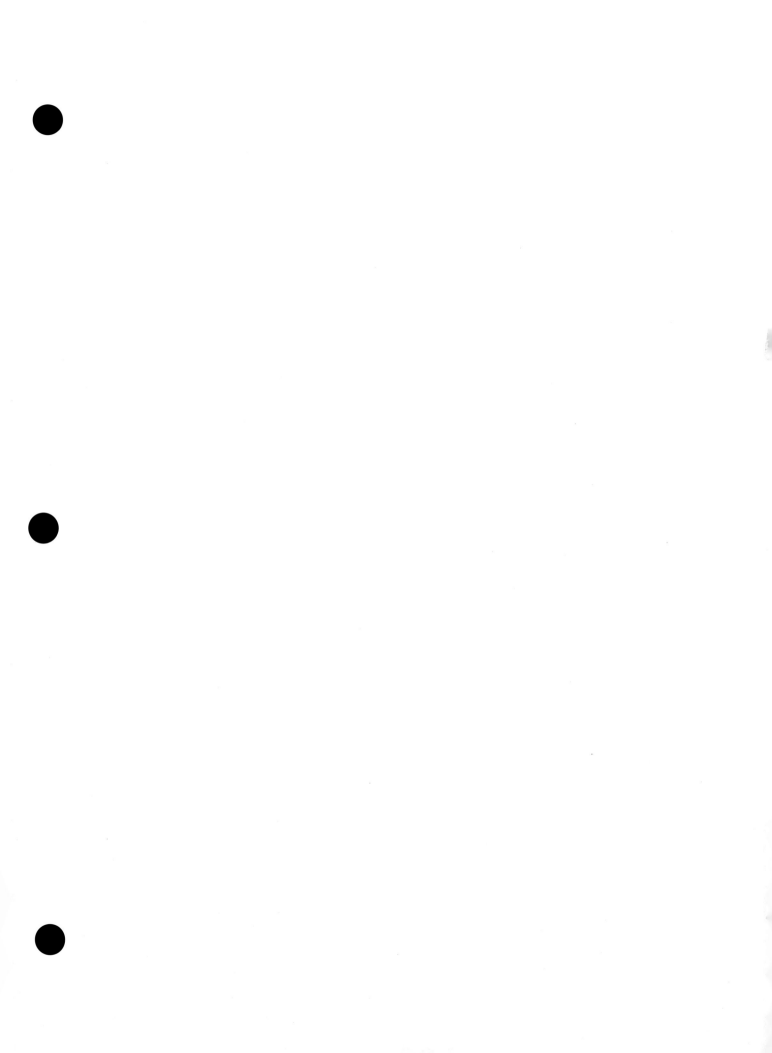